Praise for Howard Markel's

AN ANATOMY *of* ADDICTION

HOWARD MARKEL

AN ANATOMY of ADDICTION

Howard Markel, M.D., Ph.D., is the George E. Wantz
Distinguished Professor of the History of Medicine
and director of the Center for the History of Medicine
at the University of Michigan.

www.howardmarkel.com

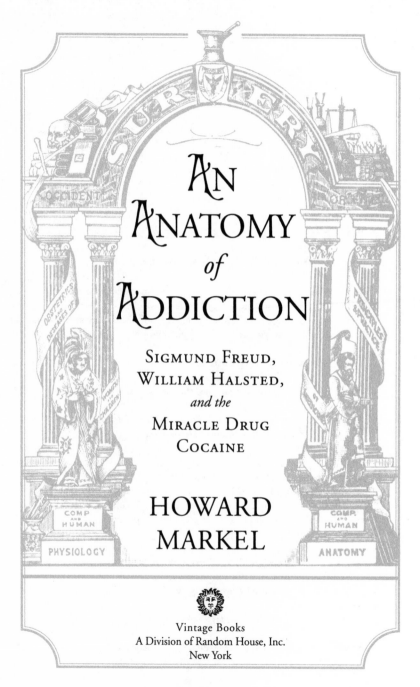

An
Anatomy
of
Addiction

Sigmund Freud,
William Halsted,
and the
Miracle Drug
Cocaine

HOWARD
MARKEL

Vintage Books
A Division of Random House, Inc.
New York

FIRST VINTAGE BOOKS EDITION, JULY 2012

Copyright © 2011 by Howard Markel

All rights reserved. Published in the United States by Vintage Books, a division of
Random House, Inc., New York, and in Canada by Random House of Canada
Limited, Toronto. Originally published in hardcover in the United States by
Pantheon Books, a division of Random House, Inc., New York, in 2011.

Vintage and colophon are registered trademarks of Random House, Inc.

The Library of Congress has catalogued the Pantheon edition as follows:
Markel, Howard.
An anatomy of addiction : Sigmund Freud, William Halsted, and the
miracle drug cocaine / Howard Markel.
p. cm.
Includes bibliographical references and index.
1. Freud, Sigmund, 1856–1939. 2. Psychoanalysts—Austria—Biography.
3. Halsted, William, 1852–1922. 4. Surgeons—United States—Biography.
5. Cocaine—History. 6. Cocaine abuse. I. Title.
BF109.A1M37 2011 362.29'80922—dc22
2010033782

Vintage ISBN: 978-1-4000-7879-0

Book design by Virginia Tan

www.vintagebooks.com

Printed in the United States of America
10 9 8 7 6 5 4 3 2 1

For Bess and Sammy,
with love from Daddy

Contents

Acknowledgments

IT IS A PLEASURE TO ACKNOWLEDGE and thank those who helped convert this book from a mere idea into an actual volume.

To begin, I am most fortunate in finding an academic home at the University of Michigan in Ann Arbor. Working with so many talented scholars, scientists, and physicians in the midst of such extraordinary resources has advanced my work in more ways than I can enumerate. At the University of Michigan Center for the History of Medicine, I am grateful to Professor Alexandra Minna Stern for her warm friendship, encouragement, and careful reading of my work; Dr. J. Alexander Navarro, who is as able a digital and computer wizard as he is a historian; Mary Beth Reilly for her superb reference and fact-checking; and Scott Oosterdorp for his helpful library searches when I was otherwise occupied. I am indebted to Professor Daniel Herwitz, who directs the University of Michigan Institute for the Humanities, where I was the John Rich Professor during the 2005–06 academic year, and who patiently read every page of the manuscript, much to my delight and this book's improvement. Similar thanks go to Professor Michael Schoenfeldt, the chairman of the University of Michigan Department of English Literature and Language. He is a treasured friend and a thoughtful reader.

From 2004 to 2010, I was fortunate to serve as a physician at the University of Michigan Addiction Treatment Service. There I saw hundreds of patients with substance abuse and addiction problems in collaboration with a dedicated and talented staff of psychiatrists, psychologists, and social workers. I thank the executive director, Dr. Kirk Brower (who also read and helped improve the scientific portions of this book), Dr. Robert Zucker, Dr. John Greden, Dr. Maher Karam-Hage, Michael Wallace, and Randall Pomeroy for teaching me so much about this stubborn and crafty disease. Although I am honor-bound to respect the anonymity of my patients and many members of the Ann Arbor recovery community whom I met along the way, I thank them as well for enriching my work and life. Their experiences, hopes, and strengths were essential in helping me to better understand Sigmund Freud and William Halsted.

I also thank Dr. David McDowell of Mount Sinai Medical School, Dr. Catherine DeAngelis, editor-in-chief of the *Journal of the American Medical Association,* Dr. James Harris of the Johns Hopkins Medical School, Dr. Sherwin B. Nuland of Yale University, Dr. Stephen Bergman (a.k.a. Samuel Shem, M.D.), Jonathan Cohn of *The New Republic,* Dr. Martin Cetron of the U.S. Centers for Disease Control and Prevention, Professor David Rosner of Columbia University, Don Bosco Hewlett, Eric Lax, and Dr. Sheldon F. Markel for taking the time to read the manuscript with careful and generous eyes.

All historians claim libraries as their workshops, but once there they rely heavily on the librarians and archivists who curate the historical collections. The staffs of the University of Michigan Libraries, the Bentley Historical Library of the University of Michigan (Francis Blouin, William Wallach, and Brian Williams), the Alan Mason Chesney Archives of the Johns Hopkins Medical Institutions (Nancy McCall and Andrew Harrison), the Weill Medical College at Cornell University/New York Hospital Archives (James Gehrlich), the Freud Museum of Vienna (Claudia Muchitsch, Christian Humber, and Martina Gasser), the Freud Museum of London (Carol Siegel), the Josephinum Medical History Museum at the University of Vienna (Dr. Ruth Koblizek), the Gesellschaft der Ärzte / Society of Physicians in Vienna (Manfred Gschwandtner), the Historical Collections of the New York Academy of Medicine, the New York Public Library, the Yale University Archives (Geoff Zonder), the F. L. Erhman Medical Library of the New York University School of Medicine (Colleen Bradley-Saunders), the Enoch Pratt Free Library of Baltimore, the National Library of Medicine, the Library of Congress, the British Library, and the Wellcome Library of the History of Medicine in London all performed their tasks with professionalism and speed. I hope that a collective thank-you will suffice.

I am also grateful to the Sigmund Freud Archives and the Sigmund

Freud Collection at the Library of Congress for allowing me to quote several short passages from letters Sigmund wrote to his then fiancée and later wife, Martha Bernays, and to many of his colleagues, including Wilhelm Fleiss.

My literary agents, Glen Hartley and Lynn Chu of Writer's Representatives, are, quite simply, the best practitioners of their profession. They believed in this project from the very start and never flagged in their encouragement, creativity, and advice. It is a pleasure to thank them, once again.

This is the second book I have completed under the tutelage of my extraordinary editor, Victoria Wilson, vice president and associate publisher of Alfred A. Knopf. She continues to hold me to the highest standards of writing, and I am grateful for her wise suggestions and counsel. I am also indebted to her editorial assistant, Carmen Johnson, for her cheerful demeanor and professionalism; to copy editor Bonnie Thompson for her superb attention to questions of language, grammar, and factual detail; and to the entire staff at Pantheon, especially Ellen Feldman, who performed their jobs with insight and ability.

I must add that while all of these people have generously given me superb assistance, any errors or defects that remain in the book are mine alone. Those flaws, I hope, are neither glaring nor fatal.

Finally, I thank my family for their support and love during the past seven years as I tracked the lives of Sigmund and William. My wife, Kate Levin Markel, scrutinized and improved every page of this book. Our daughters, Bess Rachel, age ten, and Samantha Louise, age five and who answers to "Sammy," are the lights of our lives. They never complained as I isolated myself during the throes of composition and were especially encouraging when the work was not always going smoothly. This book is dedicated to my wonderful girls and signifies my hope for their brilliant and healthy futures.

Howard Markel
Ann Arbor, Michigan
September 20, 2010

Illustrations

An
Anatomy
of
Addiction

Prologue

O N T H E M O R N I N G O F M A Y 5, 1885, in lower Manhattan, a worker fell from a building's scaffolding to the ground. A splintered bone protruded from his bloody trousers; a plaintive wail signaled his pain; and soon he was taken from the scene by horse-drawn ambulance to Bellevue Hospital. At the hospital, in the dispensary, a young surgeon named William Stewart Halsted frantically searched the shelves for a container of cocaine.

In the late nineteenth century, there were no such things as

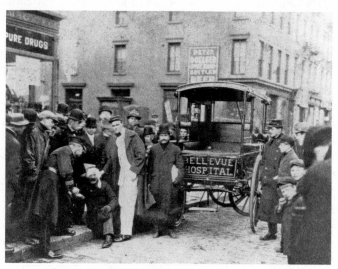

*A Bellevue ambulance arrives at an accident scene in
lower Manhattan, c. 1885.*

"controlled substances," let alone illegal drugs. Bottles of morphine, cocaine, and other powerful, habit-forming pills and tonics were easily found in virtually every hospital, clinic, drugstore, and doctor's black bag. Consequently, it took less than a few minutes for the surgeon to find a vial of cocaine. He drew a precise dose into a hypodermic syringe, rolled up his sleeve, and searched for a fresh spot on his scarred forearm. Upon doing so, he inserted the needle and pushed down on the syringe's plunger. Almost immediately, he felt a wave of relief and an overwhelming sense of euphoria. His pulse bounded and his mind raced, but his body, paradoxically, relaxed.

The orderlies rushed the laborer into Bellevue's accident room (the forerunner of today's emergency departments) for examination and treatment. A compound fracture—the breaking of a bone so severely that it pokes through the soft tissue and skin—was deadly serious in the late nineteenth century. Before X-ray technology, it was difficult to assess the full extent of a fracture other than by means of painful palpation or cutting open the body part in question for a closer look. Discounting the attendant risks of infection and subsequent amputation, even in the best of surgical hands these injuries often carried a "hopeless prognosis." At Bellevue, above the table on which these battered patients were placed, a sign painted on the wall suggested the chances of recuperation. It read, in six-inch-high black letters: PREPARE TO MEET YOUR GOD.

As the worker writhed in agony, one surgeon's name crossed the lips of every staff member working in the accident room: Halsted. When it came to a crisis of the body, few surgeons were faster or more expert than he. Leg fractures were a particular interest of his in an era when buildings were being thrown up daily and construction workers were falling off them almost as frequently. One of Dr. Halsted's earliest scientific papers assessed the surgical repair of fractured thigh, or femur, bones using a series of geometric equations based on how the leg adducted (drew toward) and abducted (drew away) from the central axis of the body. Such meticulous analysis was essential to repairing the break in a manner that accounted for the potential of the injured limb to shorten after the injury. Otherwise, the broken leg would heal in a manner that resulted in a decided limp or, given the intricate mechanics of the hip joint, much worse.

An orderly was dispatched to find Dr. Halsted as soon as possible. Running through the labyrinthine corridors of the hospital, he shouted, "Paging Dr. Halsted! Fresh fracture in the Accident Room! Paging Dr. Halsted!" Down one of these halls, in a rarely used chamber, the surgeon was entering a world of mindless bliss. He heard his name but didn't really care to answer. Yet something, perhaps a reflex ingrained by his many years of surgical training, roused him to stagger out into the hallway and make his way down-

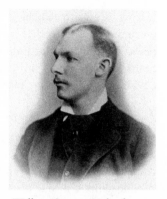

William Stewart Halsted at age twenty-eight, c. 1880.

stairs. The pupils of his eyes looked like gaping black holes, his speech was rapid-fire, and his whole body seemed to vibrate as if he were electrified.

Upon entering the accident room, Halsted was confronted with the acrid smell of blood and a maelstrom of doctors and nurses attending to the wounded worker. So intense was the pain that when Halsted gruffly demanded the patient move his leg one way or the other, the man screamed out an emphatic "No!" Passing a hand up and down the length of the laborer's lower leg, Halsted could feel the sharp ends of a shattered shinbone, or tibia, thrusting its way through the skin. It was a gory mess requiring immediate attention.

An effective surgeon must be able to visualize the three-dimensional aspects of the anatomy he is about to manipulate. He must take great care in handling sensitive structures surrounding the area in question, such as nerves and blood vessels, to prevent cutting through or destroying them entirely, lest the procedure cause more problems than it corrects. Consequently, the surgeon needs to think several steps ahead of the maneuver he is actively performing in order to achieve the best results for his patient. But the cocainized Halsted was in no shape to operate.

Halsted stepped back from the examination table while the nurses and junior physicians awaited his command, mindful that in a moment bacteria could enter the wound and wreak havoc, perhaps leaving this laborer unable to walk again—or even to die from overwhelming sepsis. To their astonishment, the surgeon turned on his heels, walked out of the hospital, and hailed a cab to gallop him to his home on East Twenty-fifth Street. Once there, he sank into a cocaine oblivion that lasted more than seven months.

FORTY-FOUR HUNDRED MILES AWAY, Sigmund Freud, an up-and-coming neurologist, toiled away in the busy wards of Vienna Krankenhaus (General Hospital). Like Halsted, he was fresh prey for cocaine's grip. On May 17, 1885, twelve days after Halsted hurried out of Bellevue, Dr. Freud boasted to his fiancée how a dose of pure cocaine vanquished his migraine and inspired him to stay up until four in the morning writing a "very important" anatomical study that "should raise my esteem again in the eyes of the public." In reality, the publication proved to be nothing more than an extraneous footnote to his literary oeuvre.

A year earlier, Freud had published an extensive review exploring cocaine's potential therapeutic uses. His central experimental subject was himself. But as impressive as his work was, Dr. Freud neglected to describe cocaine's most practical application: it was a superb anesthetic that completely numbed a living being's sensation to the sharp blade of a scalpel. In the fall of 1884, a few months after Freud's monograph appeared in print, a young ophthalmologist successfully demonstrated the drug's power to kill pain. The discovery excited the entire medical world, much to Freud's chagrin.

In the spring of 1885, the preempted Freud made plans to flee Vienna and nurse his wounded ego with a prestigious neuropathology fellowship in Paris. In the months that followed, he engaged in discussions of brain disorders, witnessed dozens of demonstrations of women and men suffering from hysteria, participated in detailed scientific research, and, too frequently, self-medicated his anxieties away.

Cocaine thrilled him in a manner that everyday life could not. He wrote romantic, often erotic letters to his fiancée, dreamed grandiose dreams of his future career, walked about the streets of Paris, visited museums and theaters, and attended sumptuous soirees—all under the influence. Even on return to his beloved Vienna in 1886, eager to embark upon his own private practice and excited about the possibility of new medical discoveries and explorations, Freud continued to take increasingly greater doses of cocaine.

THE FULL-FLEDGED diagnosis of addiction did not really exist in the medical literature until the late nineteenth century. The earliest use of the word appears in the statutes of Roman law. In antiquity, "addiction" typically referred to the bond of slavery that lenders imposed upon delinquent debtors or victims on their convicted aggressors. Such individuals were mandated to be "addicted" to the service of the person to whom they owed restitution. By the seventeenth century and extending well into the early 1800s, "addiction" described people compelled to act out any number of bad habits. Those abusing narcotics during this period were called opium and morphine "eaters." Alcohol abusers, too, had their own pejorative descriptors, such as "the drunkard," but as their problem came to the attention of physicians, the condition was often indexed in medical textbooks as dipsomania or alcoholism.

All this changed in the late nineteenth century with the overpre-

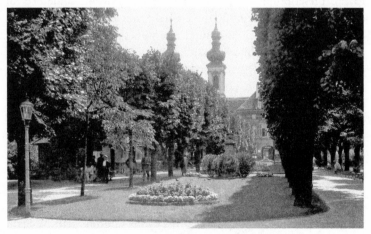

Main entrance of the Vienna General Hospital,
Allgemeines Krankenhaus, c. 1885.

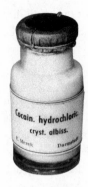

Vial of cocaine hydrochloride produced by E. Merck and Co., Darmstadt, Germany, c. 1884. This was the product Freud used in his research.

scription of narcotics by doctors to ailing and unsuspecting patients. One of the most striking measures of this era was the alarming number of male doctors who prescribed opium, morphine, and laudanum (a tincture of macerated raw opium in 50 percent alcohol) to ever greater numbers of women patients. Any female complaining to her physician about so-called women's problems was all but certain to leave the doctor's office clutching a prescription. For example, epidemiological studies conducted in Michigan, Iowa, and Chicago between 1878 and 1885 reported that at least 60 percent of the morphine or opium addicts living there were women.

Huge numbers of men and children, too, complaining of ailments ranging from acute pain to colic, heart disease, earaches, cholera, whooping cough, hemorrhoids, hysteria, and mumps were prescribed morphine and opium. A survey of Boston's drugstores published in an 1888 issue of *Popular Science Monthly* documents the ubiquity of these narcotics: of 10,200 prescriptions reviewed, 1,481, or 14.5 percent, contained an opiate. During this period in the United States and abroad, the abuse of addictive drugs such as opium, morphine, and, soon after it was introduced to the public, cocaine constituted a major public health problem.

NO EVIDENCE HAS BEEN found to demonstrate that William Halsted and Sigmund Freud ever met. Separated by physical and cultural oceans, their lives were, nevertheless, intricately braided and shaped by a handful of scientific papers on the medicinal uses of cocaine. For Sigmund Freud, the medical profession's creation of so many morphine addicts led him to experiment with cocaine as a potential antidote. In the quest to obliterate the pain incurred by the surgeon's craft, William Halsted explored the drug as a safer form of anesthesia. But because cocaine was such a relatively new drug during this period, neither

Freud nor Halsted recognized its addictive and deleterious force until it was much too late. By using themselves as guinea pigs in their research, each became dependent upon a substance that nearly destroyed their lives and the work that ultimately changed how we think, live, and heal.

CHAPTER I

Young Freud

On a June morning in 1884, eleven months before William Halsted abruptly left Bellevue Hospital, Sigmund Freud took his usual seat on a richly upholstered banquette at the Café Landtmann, a pungently academic restaurant situated on Vienna's Ringstrasse, then at its imperial peak. Freud had been studying medicine at the University of Vienna, directly across the street, since the fall of 1873, but his ascension in the arcane ranks of clinical privilege was slower than the healing of a festering wound. He was well-known to the café's impeccably attentive waitstaff. Here, as in many Viennese *kaffeehauses,* physicians congregated and pontificated with artists, philoso-

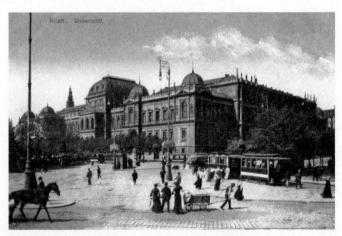

The University of Vienna, c. 1884.

phers, painters, playwrights, scientists, and poets about the latest discoveries and controversies arising in the world of ideas they inhabited. The atmosphere was thick with the exhaust of cigarettes, cigars, and inspired minds. This particular morning, however, Sigmund seemed oblivious to the chatty guests as he stroked his bushy beard and rubbed a wet, reddened nose that was the direct result of consuming too much cocaine.

The waiter asked for the doctor's order. The medico, barely looking up, responded absentmindedly, *"Einen kleinen braunen"* (a short cup of espresso that was typically accompanied by a squat pot of cream and a glass of water). Dressed in a starched white shirt, black tuxedo jacket, and black bow tie, the waiter nodded affirmatively at the request while bending over to ignite one of the small cigars the doctor habitually smoked.

Alone, tired, and agitated, Dr. Freud spent most of his days and nights at the Allgemeines Krankenhaus—the vast and malodorous Vienna General Hospital, known throughout the world as the Parnassus of medicine. The physical plant was awesome for its day: a seemingly endless complex consisting of twelve interlocking quadrangles and courtyards situated on a 250-acre campus. It boasted dozens of clinical departments, institutes, and clinics stretched across miles of connecting wards, offices, laboratories, and amphitheaters, and contained more than four thousand beds. Enclosed by an imposing stone wall, the Krankenhaus was more medical village than edifice, with its own culture, hierarchy, and water supply. More important, it was host to a series of medical discoveries that profoundly changed and improved medical practice. One of the most famous was made by a Hungarian obstetrician named Ignaz Semmelweis, who in 1847 committed the revolutionary act of urging physicians and nurses to wash their hands before examining a patient to prevent the spread of infection.

Those in charge of transforming the young Sigmund from a bright, ambitious, and socially insignificant Jewish boy into a pioneering intellectual constituted a Teutonic hall of healing fame. His physiology professor, Ernst Wilhelm von Brücke, was one of the founding fathers of his field. Brücke, along with Hermann Helmholtz, Emil du Bois-Reymond, and Carl Ludwig, is credited with initiating a now accepted tenet of medical research: every action in the human body—from the flick of a wrist to one's thoughts—has a chemical, physical, and biological foundation subject to the same laws and explanations as other physical phenomena.

In the dissection rooms, the anatomist Joseph Hyrtl elevated the preservation of human cadaver specimens to an art form by skillfully injecting wax and resins into blood vessels, lymphatic channels, and body parts. Thanks to these macabre talents, Hyrtl presided over the largest teaching collection of anatomical material on the planet. In the hospital basement, where the morgue was located, the world-renowned pathologist Carl von Rokitansky redefined his field as he performed or supervised more than thirty-two thousand autopsies, averaging two a day, seven days a week, for forty-five years.

Many mornings, Freud crossed a grand courtyard bounded by an arcade displaying busts of the University of Vienna's greatest professors. Like every medical student who gazes at such monuments to his predecessors, Sigmund looked on the statues with admiration and envy. According to his biographer Ernest Jones, the young Freud even imagined the inscription his own bust would someday bear. It was a line from Sophocles' *Oedipus Rex:* "who divined the famed riddle of the Sphinx and was a man most mighty." From the courtyard, Dr. Freud walked across the busy Ringstrasse to the Café Landtmann with a load of medical journals, which he pored over as he sipped cup after cup of expertly brewed coffee.

Freud appeared alternatively bored and distracted, nervous and phlegmatic, subdued and preoccupied. He had little appetite for the cream-filled cakes proffered by the Landtmann's pastry chef, which he had once happily consumed in two or three bites. Indeed, that pleasant June morning, Sigmund barely stomached the caffeinated beverage he had just ordered.

The waiters at Landtmann's could not help but notice the harsh odors that clung to Sigmund's black frock coat lately—sometimes, the nauseating scents of formaldehyde and ether from the laboratory; other times the aroma of sweat and disease from patients on the teeming wards. Previously, even as he'd immersed himself in the miasma of discovery and death, Sigmund had been tidy, if not splendidly attired. But on this particular morning, he looked as if he had not slept in days. It hardly required the trained eye of a Viennese physician to spot a ner-

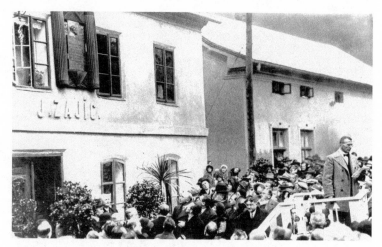

A dedication of a plaque at the Sigmund Freud birthplace in Příbor, Moravia, 1931. The Freuds lived on the second floor of this building.

vous twitch or two along his jawline as he ferociously ground down on his already tender teeth.

The twenty-eight-year-old Sigmund believed his ennui was a result of the ups and downs of his long-distance relationship with twenty-three-year-old Martha Bernays. Popular and pretty, she lived with her well-connected and well-educated Orthodox German Jewish family in Wandsbek, near Hamburg and more than five hundred miles from the Vienna city line. Like many young women of her generation, Martha centered her aspirations on raising a family and keeping a home in a comfortably bourgeois manner.

Sigmund's family, on the other hand, was not nearly as distinguished. The Freuds were a mere trickle in the steady torrent of impoverished Ostjuden (East European Jews) emi-

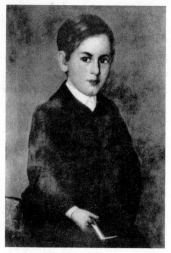

Freud as a six-year-old boy, 1862.

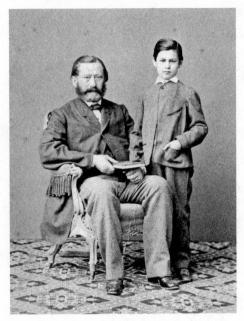

*Father Jacob, age forty-nine, and son Sigmund
Freud, age eight, 1864.*

grating west to Vienna during this period, a wave of migration that presented the city with the second-largest Jewish population in Europe
after Warsaw's. In 1855, Sigmund's father, Jacob, a forty-year-old wool
merchant with two adult sons from a previous marriage, married his
third wife, the twenty-year-old Amalia Nathansohn. The following
year, the Freuds left Brody, Galicia (now in the Ukraine), for Freiberg,
Moravia (now Příbor in the Czech Republic), where Sigmund was
born. Over the next ten years Amalia gave birth to another seven children. In 1859, the family moved to Leipzig and finally, in 1860, to
Vienna, where they struggled financially, socially, and emotionally in
the imperial city's Jewish ghetto.

In his later life, Sigmund insisted that Jacob "allowed me to grow up
in complete ignorance of everything that concerned Judaism," perhaps
as an exaggerated contrast to the more Orthodox ways of the Bernays
family. Yet even as a child, and certainly as a young man in mid-to-late-

nineteenth-century Austria, Sigmund Freud was acutely aware of the outsider status his religious and cultural background imposed. The Freud family attended synagogue services, albeit irregularly, and engaged in Jewish rituals such as celebrating the Purim and Passover holidays. One of Sigmund's most treasured heirlooms was the family's bound Pentateuch (five books of Moses, or Old Testament) that his father inscribed in Hebrew with a "memory page" (*Gedenkblatt*). Jacob frequently read aloud from the family Bible, and Sigmund remained fascinated by Old Testament lore for his entire life.

On June 17, 1882, a mere two months after they met, Sigmund impetuously asked Martha to marry him, a nuptial event that would not, and financially could not, occur until four years later, when Freud first opened his practice. Even though Martha's older brother, Eli, was engaged to Sigmund's eldest sister, Anna, and would marry her in October 1883, Sigmund was initially not the favored choice to become Martha's mate. Perhaps the most corrosive aspect of their affair of the heart was Martha's powerfully opinionated mother. A widow deeply concerned about her daughter's future, Frau Emmeline Bernays rarely missed the opportunity to inform Martha—and anyone else who

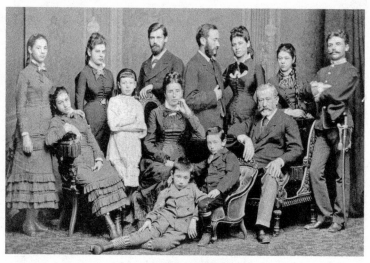

The extended Freud family, 1878.
Sigmund is in back, center, as a young medical student.

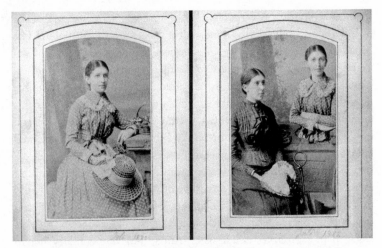

Martha Bernays, age twenty-one (left), and with her younger sister, Minna, age seventeen (Minna is seated), c. July 1882.

would listen—about Sigmund's financial unsuitability. In fact, Sigmund made his prospects even dimmer by electing to spend several years in the laboratory rather than ministering to the maladies of well-appointed and bill-paying Viennese.

SIGMUND WROTE HUNDREDS of love letters to Martha during their lengthy courtship (for most of which they were physically separated and during all of which they apparently abstained from premarital sexual relations). Throughout the correspondence, Freud employed the ingratiating methods of a doggedly attentive and hopelessly besotted suitor. Every evening, thoughts of losing the woman he habitually addressed as "my precious darling," "highly esteemed Princess," and "beloved little woman" weighed heavily upon Sigmund's already sloping shoulders. A poignant example of his longing can be found in a letter he wrote to his longtime fiancée in March 1885:

> *Now and again I see a girl in the street who looks like [Martha] in one way or another, whereupon I invariably follow her for a while to convince myself she isn't here. She probably won't see Vienna again*

until she is my wife. If only this could be soon.

But Freud's letters also describe the travails of a young doctor negotiating the turbulent waters of Vienna's medical pool. In August 1883, after returning from a month-long "country practice" clerkship, a twenty-seven-year-old Sigmund wrote Martha about the ridicule he encountered from an older colleague over the folly of marrying too early in one's career. After nearly a decade of medical training, Sigmund was still looking at an additional "eight years to get anywhere," but he also was fearful of losing Martha:

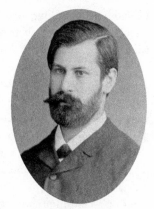

Sigmund Freud at age twenty-eight, July 26, 1884.

> *Defending my case valiantly, I told him [the doctor advising against marriage] he just doesn't know my girl, who is willing to wait for me indefinitely, that I would marry her even if she had turned thirty—a matron, he interrupted—that I would bring it off by starting work elsewhere, that a man has to take some risks and that what I stand to gain is worth any risk.*

Less than two years later, in June 1885, while preparing for an important oral examination required for a junior faculty position at the University of Vienna, Freud fretted to Martha about "the things that go with it! Top hat and gloves to be bought and then what kind of coat am I to wear? I have to appear in a dress coat—am I to hire it or have it made?"

Then as now, it was impolitic for a young doctor to admit to anyone, save a trusted lover or very close friend, that he had less interest in the hurly-burly arena of patient care than in the pristine, quiet, contemplative cocoon of the laboratory. As early as the summer of 1878, Sigmund wrote a friend about his laboratory work, "I am preparing myself for my real profession: flaying of animals or torturing of human beings and I find myself more and more in favor of the former." But in Sigmund's romantic notes to Martha he is far more introspective in explaining his calling. It was in the laboratory—and there only, it seemed at the time—where he could slake his thirst for intellectual fulfillment. The pursuit of discovery, fueled by his obsessive drive and focus, reliably numbed him to his worries; it was the perfect state for a nervous, easily excited, insecure, and prone-to-be-depressed chap like Sigmund. At the laboratory bench, specimen in hand and prepared for the microscope, he found an emollient that reliably calmed his nerves and heightened his sensations.

Yet if Freud was ever to convince Mrs. Bernays of his desirability as a son-in-law (read: his ability to provide for Martha in a manner that far exceeded his current income), he needed to bolster his career aspirations by establishing some type of carriage-trade practice. The conflict was clear. The deductive and seductive game of research was sublime but paid little. A private practice, on the other hand, did pay, but attending to an endless treadmill of Vienna's worried well was not exactly the life Sigmund envisioned for himself.

Complicating matters, Sigmund had already cast his lustrous but solemn brown eyes on the grand goal of a professorial appointment at the Vienna Medical School. Once there, he would enjoy free rein to inquire, lecture, and debate medical issues with the finest experts and scientific minds, accompanied by membership into the most elite international societies and academies. This was no mean feat for any young doctor, but Jews in particular faced significant obstacles in achieving such lofty positions. If Freud wanted to become an esteemed Viennese medical professor, he needed to mount a precipitous climb up an intellectual Everest. Foremost, he had to discover something medically earthshaking. But he also had to acquire the acumen and abilities of a world-class physician who could diagnose any illness presented to him, no matter how arcane or exotic. Such accomplishments and skills were the time-honored prerequisites for greatness at the Krankenhaus.

THE MEDICAL STUDENT'S LIFE has long been filled with anxiety punctuated by flashes of ambitious overconfidence. Sir William Osler, the eloquent physician and a founding father of the Johns Hopkins Hospital, best described their mental condition in a lecture he delivered at the University of Toronto in 1903. Medical students, he said, were prone to all forms of "ill-health of the mind." But the cause, Dr. Osler explained, was not merely hard work. Instead, "it is that foul fiend Worry." Few medical students fit this diagnostic criterion better than Sigmund Freud.

From late afternoon until well into the night, Sigmund focused on hastily written lecture notes and the thick, dog-eared tomes of anatomical structures, pathology, and chemistry he was required to memorize and regurgitate on command. The worry his medical aspirations set in motion tortured his tired neurons. Before he turned in for the night, perhaps in an effort to calm himself, Sigmund likely succumbed to a common medical student fantasy: visualizing the bright morning when he would lead a parade of interns, residents, junior physicians, nurses, and assorted acolytes down a busy hospital ward. There, his minions would troop alongside the beds of the stricken and present for his consideration a treasury of medical mysteries; in return, he would bestow upon them his latest insight of medical brilliance.

IRONIC ONLY TO THE INEXPERIENCED OBSERVER, the patient's suffering was secondary in the medical exercises conducted at the Krankenhaus. Making the right diagnosis was everything during an epoch when medicine's therapeutic arsenal was rather puny. Every morning, junior doctors reported on the details of their patients' courses along with the latest clinical tidbits culled from the piles of journals they read in the hours before rounds commenced. Their senior colleagues would then finesse, embellish, or clarify those findings.

By the close of these clinical spiels, all the heads in the crowded room would be turned to the superbly tailored attending physician, who immediately grasped what was going on with the patient, much to the amazement and admiration of his captive audiences. The cat-and-mouse games between the inquisitor-doctor and the witness-patient were composed of questions and answers, followed by more intricate questions and often vaguer answers; a dexterous dance of probing fingers; the percussion of knuckles across the patient's chest and abdomen in order to determine the consistency, shape, and size of body organs; the careful listening to, or auscultation of, the heart and lungs with a relatively new device called the stethoscope; the flick of a feather or jab of a pin and the aggressive thrust of a rubber hammer to elicit key signs of how the brain and nervous system were functioning—all of these maneuvers helped determine what ailed unfortunate denizens of the Krankenhaus.

At the inevitable autopsy, when the pathologist pronounced his measured but far-too-late medical opinion on the cause of death, no clinician wanted to be found having made an incorrect diagnosis. Failures of this magnitude were simply not an option at the Vienna Medical School. Perfection—or at least the perception of it—was demanded and expected of those bearing or coveting the title Herr Professor.

SIGMUND'S PROFESSIONAL ASCENT demanded that he become an internationally acclaimed medical investigator if he hoped to command laboratory space, financial compensation for his inquiries, and the freedom to pursue his ideas and theories. To achieve these ends, he began some of his earliest scientific work under Carl Claus, a biologist who ran the Institute of Zoology and had a long-standing fascination with hermaphroditism. Some have suggested that Sigmund was pleased neither by researching the gonads of eels nor with Professor Claus. In 1874, Sigmund left Claus for Vienna's famed Institute of Physiology, a bustling and vibrant laboratory directed by a visionary scientist named Ernst Wilhelm von Brücke. For the next six years, Sigmund would work at what was formerly a rifle factory and before that a stable alongside dozens of eager students in pursuit of scientific discovery.

When Brücke, the son of a painter, matriculated at the University of Berlin in

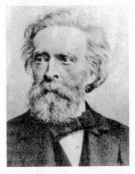

Carl Claus, Vienna Institute of Zoology, Freud's research mentor during his first year at the University of Vienna, 1873–74, when Freud was seventeen. Signaling his success there, Sigmund entered on his curriculum vitae in 1885, "I also worked a year in the laboratory of Professor C. Claus and was twice sent on vacation to the zoological station in Trieste."

1838, he secretly harbored the desire to become an artist. But Berlin was a leading capital of scientific discovery at the time, and Brücke soon fell under the spell of one of its most fertile minds, Johannes Müller (1801–1858). Müller is credited by many historians with dragging German science out of the fanciful muck and mire of *Naturphilosophie,* a now obscure theory of biology, nature, and mystical pantheism once adored by German academics.

Perhaps as a buttress against the lonely pursuits that constituted his studies, Freud bonded emotionally with Professor Brücke, the first of many teachers he latched onto during his long medical education. Sigmund's relationships with his bumbling father and his domineering, overprotective young hausfrau of a mother—not to mention the rest of his family—were, well, Freudian. With such a background, it is intriguing to focus upon Sigmund's frequent search for substitute father figures among his teachers. Too often the obscure young man experienced visceral pangs of longing, of not quite fitting in, or fears that others might declare him to be worthless that required the stern but comforting hand of a patriarch. But there were also practical reasons for Sigmund's search for the perfect parent–mentor–instructor–idea sharer. Such benevolent guides were, and are, essential ingredients in any recipe for devoting one's life to revolutionizing how the rest of the world thinks about and understands a particular corner of itself.

A small man with an oversized head, Professor Brücke was revered by his students and colleagues alike. He was obsessed with finding out precisely how the human body ticked, even as he struggled to explain how to put such a complex watch back together once he pulled it apart. Brücke was devoted to his students' professional development but was also strict and demanding. One afternoon in the late 1870s, Sigmund was tardy, resulting in a severe reprimand. Years later, Freud reported how he was "over-

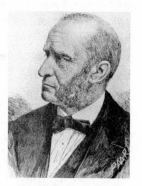

Ernst Wilhelm von Brücke, Freud's beloved mentor and director of the Vienna Institute of Physiology. The impressionable Freud worked under Professor Brücke from 1876 to 1882, between the ages of twenty and twenty-six.

whelmed by the terrible gaze of [Brücke's] eyes" and that the professor's
steely blue orbits would appear in his mind whenever the founder of
psychoanalysis was tempted to take a shortcut in his research. That one
afternoon aside, Freud was completely enamored with and inspired by
his teacher. Throughout his life, he told others that Professor Brücke
"remained the greatest authority that worked upon me." Freud also
often referred to his assistantship in Brücke's laboratory as "the happi-
est years of my youth."

The historian Peter Gay suggests another more practical attribute
that attracted Freud to Professor Brücke and, later, to his internal
medicine professor, Hermann Nothnagel: they "had no use for the
anti-Semitic agitation spreading across Vienna's culture like a stain."
Anti-Semitism remained a distressing fact of Austrian life during this
time and especially at the medical school, where Freud complained
that his "Gentile fellow students impertinently expected him to 'feel
inferior' and a stranger to the Austrian people [*nicht volkszugehörig*]
'because I was a Jew.' "

At the Vienna Institute of Physiology, students were encouraged to
conjure up original research projects and muddle through their execu-
tion. At the end of each week, armed with a sheath of notes and smoky
black kymograph tracings, the scientific novices ceremoniously presented their labors to the professor for comment, occasional praise,
and, more frequently, abrupt dismissal and immediate reassessment.
Under Brücke's exacting gaze, Freud progressed from fumbling with
the nervous systems of slimy invertebrates all the way to examining
human cadaver brains and spinal cords, in the quest to unravel the
workings of nerve cells, nerve fibers, and their far-flung connections
from the brain to the rest the body. As a result, young Sigmund completed a small corpus of competent, descriptive work, accompanied by
his own meticulous pen-and-ink drawings of what he visualized under
the microscope. A few of his studies even made their way into the
respectable typeface of the leading journals of the day.

Acquiring the skills to become a microscopic neuroanatomist in the
late nineteenth century was no simple task. The job required a strong
streak of perfectionism, a keen eye, and great attention to detail, especially when finely cutting the tissues of eels, fish, crayfish, and other
creatures so that each slice was thin enough to accommodate a gaze

through a microscope without destroying its delicate structure. One had to then carefully "fix," or harden, the intact tissue slices, typically in a pungent bath of alcohol solutions, followed by the meticulous application of stains and dyes so that the researcher could detect, as Sigmund detailed to his fiancée, "where the fibers and cells lie in relation to one another. . . . The fibers are the leading ducts of the different parts of the body, the cells are in control of them, so respect is due to these creatures."

Sigmund mastered all these chores and described them in great detail. In a few of his papers, he even suggested some fundamental points of what Santiago Ramón y Cajal, H. W. G. Waldeyer, Camillo Golgi, and others subsequently described as the "neuron doctrine," a concept that became the foundational tenet of modern neurobiology. Specifically, neurons are independent cellular structures, rather than a fused, continuous entity, that carry impulses from the central nervous system, neuron to neuron, to the peripheral parts of the body, resulting in some type of movement or action.

There was one short-lived moment, in 1883, when Sigmund

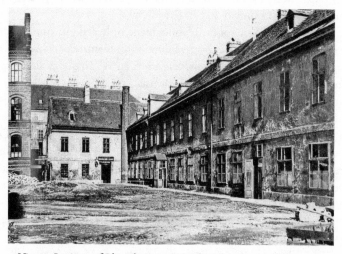

Vienna Institute of Physiology, c. 1885, when Freud worked there. The building was a former gun factory dating back to when this portion of the hospital was an armory; before that, it housed a stable.

thought a modicum of medical fame might be his, but the event quickly dissolved into professional disappointment. Brain tissue is distinctly gray in color, which makes exact visualization through a microscope difficult. During this period of intense anatomic identification, researchers played with all kinds of chemicals that might be picked up by discrete neuroanatomical structures, making them more visible. While working on the histological structure of nerves, Freud developed a novel staining technique employing potash, copper, water, and gold chloride that tinted the various neuronal fibers with red, pink, purple, black, and blue hues. He rushed his preliminary findings into print in the pages of *Centralblatt für die medizinischen Wissenschaften,* a local medical newsletter read primarily by his Viennese colleagues. He then craftily submitted a fuller, but essentially the same, account for the prestigious and widely read journal *Pflügers Archiv für Anatomie und Physiologie,* followed by still another version for the British journal *Brain.* Although this paper briefly created a mild stir among those who spent their days and evenings visualizing nervous tissue under the microscope, it lacked that essential ingredient of all good scientific research: reproducible results in the hands of others. Soon after the paper appeared in print, Sigmund's method evaporated as quickly as a rain puddle on a sunny day.

In fact, Freud's anatomical labors made only a slight ripple in an already turbulent sea of discovery. From 1873 well into the 1880s, he was firmly fixed in the fat part of his class's bell curve. To quote Sigmund's career self-assessment, at this point he was "stuck."

IN JULY 1882, a little more than a year after being awarded his M.D., Freud realized that his chances of obtaining a paying assistantship in Brücke's laboratory were less than robust. The two paid assistants already working in the laboratory—Ernst von Fleischl-Marxow and Sigmund Exner—were young and gifted, and had no intention of relinquishing their coveted posts. As a result, Professor Brücke encouraged Sigmund to complete his qualifications to become a physician and helped him secure a niche on the lowest rung of the General Hospital's steep professional ladder. The Viennese physicians called such clinicians *Aspirants;* today, they are called interns. Depending upon the medical procedure they were assisting on, these clinical subordinates were often green around the gills. But as a rule, they were ambitious, eager to please, and young of body, mind, and spirit. Sigmund was enough of a pragmatist to know that he had to find a way to earn a suitable living; but at the time, a life taking care of patients was a pale second choice to the low-paying but all-important assistantship at the Institute of Physiology. On July 31, a deeply disappointed Freud "inscribed himself in the General Hospital of Vienna."

Through the hot, steamy summer and early fall, Freud toiled on the busy surgical wards controlled by Theodor Billroth. Few young doctors would dare to touch the hem of Dr. Billroth's surgical gown. After all, Billroth had invented the procedures to circumvent age-old abdominal problems such as peptic ulcers and stomach cancer, attracting hundreds of ambitious young surgeons anxious to learn from the master. He was an enormous bear of a man with blue eyes as piercing as his surgical instruments and an imposing, luxuriant beard. But the surgeon also wielded a sharp tongue and refused to suffer fools or uncoordinated hands on his wards. Dr. Freud lasted only two months in this grueling position. Many evenings he complained about fatigue and aching muscles in his legs and arms from standing so long and so still in the operating room, where tradition and protocol dictated that he hold a senior surgeon's retractors in order to keep the surgical wound open and accessible.

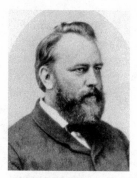

Theodor Billroth, the famed professor of surgery at the University of Vienna, c. 1880.

Freud probably had little or no contact with Billroth while serving on his clinical service, since the surgeon quit Vienna around this time for a summer holiday in Italy, leaving his chief assistant, Anton Wölfler, in command. An accomplished musician and a friend of Johannes Brahms's, Dr. Billroth was also a vociferous anti-Semite who publicly declared that Jews had no place in medicine. Evidence suggests that he was hardly shy about expressing these opinions to his students. Worse, his pedagogic bigotry was mimicked by many of his surgical assistants. As an example of this

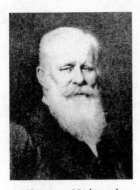

Hermann Nothnagel, professor of medicine. In 1882, at age twenty-six, Freud began working for him and spent nearly a year on the internal medicine wards of the Krankenhaus.

behavior, a few years later, in January 1885, Freud wrote to Martha describing how one of Billroth's assistants publicly berated a coreligionist as a "Jewish swine" because he failed to agree with the surgeon "about some minor technical matter."

In early October 1882, Sigmund mustered the courage to petition Hermann Nothnagel for the position of *Aspirant* on the internal medicine wards. A learned professor and internist, Dr. Nothnagel was the author of a widely used dictionary of therapeutics and an authoritative textbook on brain diseases. He was also somewhat of a clinical tyrant who exacted a commitment of time and energy from his trainees that few young doctors would ever sign up for today. Famously, Herr Professor Doktor Nothnagel admonished his medical students, "Whoever needs more than five hours of sleep should not study medicine. The medical student must attend lectures from eight in the morning until six in the evening. Then he must go home and read until late at night." Demanding he was, but Nothnagel also taught his pupils that "only a good man can become a great physician."

Freud served under Nothnagel for six and a half months, simultaneously impressing and ingratiating himself with the man who, along with the anatomist Brücke, would serve as his principal cheerleader as he advanced his career and earning power. But eventually, Dr. Freud began to appreciate that he had little interest in treating those admitted to Nothnagel's ward, let alone in studying their physical maladies.

WHAT DID INTEREST FREUD was the connection between mind and brain dysfunction. Accordingly, on May 1, 1883, he transferred from Nothnagel's internal medicine ward to the psychiatric clinic, under the direction of one of his favorite medical school lecturers, Dr. Theodor Meynert. Freud called him "the Great Meynert in whose foot-

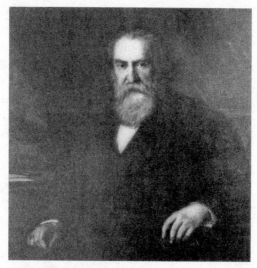

*Theodor Meynert, director of the Second Psychiatric
Clinic at the Krankenhaus. Freud worked under
"the Great Meynert" for five months beginning in
May 1883, at the age of twenty-seven.*

steps I followed with such veneration." No wonder. Professor Meynert all but ruled the fields of neuroanatomy and psychiatry in Austria, even though his university's charge to treat the mentally ill was slightly less prestigious than the chairs awarded in internal medicine or surgery. For the next five months, Freud cared for confused, psychotic, and senile patients in both the male wards (two months) and the female wards (three months). The most immediate advantage to Sigmund's career shift, however, was his promotion to the position of *Sekundararzt,* a combination of what we might today call a senior resident and a very junior attending physician or instructor. With this advance, he wrote his fiancée, Martha, he might have a decent shot at a middling career in Vienna. With perseverance—and, of course, that seminal discovery that would make his name—perhaps he could advance to a steady income that would finance the marriage and family they could now only dream about.

In October, Freud segued to the hospital's dermatology wards, which overflowed with the degenerating brains, hearts, noses, arteries,

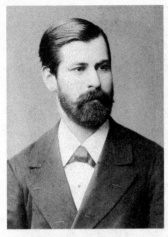

Freud as an Aspirant *at the Krankenhaus, age twenty-six, 1882–83.*

nerves, and skin of those stricken with syphilis. Dermatologists of the late nineteenth century were also known as syphilologists because their practice centered on treating the rashes and skin lesions associated with this deadly sexually transmitted infection. Sigmund complained that he saw patients only in the male wards and missed the opportunity to see the manifestations of neurosyphilis in women. He embarked on this clinical course because he knew the ability to diagnose and treat a variety of rashes was vital for a lucrative career as a general practitioner. But he also appreciated that syphilis represented one of the great puzzles of the nexus between organic and behavioral pathology. In the end, Freud did not find dermatology "a very appetizing field," and the disgust he experienced while

Vienna General Hospital, c. 1882.

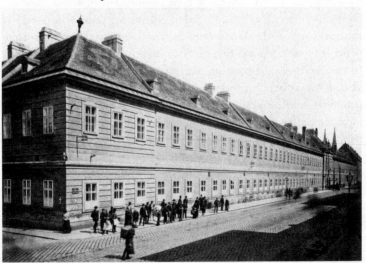

caring for the diseased and debauched permeated his letters and weighed heavily on his mind. Had he made the right choice? Was he wasting his youth? What would become of him? Such uncomfortable questions plagued his thoughts as sharply as the spiral-shaped syphilitic microbes burrowed into the brains and hearts of his patients. With resolve and focus, he managed to stifle these disturbing notions as he plied his patients with industrial-strength mercury and iodide-containing concoctions.

And rise he did. In his final full year at the Vienna General Hospital, 1883–84, Sigmund took charge of the inpatient nervous diseases ward, which comprised a typical census of 106 patients, 10 nurses, 2 junior *Sekundararzt,* and 1 *Aspirant.* Still, no aspect of his exhausting work—the long hours, the intense competition, the sordid plights of the patients he treated, his slow career progression, his self-doubt, prejudice in the workplace—could have been very soothing to Sigmund's increasingly jarred psyche. If only he could relax, rest, and refresh himself, Sigmund likely thought during those long days and nights. But how?

IN LATE JANUARY 1884, Sigmund wrote to his "Fraulein Martha" about a grand evening of papers and medical networking at the Vienna Medical Society. The still unknown physician planted himself in a seat directly behind the regal Herr Professors Billroth and Nothnagel. Sigmund silently watched and enviously stewed as they accepted the accolades and compliments of dozens of colleagues who had won their favor. To Martha, he confessed his unspoken thoughts of deep resentment: "Just you wait till you welcome me as you are welcoming the others now."

No wonder Freud was so cranky. After eleven years of training, he was facing many more years of grueling and unremunerative hospital work. A few months later, in April, the overburdened and melancholic Sigmund wrote his fiancée:

> *You will certainly be surprised, my darling, to hear that I am sitting here again after having written to you as recently as Saturday from the same spot; this is the result of my having been absent through being laid up so long, and rather awkward it is*

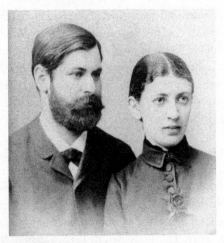

Sigmund Freud, age twenty-seven, and his fiancée,
Martha Bernays, age twenty-two, c. 1883.

too. I feel there is something altogether missing at the moment;
I cannot work at the laboratory because of the prospering practice;
work on the experiments, from which I expect little recognition,
is lying idle. It gave me quite a turn today when the proofs of
my paper on the Method arrived from Leipzig; since then, with
the exception of two small discoveries, I have done no work,
whatever.

As downcast as he may have sounded to Martha, she knew long before the rest of the world that his drive for success was indefatigable. In the years to come she would profess that she was never much of a follower of psychoanalysis, but she always believed in her Sigmund.

In many respects, his feelings would be familiar to any medical student or doctor today. If we did not know the career trajectory of the author of these many letters to Martha Bernays, one might dismiss them as a young man's means of quelling a troubled mind, literate but screaming pleas for escape from his medical Hades. But the obvious historical difference, of course, is that these were the career musings and worries of Sigmund Freud. Unlike countless other pupils who ruminate bitterly about real or perceived slights from their professors and mutter resentful vows of burying them with the attainment of fame and accomplishment, Freud actually did it.

Many medical aficionados recall the name of Billroth; far fewer recognize that of Nothnagel or Meynert; yet nearly every college graduate today has some understanding of Sigmund Freud's work. Early in his life, Freud understood that he was different from others and yet was highly desirous of being accepted into the mainstream of his professional and social sphere. Intellectually superior to many he encountered, Sigmund fantasized about greatness but had no clear idea how to achieve it. Such disquiet must have fueled his insecurity and, on many occasions, caused him to doubt the wisdom of his career choice. Sigmund was the type of genius who needed the glowing affirmation of others and yet was continually forced to hear his inner voice tell him that he was something far less. But aside from Martha, few were stroking Sigmund's battered ego.

Psychiatrists and other mental health experts have long debated the existence of what has been popularly labeled the addictive personality; yet if such characteristics could be uniformly relied upon as a diagnostic indicator, many professionals might consider Sigmund an ideal candidate. His particular constellation of bold risk taking, emotional scar tissue, and psychic turmoil would soon be put to the ultimate test. In the months that followed his experience of envy at the Vienna Medical Society, the young doctor's scientific interests and runny nose turned increasingly to an exciting new drug called cocaine hydrochloride.

CHAPTER 2

Young Halsted

L ATE IN LIFE, William Stewart Halsted recalled that his childhood was overly restrictive and occasionally nightmarish. To be sure, his living arrangements at both his family's town house on Fifth Avenue near Fourteenth Street in Manhattan and their country home in Irvington-on-Hudson, New York, were luxurious and comfortable.

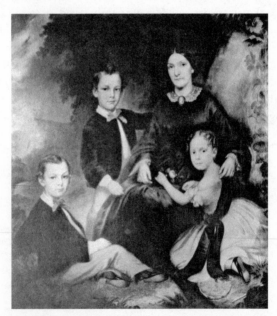

*William Halsted with his mother, sister, and older brother, c. 1860.
William is seated at left; he would have been four years old.*

But even from the distance of more than a century and a half, his parents hardly seem warm or supportive.

His father, William Mills Halsted Jr., stern, hard-nosed, and preoccupied, ran a profitable dry goods firm in Manhattan and founded the Commonwealth Fire Insurance Company. Descended from an established lineage that had first immigrated to the United States from Great Britain in the 1660s, Mr. Halsted played in the highest circles of New York City society and wielded enormous influence as a member of the Board of Trustees of the College of the City of New York, the College of Physicians and Surgeons (now part of Columbia University), and several other charitable institutions and philanthropies. William's mother, Mary Louisa Haines Halsted, was the daughter of William Sr.'s business partner, Richard Townley Haines, and hailed from a distinguished family tree that included the founders of Elizabeth, New Jersey.

Both Mary Louisa and William Jr. relegated the daily upbringing of their four children to a retinue of governesses and servants. Sadly for Halsted and his siblings, his mother preferred the company of her coiffed and powdered peers; William Jr. was most interested in the cultivation of orchids in his well-stocked greenhouse. Perhaps the singular exception to this parental distance was the father's nightly reprobation to William, filled with fire and brimstone drawn straight out of his Presbyterian code of morals, indicating disapproval of whatever his exuberant and rebellious son accomplished or avoided that day.

In 1863, at the age of eleven, William ran away from a private school in Monson, Massachusetts, only to be "captured" in Springfield, a distance of twenty-four miles, and forced to return home. Despite these hints of unhappiness at school and at home, William was accepted to Andover in the fall of 1863, where he remained an indolent if not lazy scholar, much to Mr. Halsted's chagrin.

When William graduated from the preparatory school in 1869, the father adjudged the sixteen-year-old boy too immature to go off to college. Instead, Mr. Halsted kept William close at hand and hired a series of private tutors to coach the teenaged boy for the notoriously rigorous entrance examinations at Yale. These exercises were conducted twice a year, in the three days following commencement in late July (Sundays excluded) and, eight weeks later, three days before the fall term began. William crammed for a year in order to demonstrate a yeoman's profi-

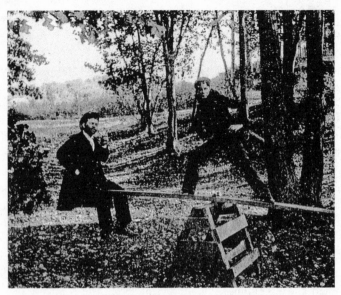

Halsted at about age fourteen, with his father, William Mills Halsted Jr.,
at the family's country home in Irvington-on-Hudson, New York, c. 1866.

ciency in Greek and Latin, a reading knowledge of Cicero, Virgil, Cae-
sar, and Homer, and a fluid recall of arithmetic, algebra, geometry, English grammar, and geography. The test cost $10 ($170 in 2010 dollars),
and roughly half of those taking it passed. Upon acceptance, the fathers
of the fortunate 151 young men admitted to the class of 1874, including
a beaming Mr. Halsted, were required to post bonds of $200 (a little
over $3,400 in 2010 dollars) "to secure the payment of all charges aris-
ing under the laws of the College."

Before the first term of his freshman year had closed, William had
abandoned Odysseus and Euclid for the playing fields. Wiry, agile,
compactly built, and muscular, William played shortstop on the college's baseball team, tumbled with the gymnastics team, and rowed
with the crew. In 1873, he served as the captain of Yale's football team,
which holds the distinction of being the first collegiate eleven-man
squad ever fielded in the nation. William's physical strength would
serve him well throughout his career, being an essential attribute for the
arduous life of a surgeon.

At Yale, William was a member of all the right fraternities and

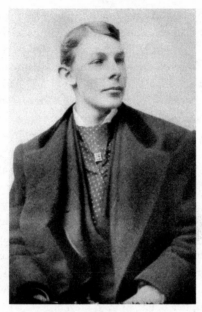

Halsted in 1868, at age sixteen,
eager to go off to college.

clubs, became proficient in French, appeared in several dramatic productions, wore bespoke suits, was an excellent dancer, and steadfastly
eschewed alcohol. His photographic portrait documents a good-
looking young man with gentle eyes, strong features, and ears the size
of jug handles.

When combing through his college transcripts, one finds little to
predict an incandescent intellectual curiosity. According to the university's library records, he didn't sign out a single volume between 1870
and 1874. Decades later, one of Halsted's classmates described William's
scholastic record as singularly undistinguished: "He was generally popular with the student body and socially minded, but gave no evidence
of unusual ability or of great ambition."

IN A LETTER WRITTEN TO HIS CLOSE FRIEND William Henry
Welch on July 14, 1922, Halsted identified the precise moment of his
intellectual awakening: "Devoted myself solely to athletics in college.

In senior year purchased Gray's Anatomy and Dalton's Physiology and studied them with interest; attended a few clinics at the Yale Medical School." The first volume William mentions was, of course, *Anatomy: Descriptive and Surgical,* the best-selling atlas of the human body by Henry Gray of London. The other book was an internationally well-regarded and authoritative physiology text, *A Treatise on Human Physiology: Designed for the Use of Students and Practitioners of Medicine.*

Physiology is the science devoted to understanding the function of living organisms and the organs, tissues, and cells that compose them. During the mid- to late nineteenth century, the field was just hitting its stride as medicine's central explanatory discipline. To put the long history of medical epistemology succinctly, one must first understand anatomy, or how the body is structured, followed by physiology, how a particular organ or structure works under normal circumstances at ever closer levels. From there, one can begin to approach studying diseased bodies and organs, what physicians call pathology, in order to assess what has changed because of a particular illness and try to develop the means to contain, treat, cure, or even prevent it.

A Treatise on Human Physiology was written by Professor John Call Dalton of New York's College of Physicians and Surgeons, a man credited as being the "first professional physiologist in the continental United States." One of the book's most glowing reviews, likely composed by the great Harvard anatomist and essayist Oliver Wendell Holmes Sr., exclaimed, "Dr. Dalton is one of the few native teachers of physiology who have made the discovery that an American has eyes, hands, organs, dimensions, senses, as well as a German or a Frenchman. He actually examines the phenomena he describes as they exist in Nature!" So persuasive were Dalton's powers as a lecturer that the famed Philadelphia neurologist and novelist S. Weir Mitchell said that he had "the rare gift of making those who listened desire to become investigators."

Gaining admission to medical school in 1874 was hardly characterized by the cutthroat competition of today. At many American medical schools, one needed only a scintilla of intellectual achievement to justify a student's berth. Few institutions even required a college diploma. But there also existed a clear-cut pecking order, from the finest academies, typically tied to established universities, such as Harvard, Yale,

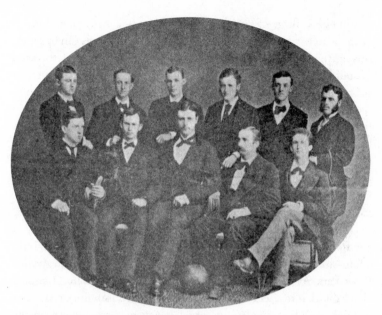

Halsted at age twenty (top row, third from left) and the 1872 Yale football team—the first eleven-man football team fielded by a U.S. college.

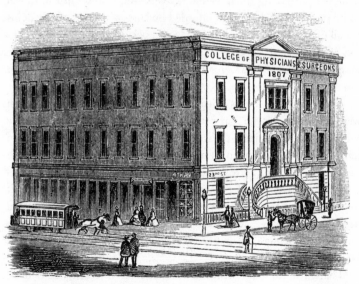

Halsted's medical school: the New York College of Physicians and Surgeons.

Columbia's College of Physicians and Surgeons, Michigan, and Pennsylvania, to less prestigious, storefront proprietary schools run by enterprising practitioners subscribing to a polyglot of medical theories, including allopathy, homeopathy, herbalism, water therapy, and eclecticism. Nevertheless, it could hardly have hurt Halsted's application to the College of Physicians and Surgeons, easily one of the best schools in the nation, to list as a reference his father, who served on the college's board of trustees. In the late spring, William was informed that he would be admitted to the class of 1876. He also secured a coveted research assistantship under his new medical hero, John Call Dalton. Given the state of medical education in late-nineteenth-century America, Halsted would have found it difficult to land in a better position.

The halls of the College of Physicians and Surgeons were hardly as austere or dignified as the decorous European medical schools. Within a four-story brick building on Twenty-third Street and Fourth Avenue (now Park Avenue South) in Manhattan, students were crammed chockablock into a series of stifling lecture rooms, amphitheaters, laboratories, and dissecting suites. The latter were always placed on the top floor of nineteenth-century medical school buildings to better ventilate the putrefying smell of the cadavers and, just as critical, to welcome in the natural daylight afforded by large windows and skylights. Yet all of the rooms at the College of Physicians and Surgeons, regardless of purpose, were smelly, smoky, dirty, and musty; in the winter months, the classrooms were blasted by the building's powerful hot-air furnace.

The medical students at the College of Physicians and Surgeons were notorious for the "cat-calls, whistles, and yells" they directed at professors as they entered the lecture hall. William scorned such sophomoric high jinks and instead hunkered down to his studies. His diligence paid off, and he rose with ease to the top of his class. Halsted delivered a sterling performance on his oral examinations, and his written thesis, "Contraindications to Operations," was awarded an academic prize and a check for $100, or more than $2,000 in 2010 dollars. In June 1876, he graduated *medicinae doctor* (M.D.), *cum laude* (with honors).

That autumn, Halsted would advance to an internship at Bellevue Hospital, a short distance on foot from his medical school. One of the

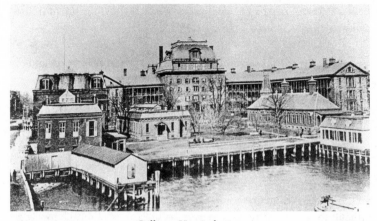

Bellevue Hospital, 1879.

oldest hospitals in the nation, it was named for a bucolic farm that once overlooked Kips Bay and the East River. Founded by a Dutch surgeon named Jacob Hendrickssen Varrenvanger in 1658, it began as an almshouse. In 1736, the Board of Aldermen of New York established a six-bed hospital. During the next century and a half, Bellevue's physical plant and medical mission grew exponentially.

Unlike today's medical centers, nineteenth-century American hospitals were charitable enterprises devoted to the care of the urban poor, orphans, widows, seamen, soldiers, and immigrants. Consequently, hospital trustees spent a great deal of effort deciding which patient was morally worthy of the healing experience they offered and, thus, should be granted admission. Drunks, criminals, unwed mothers, prostitutes, and the so-called undeserving poor need not apply. In such an institutional atmosphere, the healing process was focused less upon therapeutic medications, diagnostic tools, and invasive operations than upon improving the unhealthy living environments of patients—and their godless ways—in the hope of effecting a spiritual, if not a physical, cure.

The several blocks William traversed from his family's well-appointed town house to the hospital afforded a stunning trip into the depths of late-nineteenth-century urban squalor. For example, an 1878 *Harper's Magazine* essay explained to its well-to-do subscribers that

Bellevue was situated amid a collection of ramshackle tenement houses and that entry was no simple matter:

> [The area was] plentifully dotted with shabby little stores and corner groggeries, where the garbage is piled up in the streets, the men are idle, the women slatternly, and the children as nearly nude as the weather permits. . . . The activity at Bellevue has no end. The keeper of the lodge at the entrance is continually besought for admission, and so worried by impossible requests that one can pardon his shortness of temper.

Given the rudimentary state of medical education in this era, it was difficult for young physicians to gain the breadth of clinical knowledge and experience taken for granted today. American medical schools rarely, if ever, introduced their students to actual patients, preferring instead to pedantically lecture at them for a few years, followed by a lengthy apprenticeship with a practicing doctor. Worse, there were far more medical school graduates than there were internship slots at first-rate hospitals. Consequently, Bellevue was such a prestigious place to

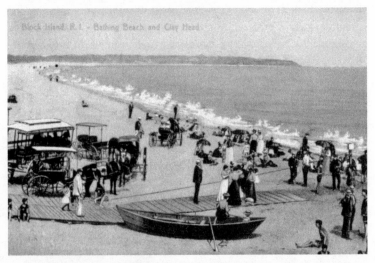

Block Island, where the Halsted family summered. Halsted studied for his internship exam at Bellevue here during the summer of 1878.

train that it required a rigorous entrance examination and selected interns from among the very highest-scoring students.

During the summer of 1876, William vacationed on Block Island, fourteen miles east of Montauk Point, Long Island, and thirteen miles south of the coast of Rhode Island. He devoted his mornings and evenings to cramming for his internship examination; his afternoons were spent swordfishing, swimming, and sailing in the Atlantic Ocean. William scored fifth among the competitive applicants and was awarded a coveted position on Bellevue's fourth surgical division. He was one of only eight interns accepted that fall. What he found within its forbidding, protective walls was a busy complex of charity wards, laboratories, and an active morgue. Docked along the East River was a funeral ferry that transported unclaimed bodies up to Potter's Field on Hart Island. Adjacent to the hospital was the Bellevue Medical College, filled to the rafters with well-dressed, well-off, young white men eager to learn how to be doctors.

The river of human pathology at Bellevue had no end, and its sources were the slums and ghettos of New York. "The picture has many changes, no reverse," William Rideing wrote about Bellevue in 1878, "it is pain, anguish, or death always. If the spectator is cynical, his morbidity is enlarged; but, if, without being an optimist, he can look at it with clear eyes, its gloom and sadness are relieved by a glimpse of the tenderness that blossoms in the hearts of the commonest poor."

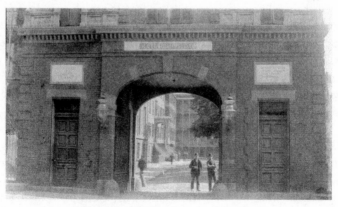

Bellevue Hospital's main gate, 1878 or 1879.

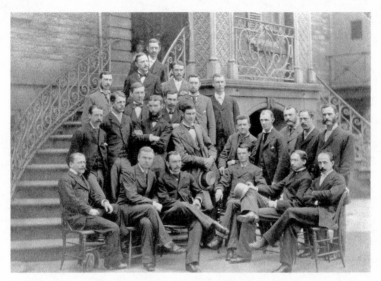

Halsted's internship class at Bellevue, 1878. Halsted, age twenty-six, is in the second row, fourth from the right, under the arch.

From morning to late at night, year after year, the sick and needy pounded on the hospital's doors, begging for admission—the victims of accidents in the building trades, the chronically and acutely ill, the hopelessly alcoholic, the insane, and the physically broken. The most desperately ill were transported in horse-drawn ambulances that received their calls through an independent telegraph wire that connected every New York City police precinct with the hospital. In 1876, 5,165 patients were admitted, most of them foreign-born; 2,215 of these patients were Irish, 1,680 American, 595 German, 256 English, and 56 French. Only 4,313 lived long enough to be discharged. With mortality rates of 16.5 percent, large numbers of former Bellevue patients were laid to rest in unmarked graves every year.

There existed a clear chain of command at Bellevue; Halsted had to ascend through job titles such as interne, junior assistant, senior assistant, and, finally, house surgeon. Internes were required to reside full-time in the hospital. Junior and senior assistants were allowed to go off duty each night at six p.m., unless an emergent case came in and the surgeon in charge felt compelled to call any and all in for help. The seven-day-a-week job (plus many nights) was "strenuous, exacting, and exhausting," according to one of Halsted's contemporaries, "but the experience was most varied and profitable."

Along the way, the impressionable young physician made medical rounds with such luminaries as Abraham Jacobi, the universally revered German émigré who established pediatrics as a bona fide medical specialty in the United States; the domineering internists Theodore Janeway and Alfred Loomis, whose textbooks and ideas on fever, practice, and therapeutics were absorbed, memorized, and communicated by generations of American medical students; and the prominent surgeons Alexander Mott, Erskine Mason, and Frank H. Hamilton. In later life Halsted noted that he learned little or nothing from the first two surgeons, while Hamilton became something of a mentor to him.

Once Halsted completed his internship at Bellevue, he ventured uptown to New York Hospital, where he served an additional six months as house physician. There he briefly flirted with studying neurology under an inspiring teacher named Edward Seguin, the distinguished son of the even more prominent French neurologist Édouard Séguin. But at New York Hospital, Halsted was biding his time for a far more important medical stepping-stone: two years of professional seasoning in the medical meccas of his day—Berlin, Würzburg, Leipzig, and Vienna.

WILLIAM WAS HARDLY ALONE in such a pursuit. For decades, young American physicians aspiring to medical greatness traveled to Europe for advanced study. In the late eighteenth and early nineteenth centuries, enormous hospitals like Guy's and St. Bartholomew's in London and the Hôtel-Dieu in Paris were the destinations of choice. By the time Halsted embarked on his postgraduate medical training, however, the German and Austrian universities dominated virtually every aspect of science and medicine. These medical and research centers beckoned eager students from around the globe to learn disciplines that were then as new, exciting, and important as genomics and stem cell biology are today. Between 1870 and 1914, more than ten thousand doctors made the medical pilgrimage; or, as one historian has estimated, approximately 40 to 50 percent of all the American physicians born between 1850 and 1890 studied in Germany. As a result, auditoriums across Germany and the Austro-Hungarian Empire were crowded with eager students kneeling or sitting at the feet of the masters, innovators, and, in many cases, founders of the modern medical research enterprise.

Like many young men who aspired to the elite ranks of academic medicine, William hailed from a wealthy family for whom money was never a concern. He simply declared his plans for the upcoming two years, drew a significant amount of money from his father's bank account, picked up a first-class-passage ticket from the steamship company, and sailed off to Europe. He arrived in Vienna on November 4, 1878.

Thereafter, for nearly a year, William stuck to a regimen of two German lessons each day so that he might better understand the countless lectures he attended at the Vienna Medical School. He focused most intently on learning about the vanguard discoveries being made at the operating table. Every evening, he washed down *Tafelspitz* with seidels of Märzen lager, exuberantly debating medical theories with his fellow students. His surgical aptitude soon caught the attention of Billroth's aide-de-camp and assistant surgeon, Anton Wölfler, who invited William to work in his laboratory. There, Wölfler provided his American protégé with unlimited access to a superb collection of expensive, powerful, and finely polished microscopes, one of the principal technological tools employed in medical research of that era but hard to come by in the United States unless specially ordered from Germany. Finally, Dr. Wölfler introduced William to Vienna's medical crème de la crème, including Theodor Billroth.

In 1878 and 1879, Halsted and Sigmund Freud orbited the same tentacular campus that was the Vienna General Hospital and Medical School. For most of that period, Freud drudged over his laboratory bench at the Institute of Physiology, while Halsted made the medical equivalent of a grand tour. Sometime during his stay, William even initiated a private course in neuroanatomy with Dr. Theodor Meynert, the university's professor of psychiatry, who a few years later would become such an important intellectual figure in Sigmund Freud's life. Halsted's tutorials were held daily at six a.m. in Meynert's apartment. Each morning, Professor Meynert insisted on conducting the lesson from his bed while still in his rumpled pajamas. Decades later, in 1922, a still disgusted Halsted recalled that because "the lesson was given in his unsavory bedroom I soon released him from his contract." Despite these near misses, no documentation exists to suggest that Freud and Halsted ever met.

For the academic year 1879–80, William traveled to several German universities and medical schools. There, he heard some of the world's leading authorities present lectures on embryology, histology (the microscopic anatomy of cells and tissues), and physiology. Until his dying days, William extolled the virtues of the German university system and its influence on his life and work. As his Johns Hopkins colleague William Osler later remarked, William returned to New York from this trip "very much *verdeutsched.*"

Halsted also returned a superbly trained surgeon, perhaps the best of his generation, firmly committed to living much of his life within the confines of the operating room. He made his career choice precisely at the time when the field was just evolving from an ancient craft to an armamentarium of miraculous cures. Even as late as 1880, the surgical enterprise overflowed with danger, during both the procedure itself and the patient's recovery thereafter. To be sure, great strides had been made with the advent of ether anesthesia, in the 1840s. But in an era before the universal acceptance of antiseptic surgery, infections ran rampant in surgical wards. Deadly surgical complications, including shock and hemorrhages, were so standard that it is little wonder some vaudevillian was inspired to remark, "The operation was a success, but the patient died!" At this point in medical history, only a consummate risk taker would devote his life to surgery.

CHAPTER 3

Über Coca

AT FIRST GLANCE, a clump of cocaine appears pearly white, crystalline, and innocuous. Lurking within, however, resides the molecular power to inhibit the human brain's uptake of dopamine, serotonin, and norepinephrine, chemical neurotransmitters essential to the governance of mood and many other mental activities. Along the way, cocaine suppresses one's appetite, speeds up thoughts and actions, races the heart, and inspires a raucous euphoria that makes the brain hungry for more and more.

There exists a long history of human encounters with cocaine's vegetative source, a rather plain-looking bush that carries the elaborate Latin name *Erythroxylum coca.* A leafy shrub of six to eighteen feet in height, it grows most potently along the eastern slopes of the Andes Mountains descending into the Amazon basin, a moist, mountainous climate, at elevations of 1,500 to 6,000 feet. Its distinctive pale green, oval leaves have been harvested there for millennia. The local Peruvian Indians, or *coqueros,* who used it on a daily basis, called it *cuca.* Their Inca forebears venerated it as "the divine plant" and incorporated it into many religious rituals and initiation rites. So cherished a staple were these *cuca* leaves that virtually every man and woman in the region carried a small pouch filled with them, always ready for a chew and typically empty by nightfall.

FREUD'S FIRST ENCOUNTERS with cocaine were on the written page. Ever the obsessive-compulsive scholar, Sigmund gathered stacks of papers and books on cocaine, many of which he borrowed from a distinguished Viennese pharmacologist named August Vogl, all neatly piled on the small worktable of his hospital quarters.

He devoured every paragraph of these documents. Long fascinated by myths and saga, Freud thrilled while reading about Manco Cápac, Incan mythology's son of the Sun God, who descended from the cliffs of Lake Titicaca to deliver his father's light to the "wretched inhabitants of the country." Manco Cápac's other gift to humankind, as Freud later noted, was the "coca leaf, this divine plant which satisfies the hungry, strengthens the weak, and causes them to forget their misfortune."

Sigmund also read about the explorers who traveled from Spain to the New World during the sixteenth and seventeenth centuries. In

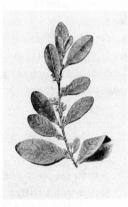

Coca leaves
(Erythroxylum coca).

places we now know as Peru, Colombia, Bolivia, the Amazon basin, and the Andean mountainsides, the Spaniards raped, pillaged, and plundered for gold, silver, and other riches, proudly proclaiming themselves masters of all they surveyed. They brought with them many deadly infectious diseases, including measles, smallpox, and diphtheria. The result was an infectious, economic, and cultural devastation of these indigenous communities—a swift, fatal erosion, if not erasure, of centuries of progress and civilization. To make matters worse, the conquistadors subjugated those who survived into a brutal slavery, forcing them to labor in a wide range of agricultural, mining, and exporting ventures, all in the name—and for the profit—of the queen and king of Spain.

Most conquistadors looked askance at the natives' *cuca* habit. Those most faithful to the Catholic Church condemned its use as a sin. The indigenous people hardly listened, let alone cared. They had long since become accustomed to living in the glow of a mild euphoria and sense of purpose that chewing these leaves reliably produced.

With the passage of time, however, many of the Spaniards who initially dismissed *cuca* as the work of the devil tried chewing a few, or a lot, of the leaves themselves. And they, too, became impressed by and reliant upon the plant's powers. Those doing the governing and enslaving in the New World recognized far more practical reasons to encourage the Indians toiling in their mines to chew *cuca:* in higher doses, it has the remarkable ability to suppress hunger, increase tolerance for cold weather, and stretch the bounds of human endurance. An agent that encouraged a person to work harder was considered ideal for forcing others into physical labor in a high mountain climate where the oxygen content is palpably thin. The Spanish conquerors of Peru went as far as to create a legal framework for the sale and taxing of coca, insisting on a 10 percent cut of the sales of each crop. Such schemes helped set in motion an endless trail of misery for many involved in the cultivation, processing, and sale of its by-products and, more directly, for those succumbing to its pharmacological allure.

At the beginning of the nineteenth century, several intrepid Europeans embarked on prolonged explorations of the New World in search of glory and fortune. Most of them wrote excitedly to their loved ones back home about the region's beauty and natural riches. One of the adventurers Sigmund read about was the brave and curious German traveler Alexander von Humboldt. The twenty-nine-year-old Humboldt set out on a pathbreaking scientific expedition of the New World in early June 1799. As he sat in his cabin in a ship named the *Pizarro,* docked in the Spanish port of La Coruña before setting off across the Atlantic abyss, Humboldt wrote several farewell letters to his friends. Fearing that he might not return from the dangerous trip, he explained what motivated his peripatetic pilgrimage: "I shall collect plants and fossils and make astronomic observations. But that's not the main purpose of my expedition—I shall try to find out how the forces of nature interact upon one another and how the geographic environment influences plant and animal life. In other words, I must find out about the unity of nature."

Humboldt and his traveling companion, Aimé Bonpland, safely crossed the Atlantic Ocean and landed in Venezuela. The two men forged ahead on foot and horseback, by boat and dugout canoe, across the plains of Venezuela, along the length of the Orinoco River, the waterway Christopher Columbus thought led to paradise, up into the Andes Mountains, and down trails, passes, and valleys that stretched into Bogotá, Quito, and Lima. From there they crossed the Columbian

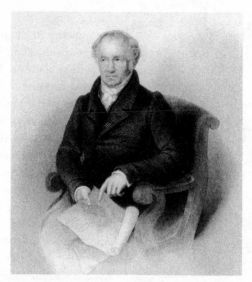

*The German naturalist Alexander von Humboldt
in 1840, at age seventy-one, forty-one years after
making his famous journey to the New World.*

isthmus and sailed to Mexico, Cuba, and the United States before finally returning to Europe in August 1804.

Along this dangerous journey, Humboldt meticulously described his observations in dozens of field notebooks, published under the title *Personal Narrative of a Journey to the Equinoctial Regions of the New Continent.* The work became one of the most popular travelogues of the nineteenth century. On its pages appear a comprehensive account of South America's climate, geology, geography, botany, zoology, political economy, and anthropology, guaranteeing Humboldt a reputation as an adventurer and scholar that, unlike those of many who preceded him, remains intact more than two centuries after the expedition ended.

In 1801, while tramping through the mountainous terrain of Peru, Humboldt was introduced to the buzzy sensations brought on by chewing coca leaves. He was impressed, to say the least, writing, "It is well known that Indian messengers take no other aliment for whole days than lime and coca; both excite the secretion of saliva and

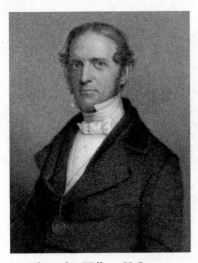

The author William H. Prescott, c. 1840.

gastric juice; they take away the appetite, without affording any nourishment to the body." Parenthetically, Humboldt erroneously hypothesized that the secret ingredient of this concoction was an alkaline ash, or lime, called *llipta* that the natives chewed with the leaves, rather than the leaves themselves.

Before long Humboldt's fascination with coca leaves was echoed by several other explorers who followed in his path and described how the leaves gave the Indians who chewed them superhuman powers of endurance and strength. As a result of such fantastic reports, coca was heralded across the popular press of the day. For example, an 1817 article published in the *Gentleman's Magazine,* a periodical read in London's finest clubs, breathlessly declared, "[The Indians] masticate Coca and undergo the greatest fatigue without any injury to health or bodily vigor. They want neither butcher nor baker, nor brewer, nor distiller, nor fuel, nor culinary utensils." The article went on to exhort Sir Humphrey Davy, England's greatest chemist, to drop everything and figure out the plant's secret, urging, "it would be the greatest achievement—whatever a London alderman might think—ever attained by human wisdom." Davy, unimpressed, stuck to his own research, elucidating the chemistry of several elements of the periodic table as well as the anesthetic properties of nitrous oxide, or laughing gas.

THE CURIOSITY ABOUT COCA among well-read Europeans and North Americans of the early nineteenth century was further advanced by one of the oddest historians ever to practice that bookish craft. He was a Boston Brahmin and Harvard graduate named William Hickling Prescott, whose work Sigmund likely read with great pleasure. One winter evening while still an undergraduate at Harvard, Prescott made his way across the Yard after eating dinner in the Commons with his school chums. College boys being college boys, a snowball fight soon ensued. A few of the students secreted out some stale bread from the dining room and buried the crusts in the snowballs about to become airborne. As Prescott turned his head to observe the commotion that accompanied this early-nineteenth-century version of a frosty food fight, he was struck in the left eye. So severe was the injury that he lost most of his vision on that side. A few years later, he developed an acute inflammation of his right eye and rheumatism, leaving him severely visually impaired and with debilitating joint pain for the remainder of his life.

Prescott's physical deficits forced him to give up his legal studies and dreams of joining his father's law firm. Instead, he retreated into the cloistered life of a writer focusing upon the storied past of Spain and its vast empire. Using his well-connected friends to gather bibliographic materials from the leading libraries of the world, along with the travel notes of those better equipped to see, explore, and characterize what he could not, Prescott produced a series of bulky tomes. He became a best-selling author in 1837 with a magisterial account of the reign of Spain's Ferdinand and Isabella. From there, he turned to writing a two-volume history of the conquests of Mexico and Peru, each of which surpassed his previous work in terms of sales and prestige when published in 1847.

Incredibly, this man, who made only occasional trips to London and the Continent, never actually visited the regions he wrote about so penetratingly for his legion of readers. Physical and geographical disabilities aside, Prescott managed to describe the climate, terrain, and culture of Peru in copious detail. He was particularly clear in stressing the brawny appeal coca leaves held for the *coqueros:*

> Even food the most invigorating is less grateful to him than his beloved narcotic. Under the Incas, it is said to have been exclusively reserved for the noble orders. If so, the people gained one luxury by the Conquest; and after that period, it was so extensively used by them, that this article constituted a most important colonial item of revenue of Spain.

Remarkably for so early in the history of Western civilization's awareness of coca, Prescott admonished, "Yet, with the soothing charms of an opiate, this weed so much vaunted by the natives, when used to excess, is said to be attended with all the mischievous effects of habitual intoxication." Unfortunately, few who embarked on studying coca in the 1880s, including Freud and Halsted, paid much attention to Prescott's prescient warning on the leaves' addictive powers.

SOME MIND-ALTERING AGENTS, such as marijuana and tobacco, need little more processing than desiccation before they are ready to be consumed, although someone, at some point, had to figure out that the effects of these particular substances were best felt when smoked. But unleashing the active, and most potent, aspects of the coca leaf for use as a medication and, later, as a drug of abuse was hardly an accident. It was the result of an exhaustive search engaging some of the best scientists, chemists, and physicians of the nineteenth century. All of these men—and not a few of the consumers of coca leaves who commissioned their research—were eager to discover just what miraculous substance was locked into these leaves that produced an endurance, confidence, and alertness so sublimely gratifying. More to the point, they wanted to know how that active ingredient could be harnessed into a profitable, life-saving—or at least life-enhancing—agent for the chronically depressed, fatigued, and inactive, as well as for a multitude of people simply seeking an extra lift.

Before such a vexing chemical equation could be solved, the first order of business was to address the enormous difficulty of shipping coca leaves around the world. The state of travel in the early to mid-nineteenth century made it all but impossible to successfully bring load after load of fresh coca leaves to Europe and North America. Transportation of coca leaves began in the treacherous, mountainous terrain of Peru and Colombia, and most mules could carry only a few bales of leaves at a time; these were subsequently hand-carried by intrepid hikers through the jungle and valleys, to the port towns. In later decades, railroad cars and riverboats were employed, but even with these innovations exporting *cuca* remained an arduous, dangerous, and expensive proposition. Making matters of importation even more complicated, the coca leaves tended to become stale and dried out on the long voyages back to Europe, and as the plants shriveled, so, too, did their vaunted powers. Worse, if the leaves became wet en route (a definite risk), they rotted and spoiled.

Beyond the limited supply of coca leaves, however, there remained the task of figuring out how to identify, extract, and mass-produce the active ingredient of the coca leaf—a process that took several decades. During much of the 1850s, chemists on both sides of the Atlantic played with alcohol solutions of coca leaves, dried residues of coca teas, and other means of extraction, with modest success.

In 1857, at the height of this interest in coca, the prominent German chemist Friedrich Wöhler contacted Carl Scherzer, a scientist assigned to the Austrian emperor Franz Josef's exploration frigate, the *Novara*. Wöhler convinced Scherzer to locate a large supply of coca leaves during his next voyage and bring them back to the empire. If Scherzer brought enough coca back to Europe, Wöhler was certain, he and his colleagues would figure out the secret of the leaves.

When Scherzer returned in 1859, an overjoyed Wöhler signed for the receipt of a large trunk of coca. In true professorial fashion, he assigned his most able graduate student at the University of Göttingen, Albert Niemann, to work up the coca leaf assignment and figure it out. Toiling over a carefully preserved thirty-pound stash of coca leaves, the largest intact shipment of coca ever to reach European shores, Niemann produced a seminal doctoral dissertation in 1860, entitled *On a New Organic Base in the Coca Leaves*. Among the many pages of complex formulas and laboratory methods, Niemann describes how he solved the holy grail of converting coca leaves into the highly purified coca alkaloid. Sadly, Dr. Niemann died at age twenty-six, a year after the Göttingen faculty approved his dissertation, constituting an especially odd case of publishing and then perishing. Nevertheless, Niemann's chemical inquiries became the basis of deriving the addictive cocaine alkaloid crystals from coca leaves. By the close of the nineteenth century, these chemical methods would be further refined and exploited in a more profitable manner.

MOST THRILL-SEEKING EUROPEANS of the late 1850s and early 1860s found chewing on coca leaves to be déclassé, if not disgusting. As a result, infusions, or teas, of coca leaves and, later, other liquid prepa-

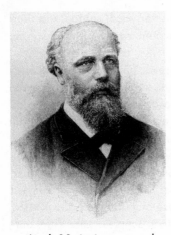

Angelo Mariani, creator and masterful marketer of Vin Mariani, c. 1890.

rations became a popular means of consuming the drug in cafés and dining establishments. The credit for introducing this fashionable craze to Western consumers belongs largely to a French chemist named Angelo Mariani, originally from Corsica, who hailed from a long line of physicians and chemists. From 1863 until well into the 1900s, Mariani and his associates concocted, manufactured, and distributed the second-most-popular coca-based beverage in human history.

In 1892, Mariani wrote a charming memoir of coca leaves as he supervised his well-stocked and bustling laboratory high above Haussmann Boulevard in Paris. In it, he credits a scientific publication entitled *On the Hygienic and Medicinal Virtues of Coca*. Even when reading this pamphlet nearly a century and a half later, one sees immediately why it proved to be so perversely inspirational. The report was written "with great difficulty" in 1859 by the eminent Italian neurologist Paolo Mantegazza, after a trip to Peru. Using himself as a subject, the neurologist describes a series of wild drug-induced experiences; most prominent is the phantasmagoria induced by consuming a walloping fifty-four grams of coca: "I sneered at all the poor mortals condemned to live in

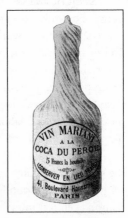

A bottle of Vin Mariani.

the valley of tears while I, carried on the wings of two leaves of coca, went flying though the spaces of 77,438 worlds, each more splendid than the one before."

Armed with his own considerable powers of verbal expression, and years of self-experimentation with coca, Monsieur Mariani recorded his own romantic account on the human propensity to indulge in mind-altering substances:

> Each race has its fashions and fancies. The Indian munches the betel; the Chinaman woos with passion the brutalizing intoxication of opium; the European occupies his idle hours or employs his leisure ones in smoking, chewing or snuffing tobacco. Guided by a happier instinct, the native of South America has adopted Coca. When young, he robs his father of it; later on, he devotes his first savings to its purchase. Without it he would fear vertigo on the summit of the Andes, and weaken at his severe labor in the mines. It is with him everywhere; even in his sleep he keeps his precious quid in his mouth. But should Coca be regarded merely as masticatory? And must we accept as irrevocable the decision of certain therapeutists: "Cocaine, worthless; coca, superfluous drug"?

Undaunted neither by pooh-poohing medical experts nor by the difficulties of chemical production, Mariani worked day and night to manufacture palatable coca-laced beverages. His great eureka moment arrived when he mixed ground coca leaves with a far more traditional French intoxicant, Bordeaux wine. Through careful experimentation and measurement, the chemist realized that the alcohol in the red wine acted to unleash the power of the coca leaves. In the decades that followed, scientists discovered that when alcohol and cocaine are combined a new, even more intoxicating compound, called cocaethlyene, is formed in the liver. After months of research and quality control, Mariani could guarantee his customers that each fluid ounce of his wine contained precisely 6 milligrams of cocaine, with the exception of those bottles exported to the United States, which were moderately more powerful at 7.2 milligrams of cocaine per ounce of wine. Angelo called his elixir Vin Mariani and, not surprisingly for a beverage that contains two very addictive components, it soon became enormously popular. In later years, he came out with a wide menu of coca-containing products, including Mariani teas, Mariani throat lozenges, Mariani cigars and cigarettes, and even Mariani margarine.

Mariani ingeniously approached several leading Parisian ear, nose, and throat doctors in search of soothing tonics to prescribe for their patients suffering from postnasal drip and sore throats. Product in hand, the Corsican provided them with complimentary samples of his bottled coca elixirs. In so doing, Mariani predated by more than a century and a half the unholy alliance of pharmaceutical houses and too many practicing doctors, a partnership that continues to conspire, inundate, and overmedicate us all in the twenty-first century.

Ever the savvy medicinal magnate, Mariani extolled his product to the general public in colorful advertisements and pamphlets. "It nourishes, fortifies, refreshes, aids digestion, strengthens the system," the advertisements declared; "it is unequaled as a tonic, it is a stimulant for the fatigued and over worked body and brain, it prevents malaria, influenza and wasting diseases." Well, perhaps he oversold it a bit.

Legend has it that one of Mariani's first important customers was a neurasthenic Parisian actress. She became so enamored with the drink that every evening as she took her curtain call, she crossed the footlights and told her audiences about the muse behind her spectacular performances.

Appreciation of the beverage apparently crossed religious boundaries as well. During the late 1880s, the grand rabbi of France, Zadoc Kahn, announced, "My conversion is complete. Praise be to Mariani's wine." Around the same time, Pope Leo XIII awarded the Mariani Company a special Vatican gold medal, allowed his face and name to be featured on a Vin Mariani advertisement, and was said to have carried around, under his cassock, a flask filled with the wine that was, "like the widow's cruse, never empty."

World leaders, too, loved the drink. For example, in 1885, former president Ulysses S. Grant was suffering from the end stages of throat cancer (itself likely caused by an unhealthy devotion to alcohol and tobacco) and eking out the last chapters of his autobiography for Mark Twain's ill-fated publishing house. It became a book many historians laud as one of the best memoirs ever penned by an ex-president. Yet even as he scribbled down his thoughts about the Civil War, Grant was swilling bottle after bottle of Mariani's wine. By the close of the nineteenth century, Queen Victoria, the shah of Persia, and President William McKinley had publicly declared their appreciation for Mariani's cocaine-enhanced tonic.

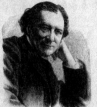

VICTORIEN SARDOU
The Distinguished Dramatist

VICTORIEN SARDOU Writes:
In truth, Vin Mariani is of such excellent quality,
it is perfect, gives health, drives away the blues.
VICTORIEN SARDOU.

Never has anything been so highly and so justly praised as

VIN MARIANI

MARIANI WINE, the FAMOUS FRENCH TONIC for BODY, NERVES and BRAIN

For Overworked Men, Delicate Women, Sickly Children

Vin Mariani has written indorsements from more than 8,000
American Physicians. It is specially recommended for Nervous
Troubles, Throat and Lung Diseases, Dyspepsia, Consumption,
Wasting Diseases,

MALARIA, GENERAL DEBILITY and LA GRIPPE

Sold by all Druggists   Refuse Substitutions

VIN MARIANI GIVES STRENGTH

SPECIAL OFFER.—To all who write, mentioning SCRIBNER'S MAGAZINE, we send a book containing portraits and indorsements of EMPERORS, EMPRESS, PRINCES, CARDINALS, ARCHBISHOPS
and other distinguished personages.

MARIANI & CO., 52 WEST 15TH STREET, NEW YORK

Paris—41 Boulevard Haussmann.   London—83 Mortimer Street.   Montreal—29-31 Hospital Street.

78

*An advertisement for Vin Mariani
featuring the French playwright
Victorien Sardou, c. 1890s. Freud
saw Sarah Bernhardt in one of
Sardou's plays in 1886.*

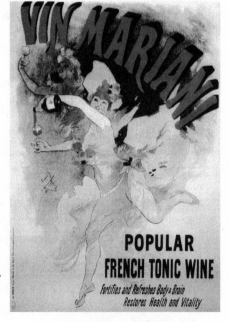

*An advertising poster
for Vin Mariani,
c. 1890s.*

Mariani further exhibited his flair for marketing by sending cases of coca wine to celebrities around the globe, requesting in return only a note expressing their thoughts on the product and an autographed picture. In the years to come, he published these celebrity endorsements in a series of albums called *Portraits from Album Mariani,* featuring some of the most prominent figures of the era. Thomas A. Edison, Auguste Rodin, Jules Verne, Arthur Conan Doyle, Robert Louis Stevenson, Henrik Ibsen, Émile Zola, Alexandre Dumas, and H. G. Wells, among others, all wrote exuberant letters about the product to their dealer, Angelo Mariani. These glowing encomiums were also prominently featured in the lush advertising materials the Mariani Company distributed throughout Europe and the United States. Such positive buzz, undoubtedly, helped to make Angelo the world's first cocaine millionaire.

MARIANI WAS HARDLY ALONE in the mass production of popular coca products during this era. Nor was he to be accorded the claim of the number one producer of cocaine-containing drinks. In fact, an even more popular version still exists (albeit in a slightly different form, sans cocaine): the ever-popular Coca-Cola, which in its original concoction was much like Vin Mariani but employed cola syrup and soda water instead of alcohol. This now ubiquitous beverage, with its biting bubbles and refreshing taste, was originally marketed as a tonic guaranteed to energize those who pulled long swigs from its bottles.

Like many men who fought in the Civil War, John Stith Pemberton was injured on the battlefield and, in search of relief from excruciating pain, became a morphine addict. Not surprisingly, he was intrigued by medical reports in the early 1880s that cocaine might be a cure for morphinism. A pharmacist and patent medicine manufacturer, he was always on the lookout for profitable drugs to sell and began producing a product similar in composition to Vin Mariani, only he called it "French Wine Coca, the ideal tonic and stimulant."

Coca-Cola's illustrious history began in 1886, soon after the citizens of Fulton County, Georgia, voted to ban the sale of alcohol. The local prohibition law proved to be the mother of invention as Pemberton scrambled to come up with something new and legal. Creating a recipe that included coca leaves and kola nuts (in proportions that to this day remain a closely guarded secret), Pemberton concocted his now famous drink. The first "Coke" was served in Atlanta, at the Jacob's Pharmacy soda fountain, on May 8, 1886. Originally selling the product as a patent medicine for 5 cents a glass, Mr. Jacob moved only ten Coca-Colas a day. Undaunted, Pemberton was relentless in his promotion of the "health drink" he claimed was a cure for neurasthenia, impotence, headaches, and morphine addiction. That first year, Pemberton cleared gross sales of $50 (or more than $1,180 in 2010 dollars), but his expenses were more than $70 (or more than $1,650 in 2010 dollars).

Eventually, the drink began to gain favor. Pemberton sold Coca-Cola syrup in bulk to pharmacists around Georgia and beyond. Soda jerks took dollops of the dark brown syrup and added the "2 cents plain," or carbonated water, drawn from their soda fountains. Thousands of drugstores served it daily to clamoring customers, all eager to quench their physical and, with successive ingestion, addictive thirsts.

Although the beverage's popularity was on the ascent, Pemberton grew impatient with the returns on his investment. In 1887, he abruptly sold the recipe for Coca-Cola to a lapsed medical student named Asa Griggs Candler for the then remarkable sum of $2,300 (more than $54,000 in 2010 dollars), constituting one of the greatest blunders in the history of the soft-drink industry.

Cynically, Pemberton also sold the rights to Coca-Cola to a few other investors, and for a brief period there were at least three different versions of the soft drink on the market. As the sales of Coke increased throughout the 1880s and 1890s, scores of "copycat" products cluttered grocers' and druggists' shelves. Their labels displayed such enticing names as Inca Cola, Roco Cola, Kola Ade, and the like. All were basically similar to Coca-Cola and contained either extract of coca leaves or small amounts of cocaine mixed with syrup and soda. In 1892, Candler prevailed over his competitors and incorporated what is today known as the Coca-Cola Company, the leading purveyor of soda pop in the world.

BY THE EARLY 1880S, a gaggle of pioneering pharmaceutical manufacturers, too, had entered the cocaine market. They ordered their armies of chemists to take batches of coca leaves, add touches of

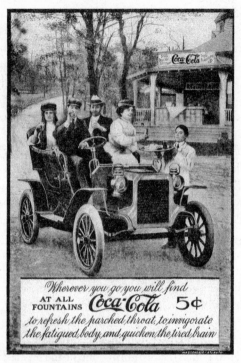

"To refresh the parched throat, to invigorate
the fatigued body, and quicken the tired brain."
Coca-Cola advertisement, c. 1905.

hydrochloric or sulfuric acid here, solutions of bicarbonate of soda and alcohol there, followed by careful extractions, distillations, and crystallizations. And tinker they did, until eventually emerging from their laboratories with the means to mass-produce a pure substance known as cocaine hydrochloride. Such complex chemical machinations facilitated the combination of the active ingredient of the coca leaf with a chloride salt, producing a product that could then be easily crystallized as a powder, measured, weighed, and dispensed. These critical accomplishments allowed the drug to be successfully marketed and distributed to physicians, pharmacists, and patients as a modern medication. Such chemical developments were underwritten by several firms, including G. D. Searle and E. R. Squibb, both based in New York, and

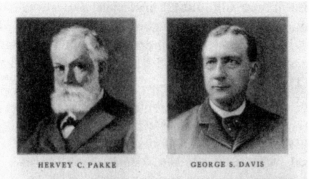

HERVEY C. PARKE   GEORGE S. DAVIS

Hervey Parke, a savvy Detroit businessman (left) and George Davis, a brilliant salesman (right), founded the pharmaceutical company Parke, Davis and Company in 1873. Portraits are c. 1890.

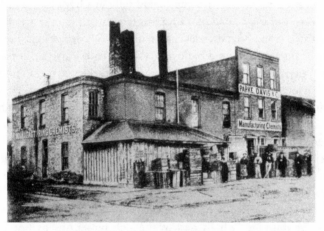

Parke, Davis and Company of Detroit, c. 1875.

Boehringer and Merck, a company with factories in Germany, New Jersey, and St. Louis. But while they all became adept at making and selling pure cocaine hydrochloride, none was as proficient as Parke, Davis and Company of Detroit.

Built on the banks of the Detroit River, the firm opened its doors in 1866. Its original partners included a Michigan businessman named Hervey C. Parke and a physician and German-trained Ph.D. in medicinal chemistry named Samuel P. Duffield. Joining them a year later was George S. Davis, an energetic and creative salesman credited by many with making Parke, Davis the pharmaceutical powerhouse it was for nearly a century, before being bought out by larger and larger corporations beginning in 1970. In the decades before Henry Ford ever dreamed of assembly lines manufacturing millions of Model T's and Detroit became the "Motor City," Parke, Davis and Company constituted one of the city's biggest industries.

Initially, Parke, Davis specialized in marketing a number of medicinal herbs. One of the firm's major products was an extract of the purple-flowered foxglove plant called digitalis, which helped failing hearts beat more strongly. By 1884, however, the company had turned its attention to the uses of cocaine. In the competitive world of selling medicine, the principals at Parke, Davis determined to place a lock on the coca-leaf market, so that they could roll out a huge line of cocaine products. But the demand for coca was far greater than the actual supply. Just as it had been decades earlier, in the 1880s delivering large supplies of intact, fresh, and biologically active coca leaves to European and American pharmaceutical houses for further refinement and processing remained the rate-limiting step in this chemical bonanza.

Instrumental to Parke, Davis and Company's attempt to assume a cocaine monopoly was Henry Hurd Rusby, an intrepid physician and botanist described by one historian of narcotics as "the Theodore Roosevelt of bio-imperialism." As Rusby recounted in his 1933 memoir, *Jungle Memories,* he was invited to the office of George S. Davis in the fall of 1884, only months after receiving his medical diploma from New York University. Nearly half a century later, Dr. Rusby recalled how cocaine's ability to "wholly destroy the local power of sensation in an eye, on coming in contact with the eyeball" had inspired his future bosses "to investigate it thoroughly." In other words, Parke, Davis executives sensed what pharmaceutical companies today call a "blockbuster drug" and promptly positioned themselves for a profitable windfall. The very afternoon they met, an impatient Davis gave Rusby his travel orders from Detroit to Bolivia, with the mission of securing the largest possible supply of coca leaves.

Over the next few years, Dr. Rusby made seven journeys to Central and South America on behalf of Parke, Davis, collecting 35,000 to

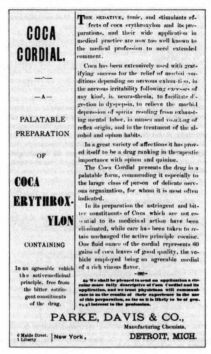

A Parke, Davis advertisement, c. 1880s.

40,000 different biological specimens. On the first trip alone, he gathered together 20,000 pounds of coca leaves, but they spoiled while enduring the rain, mud, and long delays encountered in crossing the Colombian isthmus. It was, as Rusby later described, an "insane journey"—accompanied by hostile encounters with indigenous people and a host of pestilential swamp diseases. He subsequently recommended to his employers that it made much better business sense to extract a crude but stable version of the alkaloid from the coca leaves in South America and then ship it back to Detroit for further chemical refinement. Mr. Parke and Mr. Davis listened carefully to their employee's advice from the field and soon became one of the largest suppliers of pharmaceutical-grade cocaine in the world.

To amplify their sales, Parke, Davis and Company worked hard at encouraging doctors to recommend the new product to their patients.

The nineteenth-century equivalent of "detail men" enticed physicians and patients on both sides of the Atlantic to give cocaine a try by offering them impressive publications replete with descriptions of the "drug's history, botanical origin, production and cultivation, chemical consumption, therapeutic action, physiological action and medical preparation." These reports also featured, if not exaggerated, cocaine's ability to energize the most indolent of patients and to cure a wide variety of chronic maladies such as dyspepsia, flatulence, colic, hysteria, hypochondria, back pain, muscle aches, nervous dispositions, pain resulting from dental, eye, or nose surgery, and the fatigue that often followed acute infections such as influenza. Similar advertisements were aimed directly at medical consumers. As was true of morphine, opium, and cannabis during this era, patients themselves could easily purchase cocaine products from their local druggist without a prescription or medical supervision. With such ready access to addictive substances, subsequent sales rates skyrocketed.

George Davis's genius as a pharmaceutical salesman was amply demonstrated in the many highly regarded medical journals he edited and published, which were prominently displayed in medical libraries across the United States and as far away as the august reading rooms of the University of Vienna. Inquiring doctors eagerly awaited and avidly leafed through each month's issue of *Detroit Lancet, American Lancet, New Preparations, Medical Age,* and *Therapeutic Gazette.*

During the early 1880s, cocaine was one of the most exciting medical topics reported in Europe and North America. But by far, the best place to read the latest invited reviews and clinical studies on cocaine was George Davis's attentively packaged and widely distributed *Therapeutic Gazette.* Indeed, this now forgotten and crumbling periodical loomed largest among Sigmund Freud's many sources of information on cocaine.

For a brief period, beginning in 1885, Davis went as far as to take control of the publication of *Index Medicus,* which would later become the leading print index of every medical publication in the world. This multivolume set of catalogs represented a rather laborious but reliable search engine. Doctors who needed to research a particular medical topic turned to thick, dog-eared copies of the *Index Medicus* to see what had recently been published on it and then proceeded through the stacks of their local medical libraries to dig up the actual papers. The idea of one pharmaceutical company controlling and publishing one of the dominant indexes of the world's medical literature constitutes a definite conflict of interest. But Davis conveniently chose to ignore such ethical niceties because the endeavor resulted in a veritable gold mine of advertising opportunities. Incidentally, many an issue of *Index Medicus* during this period contained Parke, Davis and Company's illustrated pitches for cocaine.

In light of all these factors, underscored by the drug's enticing and miraculous powers, the desire for cocaine traveled fast and wide. Like an influenza epidemic that starts with merely a few sniffling or sneezing people before spreading like wildfire to those around them, the abuse of cocaine hydrochloride was quickly taken up from person to person and across national borders. Unwittingly or not, the medical profession, pharmaceutical companies, and too many patients entered into a decades-long toxic relationship with cocaine abuse and addiction.

CHAPTER 4

An Addict's Death

D R. FREUD'S SECOND-FLOOR, twelve-foot-by-twenty-foot cell in Courtyard 6 of the Krankenhaus represented a significant accomplishment in his career advancement. Along with its newly whitewashed plaster walls and eleven-foot-high ceiling, its most *haimish* feature was an arched window complete with a seat and southern exposure. The furnishings consisted of a narrow bed near the window, a pitcher and water bowl placed on a thin marble shelf, a bureau and mirror, a few shelves for his books, a desk and chair, coat hooks for

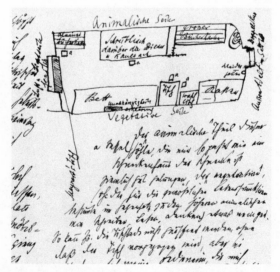

Freud's sketch of his room at the Krankenhaus, October 5, 1883.

his clothes, and an erratic stove for heat. Above his cluttered desk, the young physician hung pictures of Goethe and Alexander the Great; he adorned the wall closest to his bed with embroidered votive panels lovingly sewn by Martha. They were inscribed with lines written by Saint Augustine and Voltaire declaring, respectively: "When in doubt, abstain," and "Let us work without philosophizing." Sigmund needed these sustaining homilies, considering that he slept, studied, and ate within earshot of the screaming and insane patients assigned to the nervous diseases ward.

Freud's accommodations were spartan, but living conditions for patients at the Krankenhaus were appalling. Cleanliness was less a concern than an absolute impossibility. The sweat-soaked mattresses were infested with bedbugs and vermin; the sheets were filthy and the floors slick with rancid blood, urine, vomit, and feces. During the day, the long, interconnected dank wards were illuminated by trickles of sunlight piercing through blackened and smudged windows. By dusk, a paucity of gaslights and candles forced many patients to remain in bed cursing the darkness. When called for a late-night request, doctors often stumbled over both beds and bones for want of a much-needed lantern.

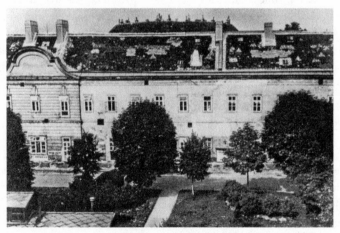

The First Psychiatric Clinic of the Vienna General Hospital,
where Freud was a resident physician.

Dr. Franz Scholz, the superintendent of the psychiatric clinic's nervous diseases ward, only exacerbated matters of hospitality by devising all sorts of ways to keep costs down, resulting in insufficient food, supplies, and medications for the patients. Penury aside, Dr. Scholz encouraged his underlings to take up any and all medical research in their limited spare time, with the tacit understanding that he would receive some of the credit. Sigmund, who hardly needed any incentive in his quest for a slice of medical fame, added a few hours of scientific pursuits each night to his already exhausting twelve- to fourteen-hour schedule. The task he chose for himself was nothing less than composing a seminal synthesis of the world's medical literature on the uses and actions of cocaine. Freud's initial attraction to cocaine was motivated by far more than an impulse to climb up a few rungs on the career ladder. Instead, his main inspiration for researching cocaine's powers was Dr. Ernst von Fleischl-Marxow, a treasured friend and desperate morphine addict whom Sigmund hoped to cure.

FLEISCHL-MARXOW WAS BRILLIANT, charismatic, and well mannered, easily one of the best in Vienna's crop of talented doctors and the first assistant (or junior professor) in Brücke's laboratory. At the age of twenty-five, while conducting anatomical pathology research under the great Carl von Rokitansky, Fleischl-Marxow accidentally nicked his right thumb with a scalpel he was applying to a cadaver. What began as an annoying wound rapidly progressed into a raging infection that ultimately led to an amputation. The procedure may have prolonged his life, but it effectively ended his medical career.

The wound never properly healed, resulting in a tangle of red, heaped, fragile, and easily irritated scar, or granulation, tissue. Nineteenth-century surgeons applied a descriptive bit of clinical nomenclature to this condition: "proud flesh." Healthy skin had a difficult time filling in the ends of the opening of the incision line, setting up a vicious cycle of skin ulceration, infection, and more surgery. To make matters worse, below the gnarled scar tissue, abnormal growths of sensory nerve endings called neuromata formed around the stump of what had formerly been his opposable digit. To say that neuromata are painful is an insult to the power of pain. They are excruciating, inescapable, and unrelent-

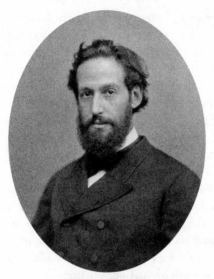

A portrait of Ernst von Fleischl-Marxow at about age thirty-six, c. 1882. After Fleischl-Marxow's death in 1891, Freud hung this portrait in his study as a reminder of his beloved friend.

ing in their ability to burn and sting the flesh. Despite a series of operations by the great Billroth to revise the wound and remove the errant nerve fibers nestled within, the lesions had a life of their own and kept growing back, enlarging and multiplying, leading only to more pain and, ultimately, Fleischl-Marxow's demise in 1891, at the age of forty-five.

Dr. Fleischl-Marxow rarely complained about his condition; repulsed by the slightest hint of pity, he was determined not to let his disability interfere with his academic responsibilities or progress. Indeed, after his injury he was more productive than ever, taking on a multitude of students and publishing a raft of important neurophysiological studies. But on many nights, Fleischl-Marxow's discomfort was so intense that he was unable to sleep. As the rest of Vienna retired for the evening, he pored over precariously perched textbooks while soaking in a hot tub. At first, he studied mathematics to keep his mind occupied. After he had mastered the intricacies of trigonometry and calculus, he turned to classical physics. Once adept at Newtonian principles of gravity and other physical facts, he pondered the ancient language of Sanskrit; and so it went, in the secluded chambers of this determined, stoic young man, until the pain finally proved unbearable. In fact, his life was "an unending torture of pain and of slowly approaching death." Such courageous behavior only served to inspire Sigmund to admire Fleischl-Marxow all the more, or as he explained to Martha: "I could not rest until we became friends and I could experience pure joy in his ability and reputation."

With a slow accumulation of deductive dribs, drabs, and diagnostic clues, sometime in late 1883 or early 1884 Sigmund realized that Fleischl-Marxow's only respite for his constant pain was a hypodermic syringe filled with morphine. Such a protracted process of discovery underscores one of the great conundrums of addiction: many addicts learn to hide the truth of their malady from those around them while actively pursuing their drug of choice.

In many cultures across time, physicians have often anthropomorphized the diseases they battled. Such identifications, undoubtedly, help put a human face or character on the sworn enemies of both doctor and patient. In the modern Western world, this custom has lost favor when confronted by modern, scientific understandings of the precise workings of the human body. One wonders what we have lost by embracing this form of intellectual sophistication. As a physician who has long treated substance-abusing patients, I have learned all too well that addiction is one of the most recalcitrant diseases known to humankind. "Cunning, baffling, and powerful" is how the *Big Book* of Alcoholics Anonymous describes it. These three simple words carry a great deal of weight for anyone who has suffered from it or who cares for an addict or alcoholic. One of the most maddening features is the malady's stealthy ability to convince the sufferer and his family that nothing, nothing at all, is askew or dangerous about something that most decidedly is. Indeed, if you were going to design addiction as a disease, one that conspires within the brain for long periods before eventually killing that person off and proceeding on to the next vulnerable victim, you would be hard-pressed to come up with a more diabolical symptom than denial, the need to lead a double life; the subject feeds the addiction in private while struggling to starve, or at least conceal, it in public. Until, that is, the addiction completely takes over, with disastrous results, and public masquerade is no longer possible.

IN A MATTER OF TIME, thanks to more and larger self-injections of morphine, Fleischl-Marxow watched his life sink with the force of a lead bucket dropped into a lake. His was an addiction that was becoming increasingly common and was often provoked, if not caused, by physicians. Most of these medical doctors were well-intentioned and merely hoped to alleviate pain without a wide menu of therapies to do so. When it came to the effective control of severe pain, from antiquity through the nineteenth century, the options were limited to the highly habit-forming opium and, later, morphine and its pharmacological relatives.

Opium was the first global pharmaceutical agent in the history of medicine. It is a sticky, bitter brown sap produced by the poppy (*Papaver somniferum*), a red wildflower that flourishes in Turkey, Afghanistan, China, India, and the Middle East. The plant may have originated along the western Mediterranean near southern France and Italy. By the Roman era, however, it had been transplanted in Egypt, and its use as a pain medication soon spread from the Middle East to Asia and Europe. Although highly valued by physicians of the Middle Ages, opium fell out of favor, its use in Europe declining precipitously during the Renaissance and the Inquisition. Beginning in the early sixteenth century, however, the seafaring Portuguese reaped great fortunes by importing opium from India. Britain's expanding imperial influence in India during the seventeenth and eighteenth centuries, its growing wariness of and competition with nearby China, and a burgeoning opium trade ushered in the infamous Opium Wars of the nineteenth century. During the mid-1800s, opium was, once again, the doctor's drug of choice for treating all forms of severe pain.

For example, in 1860, the Harvard Medical School professor and literary superstar Oliver Wendell Holmes Sr. described the dangerous purgatives, emetics, and other industrial-strength agents then widely in use in the United States: "If the whole *materia medica,* as now used, could be sunk to the bottom of the sea, it would be all the better for mankind—and all the worse for the fishes." The only agents Dr. Holmes exempted from this water dump were opium, "which the Creator himself seems to prescribe," wine, "which is a food, and the vapors [ether] which produce the miracle of anesthesia." Holmes was hardly alone in ascribing to opium a divine conception.

Even more potent and convenient to use was morphine, the active alkaloid compound chemically derived from opium or poppy sap. A German pharmacist named Friedrich Wilhelm Adam Sertürner was the first to isolate the alkaloid, in 1803; he called it "morphium" after Morpheus, the Greek god of dreams. The drug was produced and mass-marketed beginning in the 1820s. Morphine's popularity and profitability eventually inspired pharmaceutical manufacturers to introduce synthetic versions of the drug, beginning with codeine, in 1830, and, in 1898, heroin. Especially in the decades after the development of the hypodermic needle and syringe in 1853, there was an explosion of doctors freely prescribing and patients readily taking it. Many of the latter, unfortunately, became addicts.

A superb example of the physician-created morphine addict of this era was presented in Eugene O'Neill's *Long Day's Journey into Night*. The playwright's mother, Mary Ellen, first encountered opiate narcotics after a difficult pregnancy and the delivery of Eugene in 1888. Mrs. O'Neill fell into a serious postpartum depression, and within months her well-intentioned doctor had inadvertently transformed the grieving woman into a full-blown addict. In O'Neill's play, Mary Tyrone, the character based on his mother, suffers relapse after relapse, no matter how hard she tries to abstain, much to the consternation, disappointment, and disgust of her husband and two sons.

Interestingly, morphine addicts who self-injected the drug or sipped bottles of laudanum considered their habit to be more legitimate and less problematic than those who smoked opium in dens of iniquity. Regardless of the mode of administration, however, physicians at the close of the nineteenth century grew increasingly concerned about the cases of "opium invalidism" or "morphinism" that they were creating on an ever-increasing basis.

ALTHOUGH MORPHINE CAN BE TAKEN orally or rectally, most avid addicts soon abandon these routes. This is because the drug is poorly absorbed by the gut and rarely produces the type of euphoric experience addicts crave. Some people will sniff it or smoke it in an opium pipe or cigarette. But the best way to consume the drug is to inject it into one's veins using a hypodermic syringe. "Shooting up" gives these psychoactive molecules free rein in the bloodstream, so that more of the dose is quickly available to the brain, where the action is. Once a dose crosses the blood-brain barrier, it interacts predominantly with mu neuroreceptors, the same receptors that interact with the naturally occurring painkillers avid athletes know as endorphins. Opiates reinforce their power by inducing the increased release of dopamine, one of the central neurotransmitters the brain uses to interpret pleasure. Such chemical manipulations bring on a rapid relief from physical and even psychic pain—an indifference to it, really—even though the recipient is often awake and conscious. As the late comedian and heroin addict Lenny Bruce once said about his frequent drug-induced swoons, "I'll die young but it's like kissing God."

The so-called rush of morphine, opium, and heroin begins shortly after its injection. One of the first signs is the rapid constriction of the pupils. As those black dots dominating the eyes grow smaller and smaller, practically to pinpoints, one is less able to accommodate light and visual cues. So, too, does the outlook of an individual transform from an outward glance into an inward and transfixed stare. Warm sensations in the stomach progress to erotic stirrings and tingling in the genitals; the feeling has been described as better than the most extraordinary of sexual orgasms. Once the sensual fireworks subside, however, a stage even more highly coveted by addicts emerges, a first-class, high-speed ticket to temporary oblivion. Time appears to come to a halt and the junkie can pose as still as an accomplished yoga practitioner: silently sitting or lying on the floor, hugging his knees, or crouched in a fetal position. For the next few hours, the opiate-dominated mind is embraced in a silky, dreamy envelope of comfort that promises escape from the hardships, stresses, and trials of daily life.

There are, of course, many negative side effects to opiate agents. Taken in excess, they constipate by retarding the movement of the gastrointestinal tract; for some people, these drugs can induce outright nausea and vomiting. At too high a dose, or overdose, morphine and its relatives profoundly depress the impulse to breathe by lulling the brain's respiratory center into total complacence. Normally, this neurological center closely monitors levels of oxygen and carbon dioxide in the blood and, in response, sends messages to the lungs to breathe faster and deeper or slow and shallow, depending on what chemical mix it discerns. Under the influence of opiates, however, the brain's oxygen receptors simply take a holiday. The subjective experience of the addict, as he delays taking each succeeding breath for just a bit longer than the last, is an intoxicating game of anticipation. As the level of carbon dioxide in his blood rises, he tumbles into an ecstatic but deadly bliss called narcosis. Such physiological perversion, incidentally, is one of the major reasons why the coda to so many opiate overdoses is death by respiratory failure.

Long-term abuse of morphine and its pharmacological relatives essentially resets the rheostats of the brain. And because its frequent use leads to a rapidly increasing tolerance—meaning you need more and more drug to achieve the same desired results—a profound physical dependence rears its ugly head whenever the addicted body perceives that it is not getting enough of the stuff it craves. Ramped-up versions of restlessness, irritability and depression, anxiety, panting, cramping, insomnia, explosive diarrhea, intense aches and pains: these are the symptoms of withdrawal that most morphine and heroin addicts avoid like the plague and that every young physician learns to diagnose the moment a withdrawing patient enters an emergency room.

AS HE SEARCHED FOR a medicinal agent to rid Fleischl-Marxow of his morphine addiction, Freud hit upon the idea of trying cocaine. One of the earliest records of this therapeutic misadventure is documented in a letter Sigmund wrote to his Martha on April 21, 1884. That evening, he was assigned to cover the main hospital's patient reception desk on what must have been a slow night. Instead of being swamped with composing the long and careful case histories that accompanied the admission of patients, the devoted Sigmund described his latest findings about cocaine's alleged therapeutic powers:

> I am also toying with a project and a hope which I will tell you about; perhaps nothing will come of this either. It is a therapeutic experiment. I have been reading about cocaine, the effective

ingredient of coca leaves, which some Indian tribes chew in order to make themselves resistant to privation and fatigue. A German has tested this stuff on soldiers and reported that it has really rendered them strong and capable of endurance. I have now ordered some of it and for obvious reasons am going to try it out on cases of heart disease, then on nervous exhaustion particularly in the awful condition following withdrawal of morphine (as in the case of Dr. Fleischl). There may be any number of other people experimenting on it already; perhaps it won't work. But I am certainly going to try it and, as you know, if one tries something often enough and goes on wanting it, one day it may succeed. We need no more than one stroke of luck of this kind to consider setting up house. But, my little woman, do not be too convinced that it will come off this time. As you know, an explorer's temperament requires two basic qualities: optimism in attempt, criticism in work.

Elsewhere in this letter Freud demonstrates mastery of the extant medical literature, in English, French, and German, on the subject of cocaine. For example, he refers to the same article by Italian neurologist Paolo Mantegazza that so fascinated Angelo Mariani, the coca-wine king; it reported how cocaine enhanced strength and sexual potency among the Peruvian Indians who chewed coca leaves well into old age. He also describes a well-regarded 1883 medical report written by the German physician Theodor Aschenbrandt, suggesting that cocaine be prescribed for soldiers to improve their performance on the battlefield.

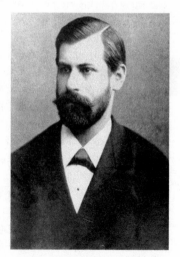

Sigmund Freud at the time of writing Über Coca, *1884.*

Even more intriguing to Freud were a series of clinical papers published in George Parke's house organ, the *Therapeutic Gazette*. In 1878, an American physician named W. H. Bentley described successfully treating a patient addicted to the "opium habit" with coca. Two years later, in 1880, Bentley reported his success in treating both opium and alcohol abusers with cocaine. With the twenty-twenty vision of historical hindsight, it is easy to shake one's head at such a harebrained theory. Substituting one addictive drug for another was a common medical means of treating substance abuse in the late nineteenth century and, in fact, remains so to this day. It is impossible to give an accurate number of how many morphine addicts were unwittingly turned into cocaine addicts by well-intentioned physicians during this era; similarly, alcoholics were often prescribed morphine to the point of addiction and, later, cocaine and even nicotine to help them kick their drinking habits. At the dawn of doctors' recognition of addiction as a disease, what all these games of medical musical chairs most reliably did was to create "new and improved" addicts.

THE GREAT MICROBIOLOGIST Louis Pasteur declared that when it came to conducting scientific research, "chance favors only the mind that is prepared." History shows that desperation can be a stimulant to such inspired activities as well. Sigmund Freud first encountered cocaine when his medical-career blues were playing cacophonous riffs in his head. Everything he worked for or aspired to seemed so tentative, so out of reach. Like Moses, the biblical figure who fascinated him throughout his life, Sigmund must have felt as if confined to Mount Nebo. He could see the Promised Land, which for him was a professorial appointment at the Vienna Medical School, but it looked as if he would never get there. In late May 1884, he reported to Martha about a meeting with his former teacher Hermann Nothnagel; the tête-à-tête was hardly encouraging. Writing about the conversation as if it were a one-act play, Sigmund recorded several of the internal medicine professor's deflating observations, none more cutting than the comment "You know how hard it is to get along in Vienna, how hard our colleagues work from morning to night and still barely eke out a living." Nothnagel also made a far from appealing offer: "I could give you some recommendations to Buenos Aires, where a former assistant of mine has a practice; or to Madrid, where I have any number of connections."

The surgeon general's catalog entry on cocaine,
1883. Freud consulted this volume when
beginning to write Über Coca.

Sigmund quickly dismissed this depressing conversation because he was so busy looking after Fleischl-Marxow. On the nights he sat at his friend's bedside, "every note of the profoundest despair was sounded." As he worriedly wrote Martha: "I admire and love him with an intellectual passion, if you will allow such a phrase. His destruction will move me as the destruction of a sacred and famous temple would have affected an ancient Greek."

In May 1884, Freud explained to Fleischl-Marxow his idea about trying cocaine as a means to break the surgeon free from morphine. Fleischl-Marxow eagerly consented and embarked on a path that made him, quite possibly, the first morphine addict in Europe to be treated with this new therapeutic. The initial results were nothing short of miraculous. During the first three weeks of the "cocaine therapy," Fleishel-Marxow's morphine intake drastically fell to minute doses.

Sadly, his condition soon plummeted. One night several weeks

later, Freud; Sigmund Exner, Brücke's other assistant; the neurologist
Heinrich Obersteiner; and Fleischl-Marxow's physician, Joseph Breuer,
visited Fleischl-Marxow's apartment only to find the door locked. The
four men eventually procured a master key from the landlord. Once
inside, they discovered their beloved colleague writhing on the floor,
unwashed, naked, and delirious from pain. After the administration of
large injections of morphine, Fleischl-Marxow finally collapsed into a
narcotic-induced sleep. A few days later, the surgeon Theodor Billroth
attempted an electrical stimulation of the stump, with disastrous
results.

By now, Fleischl-Marxow was consuming more than a gram of pure
cocaine a day, along with enormous amounts of morphine. Addicts
who mix opiates and cocaine enthusiastically endorse this combination because it produces a far more stunning high than either agent
can produce alone. Following an injection of the ecstasy-producing
morphine, Fleischl-Marxow added a chaser of cocaine to inspire a
rush of electric-like waves of pleasure throughout his body. In the time
span of less than three months, Fleischl-Marxow spent 1,800 marks
(more than $3,300 in 2010) on cocaine hydrochloride, a sum that was
a hundred times greater than Sigmund's outlay of cash for cocaine
during the same period. This does not even account for the money
Fleischl-Marxow was regularly spending on his multiple daily fixes of
morphine.

Money for drugs aside, there was a higher price to pay. Eventually,
Fleischl-Marxow's copious substance abuse brought on severe fainting
spells, convulsions, insomnia, hallucinations, and increasingly odd
behaviors. As his addiction raged, his brain demanded more doses of
the very drugs that were killing him. What followed were many more
crisis-filled nights when Sigmund was urgently called to Fleischl-
Marxow's flat to nurse his drug-addled friend, only to repeat the whole
horrible affair again the next evening. On June 4, 1885, Sigmund discovered Fleischl-Marxow in a state of "delirium tremens with white
snakes creeping over his skin"—a result of cocaine intoxication and
psychosis. Freud recalled it as "the most frightful night he had ever
spent." Although Sigmund predicted that his friend would live only
another six months, it took six years before this "Greek temple" of a
man was dead. A guilt-ridden Sigmund kept a photograph of Fleischl-
Marxow hanging on the wall of his study for the remainder of his life.

IN THE DAYS IMMEDIATELY FOLLOWING his initial "cocaine success" with Fleischl-Marxow, however, Freud was absolutely convinced that cocaine would prove to be a valuable therapeutic for addiction, depression, and neurasthenia, an exhausting condition defined by late-nineteenth-century physicians as an ambiguous type of nerve-cell fatigue. It was, unfortunately, an erroneous theory he would hold for some time even after Fleischl-Marxow's descent, and with strikingly bad results. Soon after administering the first restorative doses to his friend, Sigmund set out to write the definitive monograph on cocaine. This project was conducted with the encouragement of the temporarily stable Fleischl-Marxow, who insisted that Sigmund get his findings into print as soon as possible.

In order to produce more scientific data, however, Sigmund needed more cocaine. Consequently, he made a significant monetary investment by ordering a gram of cocaine hydrochloride from the Merck Company of Darmstadt. Like its American counterpart, Parke, Davis and Company of Detroit, Merck advertised its product with authoritative reviews on cocaine that were widely distributed to German physicians and, a few months later, American doctors. In one 1884 publication, for example, Merck methodically describes cocaine's molecular structure, chemical properties, and physiological effects in animals ranging from puppies to humans, stipulating that all of the experiments reported, "without exception," were conducted using " '*Cocain mur. Solut. Merck,*' " and noting that "only for these are the doses and action, as above stated, to be relied upon." Before long, Dr. Freud became a regular customer of the Merck firm.

Even if Sigmund did not appreciate cocaine's addictive properties, he did quickly realize that it was an expensive drug. Budgeting 33 kreuzer (nearly $3 in 2010) for his first cocaine purchase, the pfennig-pinching Sigmund was astounded when he received a bill from the Merck firm for 3 gulden, 33 kreuzer (roughly $30 in 2010). This sum represented a huge outlay for Freud. As a *Sekundararzt,* he earned 30 gulden a month (a little more than $90 in 2010), which barely paid for the cost of his meals. Additional expenditures would have to be covered by tutoring whining medical students who could not or would not commit their studies to absolute memory with rapid recall, a task that

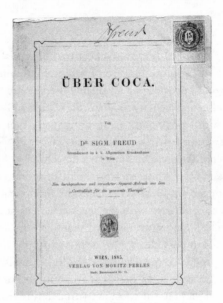

The title page of Über Coca, *1885.*

paid 3 gulden an hour. When he received his first shipment of cocaine in late April 1884, Sigmund allayed his financial worries by immediately ingesting 200 milligrams mixed into a glass of water. His bad mood was instantly transformed into one of cheerfulness; he was filled with the rare and incomparable feeling "that there is nothing at all one need bother about."

Like many inquiring doctors of his generation, Freud grounded his scientific studies by experimenting on himself. After consuming a few doses of cocaine, he was hopelessly enamored of its ability to cure indigestion, soothe aches and pains, and, perhaps more important, relieve depression and anxieties. Freud even purchased some to distribute to his friends, colleagues, and sisters. In May 1884, he sent several doses of cocaine to his fiancée to "make her strong and give her cheeks some color." Around the same time, Sigmund expressed to Martha his high expectations for the drug and what it would do for his patients, his career, and their lives together:

> *If all goes well I will write an essay on it and I expect it will win its place in therapeutics by the side of morphium and superior to it.*

I have other hopes and intentions about it. I take very small doses of it regularly against depression and against indigestion and with the most brilliant of success. I hope it will be able to abolish the most intractable vomiting, even when this is due to severe pain; in short it is only now that I feel I am a doctor, since I have helped one patient and hope to help more. If things go on in this way we need have no concern about being able to come together and to stay in Vienna.

A few weeks later, on June 2, 1884, Sigmund exhibited both concern for Martha's poor health and evidence of the drug's sexually thrilling effects. He also demonstrates a loquacious, if not reckless, style of writing he adopted when under the influence during this period:

Woe to you, my Princess, when I come, I will kiss you quite red and feed you till you are plump. And if you are forward you shall see who is the stronger, a gentle little girl who doesn't eat enough or a big wild man who has cocaine in his body. In my last severe depression, I took coca again, and a small dose lifted me to the heights in a wonderful fashion. I am just now busy collecting the literature for a song of praise to this magical substance.

During the summer of 1884 and after, Freud wrote many more cocaine-fueled encomiums to his fiancée. No matter what the reason, the need for relief from a migraine or a stomachache, an attack of sinusitis, the lows of his melancholia, or simply to daydream about his beloved Martha, Sigmund continued to use cocaine to make bad days good and good days better. The turmoil and uncertainty that framed his professional and romantic life demanded a potent tonic to calm his state of agitation and restore the stamina he desperately needed to make history. Ever sneaky and seductive, cocaine appealed to his psychic needs at his most vulnerable moments. And as his use of cocaine progressed, he required more of the stuff to satisfy his brain's urgent pleas.

Between April and July 1884, the young neurologist researched and completed what would become *Über Coca* (On Coca), a treatise filled with adulatory descriptions of the "magical drug" and his "most gorgeous excitement." Freud's biographer Ernest Jones described the text as "a remarkable combination of objectivity with a personal warmth, as if he were in love with the content." Hyperbolic phrasing aside, the bulk of *Über Coca* is a well-written, comprehensive review of cocaine in concert with substantive, original scientific data on its physiological effects.

The monograph signals a striking shift in Freud's scientific modus operandi. No longer is he content to work exclusively on laboratory animals or the brains of cadavers. He now begins to explore living human beings or, as he tells the reader of *Über Coca*, "I have carried out experiments and studied, in myself and others, the effect of coca on the healthy human body."

Over the span of several weeks, Sigmund swallowed cocaine dozens of times, in doses ranging from .05 to .10 grams. From these experiences, he was able to compose an accurate précis of the drug's immediate effects:

> A few minutes after taking cocaine, one experiences a sudden exhilaration and feeling of lightness. One feels a certain furriness on the lips and palate, followed by a feeling of warmth in the same areas; if one now drinks cold water, it feels warm on the lips and cold in the throat. On other occasions the predominant feeling is a rather pleasant coolness in the mouth and throat.

In the pages that follow, the text becomes exclusively centered on how the drug altered his body and mind, including such effects as a rapid heartbeat, euphoria, and sleeplessness.

Prior to his cocaine studies, Freud's scientific work had focused on the quantitative, fact-based research he conducted in the laboratory. What was the precise relationship of one anatomic structure to another? How did manipulating that structure alter its function in terms of measurable criteria such as blood pressure or heart rate? These were the questions upon which Sigmund and his medical peers typically confined their gaze, if they were to have any hope of publishing their work, let alone impressing their teachers and the medical world at large.

Yet the most striking feature of *Über Coca* is how Sigmund incorporates his own feelings, sensations, and experiences into his scientific observations. Throughout the monograph, Sigmund is careful to present his findings in language that generalizes the experience for a medical audience. But the "n of 1" in these experiments, the "one" who experienced these effects, was clearly Sigmund Freud. When comparing this study with his previous works, a reader cannot help but be struck by the vast transition he makes from recording reproducible, quantitatively measurable, controlled laboratory observations to exploring thoughts and feelings. In essence, *Über Coca* introduces a literary character that would become a standard feature in Sigmund's work: himself. From this point on, Freud often applies his own (and later his patients') experiences and thoughts in his writings as he works to create a universal theory of the mind and human nature. It was a method that for its time would prove scientifically daring, at times somewhat incautious, and, in terms of the creation of psychoanalysis, strikingly productive.

The cocaine study first appeared in the July 1884 issue of *Central-blatt für die gesammte Therapie,* a medical journal published by Verlag von Moritz Perles of Vienna. By midsummer, Freud saw a financial return on his intellectual investment in the form of an offer of 60 gulden from Parke, Davis and Company to compare its product to Merck's.

ÜBER COCA SIGNIFIED MANY THINGS for Sigmund. It was his first major scientific publication. It boldly announced his industry and presence to the world of academic medicine. At the same time, it erroneously described the drug as an effective antidote to serious morphine and alcohol abuse. And it facilitated, if not encouraged, his consumption of the drug.

Über Coca also represented a missed opportunity. As Sigmund raced to compile the drug's history, uses, and therapeutic effects, he skimmed over cocaine's most important clinical use as a local anesthetic. In a hurried last paragraph of his monograph—a postscript, really—Freud noted that "cocaine and its salts have a marked anesthetizing effect when brought into contact with the skin and mucous membrane in concentrated solution." Without offering any additional data or experiments, Freud merely concluded that these properties "should make it suitable for a good many applications."

It is not surprising that, as a physician specializing in nervous dis-

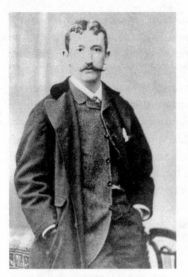

Carl Koller, the ophthalmologist who bested Freud with his "discovery" of cocaine anesthesia, in 1884, when Koller was twenty-seven.

eases and as the concerned friend of an addict, Sigmund focused primarily upon the uses of cocaine as a treatment for depression and morphinism. But it hardly required the genius of a Freud to inquire in detail why touching his tongue and lips with the smallest amount of cocaine powder created such powerfully numbing sensations; this is, after all, a key characteristic of ingesting cocaine. Considering his frequent use of cocaine, it is difficult to explain why Sigmund did not value this particular action of the drug as much as he did the drug's ability to alter one's mood, blood pressure, breathing rate, and any number of physiological and sensational parameters.

Perhaps Freud was so preoccupied with completing his paper and rushing it into print that he simply neglected it. Perhaps his lack of interest in pain-inducing surgical procedures blocked his view to such a critical finding. An even more probable explanation might be that the deliciously exhilarating effects of cocaine—the high rather than the physical numbness—dominated his thoughts and actions. Whatever the precise reason, he made a colossal mistake by overlooking what would have been a historic description of the drug's anesthetic properties.

DISCOVERY, OF COURSE, is a relative term, especially when one is contemplating the world of science and medicine. As a rule, doctors and scientists are driven, determined, and obsessed with primacy of discovery. To the victors belongs more than mere mention in a textbook; discovering something represents a research investigator's best shot at immortality. One wonders whether medical discovery would advance so quickly were doctors not all chasing their version of a holy grail that allows them to boast "I was there first." Even the most cursory review of the historical record amply demonstrates that the quest to discover—and, at times, the outright bad conduct it can enable—is probably as old as scientific inquiry itself. As early as the second century A.D., the eminent physician and anatomist Galen of Pergamon derided his intellectual rivals as "lazy" and "ignorant" and refused to explain his discoveries to them because such knowledge would prove "as superfluous to them as a tale told to an ass."

The person who did capitalize on first reporting cocaine's anesthetic properties was Sigmund's colleague Dr. Carl Koller, an *Aspirant* in ophthalmology at the Vienna General Hospital. The two had known each other since medical school and, because of similar backgrounds and ambitions, tended to understand, envy, admire, and, alternatively, barely tolerate each other. On many occasions Sigmund considered his friend's narrow devotion to all things optical tiresome. Carl, incidentally, was the young physician berated in Billroth's clinic as a "Jewish swine" who'd inspired a touching defense from Freud in a letter to Martha. Yet while both of these men tasted cocaine on their lips, its ability to numb the mouth proved far more inspiring to the budding ophthalmologist than to the eventual founder of psychoanalysis.

In July 1884, around the time of the publication of Freud's cocaine paper, Koller began some experiments of his own, applying solutions of water and the white powder to the eyes of frogs, rabbits, and dogs before concluding it was an excellent anesthetic for operations on the human eye.

As eager for professional accomplishment as Sigmund, Carl Koller scrambled to complete his experiments and prepare a formal address at the Ophthalmological Congress in Heidelberg slated to commence in early September 1884. After being awarded a prominent spot on the program, however, Koller ran into some difficulties not entirely biological in nature. Around this time, he was estranged from his father and stepmother (who apparently lived up to all the negative connotations of such a relation). As a result, Koller was subsisting solely on his paltry salary as a training physician at the Vienna General Hospital. Too poor to afford the travel expenses to the Heidelberg meeting, he asked a forty-nine-year-old ophthalmologist named Josef Brettauer to read the paper and demonstrate the experiments—a rather common practice in an era when travel was both expensive and arduous. The presentation was nothing short of spectacular.

As the world's most distinguished eye surgeons took their seats in the crowded and stuffy auditorium, Brettauer approached the podium and cleared his throat. He knew the data cold and was quite comfortable demonstrating cocaine's effects before an audience. He enjoyed the advantage of knowing that it was not his career that teetered on the brink of this presentation's success or failure; he was merely filling in for Koller, and this, no doubt, added to his confidence level as he began to speak.

After explaining what Dr. Koller had been working on for the past few months, Brettauer snapped his fingers. On cue, a laboratory assistant wheeled in a large dog that had been waiting patiently in the wings of the amphitheater. Once on the stage, Brettauer displayed the mutt to the audience to show that the animal was alert, comfortably seated on a cushion, and loosely tied down to the gurney. He then picked up a carefully calibrated dropper full of cocaine solution, delicately held the canine's left eye open with his thumb and forefinger, and introduced three or four drops of the elixir. Dramatically, the physician let one, then two minutes pass by in silence—a period that seems like a lifetime when giving a lecture before a crowded room. Once satisfied that the cocaine had taken effect, he thrust a forceps toward the dog's eye. While the animal's right eye blinked in response to such a threat, the left eye remained still. Deftly, Brettauer touched the canine's left eye with the surgical instrument, and the results were astonishing: nothing happened! No whimpering, no barking, not even a flinch— that is, until the crowd sighed in relief that no harm had come to the dog and burst into uproarious applause.

A month later, on October 17, 1884, Carl Koller read his paper before the prestigious Gesellschaft der Ärzte (Vienna Medical Society). But as Koller's daughter Hortense recalled several decades later: "By this time, however, the news had already spread like wildfire (so great had been the need for this remedy) and experiments were under way all over continental Europe, England and across the Atlantic, wherever doctors gathered."

Freud, of course, was far from thrilled about Koller's paper and its aftereffects. The fact that they both worked in the same hospital, where gossip of successes and failures traveled quickly, could not have been an easy cross for the always sensitive Sigmund to bear. Whenever the word "cocaine" came up in medical circles, it was Koller's name and not Freud's that generated great admiration. Consequently, Freud moped and complained about how still one more chance at medical immortality had passed him by.

There are many different accounts of how Freud tolerated his usurpation by a junior colleague. In 1963, Koller's daughter reported that Sigmund had taken the news in good stride. The historical record, however, reveals a more complicated tale. In late 1884, still possessed by what he misinterpreted as being scooped on the discovery of his career, Freud declared that he and several other medical scientists had long wondered about the drug's anesthetic properties. Freud also claimed, without much evidence, that he and a Viennese eye surgeon named Leopold Königstein had been working on some unpublished investigations into cocaine's pain-deadening effects on the cornea prior to Koller's monumental announcement.

Perhaps his most pitiful assertion of primacy occurred in early 1885. To several colleagues, Freud asserted that Carl Koller was present months earlier when he prescribed a 5 percent solution of cocaine to a Krankenhaus patient complaining of intestinal pain and that the administered drug produced a side effect of numbness to the lips and tongue. This episode, Sigmund insisted, was when Koller made his "first acquaintance" with the anesthetic properties of cocaine, which he then applied to his work as an eye surgeon. It was an attractive, but not widely accepted, version that Sigmund had great difficulty relinquishing from his mind.

Another barometer of Freud's feelings about his scientific rival can be summarized by his now famous contention that a joke is never really a mere joke. To Martha, in January 1885, Sigmund blithely dismissed the cocaine work as a scientific trifle he executed in the "chase after money, position and reputation." Later, Freud was said to have inscribed a copy of his *Über Coca* to Koller with the words "To my dear friend, Coca Koller, from Sigmund Freud"; the mildly demeaning sobriquet, much to the ophthalmologist's chagrin, followed him for the remainder of his life and extended well after his death in New York City in 1944.

Nor did it end there. In 1895, Sigmund reported a dream that awarded him due credit for the medicinal uses of cocaine. It occurred at a time when his father was suffering from glaucoma and required an ocular operation. The dutiful Sigmund had just arranged the procedure for his father with the benefit of cocaine anesthesia. Sigmund later noted that in his unconscious reflections on these events, Koller congratulated both him and his colleague Leopold Königstein for being members of the medical triumvirate that introduced local anesthesia to the world. The dream may have been based on a real experience; more likely, it was merely a wish.

Freud's subsequent memories as recorded in his brief 1925 autobiography prove even more entangled. In that volume, he blames his failure to recognize cocaine's anesthetic properties on the distracting influences of Martha. Acting more like a repressed patient than the acclaimed psychoanalyst he was, Freud recalled the events with great, albeit questionable, detail:

> *I may here go back a little and explain how it was the fault of my fiancée that I was not already famous at that early age. A side interest, though it was a deep one, had led me in 1884 to obtain from Merck some of what was then the little-known alkaloid cocaine and to study its physiological action. While I was in the middle of this work, an opportunity arose for making a journey to visit my fiancée, from whom I had been parted for two years. I hastily wound up my investigation of cocaine and contented myself in my book on the subject with prophesying that further uses would soon be found. I suggested, however, to my friend Königstein, the ophthalmologist, that he should investigate the question of how far the anesthetizing properties of cocaine were applicable in diseases of the eye. When I returned from my holiday I found that not he, but another of my friends, Carl Koller (now in New York), whom I had also spoken to about cocaine, had made the decisive experiment upon animals' eyes and had demonstrated them at the Ophthalmological Congress in Heidelberg. Koller is therefore rightly regarded as the discoverer of local anesthesia by cocaine, which has become so important in minor surgery; but I bore my fiancée no grudge for her interruption of my work.*

. . .

A FEW YEARS LATER, while reading the 1931 biography of his life by Fritz Wittels, Freud still felt a need to deny cocaine's negative impact on his career. As he read the passage describing the cocaine episode, where Wittels suggested that Sigmund had "thought long and painfully just how this could have happened to him," the psychoanalyst wrote an ink-stained "False" in the book's margin. Almost a decade earlier, in 1923, an irritated Freud had written to Wittels, "I know very well how it [the cocaine episode] happened to me. The study on coca was an allotrion [an idle pursuit that takes one from the fulfillment of serious responsibilities] which I was eager to conclude."

Regardless of the compliments Freud might pay to Carl Koller or the altered versions of events and finger-pointing he would later concoct for the sake of his future biographers and students, Freud completely missed recognizing the most important therapeutic use of cocaine, and it upset him greatly.

CHAPTER 5

The Accidental Addict

IN 1844, AFTER MORE than a decade of perfecting a long-distance communication device he called the telegraph, Samuel F. B. Morse convinced the U.S. government to fund the construction of a line of wires between Washington, D.C., and Baltimore. At the system's official opening on May 24 of that year, Morse sent the most famous telegram in history: "What hath God wrought!" In the decades that followed, his technological marvel of hardware, dots, and dashes, along with new developments in wire insulation and conductor materials, led to the creation of a thick, sinewy network of cables stretching across vast swaths of countryside, extending far beneath the surface of the Atlantic and Pacific oceans, and connecting villages, towns, and cities around the world. This vast complex of wires and electronics transmitted rivers of information, which were rapidly heralded by the largest and most varied print press in our nation's history. Forty years after Morse's triumph, in the fall of 1884, this was precisely the path taken by the news of cocaine.

For months, cocaine led the discussions in the clinical societies and hospital rounds in Vienna, Paris, London, Berlin, Boston, Philadelphia, New York, and other great medical capitals. The primary focus, of course, was Koller's announcement of the drug's anesthetic potential. One of the most energized readers of these dispatches was William Halsted, the up-and-coming New York surgeon who had committed to filling his days with the pursuit of a single goal: the perfection of the art of surgery.

On October 11, 1884, a few weeks after Koller's lecture by proxy in Heidelberg and within days of his formal presentation in Vienna, Halsted sat in the library of the New York Academy of Medicine on West Forty-third Street. He was reading the latest issue of the *New York Medical Record,* a publication that reliably gathered medical news from around the world and reprinted the medical society lectures of New York's most prolix doctors. The scientific details of cocaine's anesthetic properties fired his imagination. Before the day drew to a close, William resolved to purchase some cocaine to begin an investigation of his own. And like Freud in Vienna a few months earlier, William spent a great deal of money on this brand-new pharmaceutical wonder. On October 29, 1884, the *New York Times* published a story about the cocaine craze sweeping the medical profession. The price of cocaine, the reporter noted, was $420 per ounce and $6,720 per pound (or $9,157 per ounce and $146,512 per pound in 2010 dollars).

It is critical to appreciate how dependent the advancement of surgery was on the physician's ability to render a patient unconscious to the pain of the scalpel. Modern medicine is simultaneously blessed and cursed by an endless cornucopia of pharmaceutical-grade painkillers, anxiety squashers, and pepper-uppers. But for most of human history, the mere extraction of a tooth, let alone anything that demanded invasion of the body, was a most risky business. The 1846 discovery of ether as an anesthetic and the subsequent development of antiseptic surgery allowed its practitioners to probe deeper and deeper into the recesses of the body in search of diseased organs and tissue to extirpate. Nevertheless, ether and chloroform, the primary anesthetic drugs of Halsted's era, were not without their failings. Noxious, nauseating, and heavily sedating, they rendered patients groggy and unaware of their surroundings for hours. Consequently, the development of an agent that could be safely injected under the skin, leaving a patient completely awake yet insensate to the surgeon's pointedly sharp manipulations, was earthshaking. In fact, the news captured the attention of just about every doctor keeping abreast of the medical literature.

That Koller the ophthalmologist became so interested in cocaine anesthesia was a direct result of the operation he most frequently performed: cataract removal. Although practiced since the days of antiquity, it had long remained a dreaded procedure. After all, without pharmaceutical assistance, cataract removal is not only excruciating; it packs the extra punch of requiring the patient to watch as the surgeon literally pokes him in the eye. Many observers have described this awful ordeal, yet few re-create the immediacy of the moment as well as the British novelist Thomas Hardy: "It was a like a red-hot needle in yer eye whilst he was doing it. But he wasn't long about it. Oh no. If he had been long I couldn't ha' beared it. He wasn't a minute more than three quarters of an hour at the outside."

With the advent of ether and chloroform in the mid-nineteenth century came great hopes for making cataract removal less painful. But these anesthetics often induced vomiting in patients—and this, in turn, created a cascade of alarmingly high pressures in the abdomen, chest, and head, which are not conducive to performing delicate eye surgery.

In late October 1884, when cocaine first captured Halsted's attention and time, he was making quite the name for himself in New York medical circles. Upon his return from Vienna in 1880, he joined the faculty of the College of Physicians and Surgeons and soon after assumed important surgical posts at several New York City hospitals. While simultaneously serving as attending surgeon at the Charity Hospital on Blackwell's Island, the Emigrant Hospital on Ward's Island, and the Roosevelt, Bellevue, and St. Luke's hospitals in Manhattan, Halsted demonstrated his talents as an operator on a daily (and often nightly) basis. "He worked with superhuman energy and endurance of ten men," wrote one biographer, the Johns Hopkins pathologist W. G. MacCallum. So frenetic was Halsted's daily schedule between 1880 and 1885 that it led MacCallum to ponder:

> One can perhaps imagine the extent of the task with the outpatient department of Roosevelt occupying the morning, five other hospitals demanding his services in the wards and operating room at any time, and especially at night, with regular hours of teaching in the dissection rooms at the College and with his quiz of sixty-five or more students at his house. What leisure he could ever have with his programme it is hard to tell.

By all accounts, Halsted had found his true calling. In 1881 his sister had delivered her first child. While visiting her, Halsted found her to be "ghastly white, pulseless, and unconscious." So, focused on his craft and smooth in professional demeanor, Halsted used a hypodermic needle to withdraw blood from his own arm and transfuse his moribund sibling. Luckily for her, in an era before the discovery of blood groups and blood incompatibility, Halsted's and his sister's blood type matched perfectly, and he saved her life. A year later, he performed a cholecystostomy on his ailing mother after diagnosing a potentially fatal case of gallstones and ascending cholangitis (an inflammation and possible infection of the bile ducts caused by blockage). He performed the death-defying procedure on the family's kitchen table at two in the morning, with his father and siblings as assistants.

The gregarious William enjoyed a long waiting list of students eager to learn from him. His formal lectures on surgery at the medical school were fully subscribed. In addition, each academic year he held special "quizzes," or tutorials, on surgery at his home for those pupils desperate to master the many arcane questions their professors would ask them on the examinations that determined class rank and, in a real sense, their careers. And to sate his own scientific curiosity, the young surgeon was constantly searching for ways to apply the medical miracles unfolding in Vienna, Berlin, Leipzig, and elsewhere to his operating room.

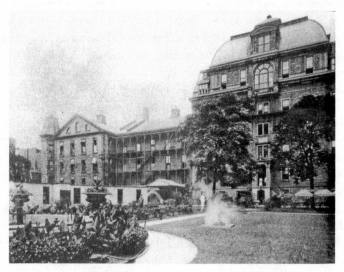

The Bellevue Hospital grounds, c. 1880.

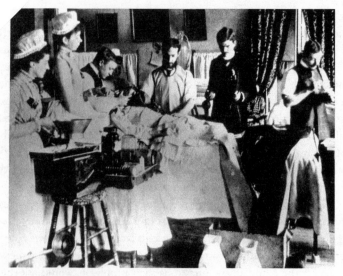

A surgical operation at Bellevue Hospital under less than hygienic conditions, c. 1880.

William's principal workshop, Bellevue Hospital, was a place filled with disease, discussion, and doctoring. It contained more than eight hundred beds and admitted more than twenty thousand patients per year. When he returned to Bellevue from Vienna in 1880, the ethos of saving the poor from themselves still permeated the wards, but so, too, did the spirit of discovery and medical professionalism. Without question, Bellevue was internationally known as a first-rate medical center. Yet the permanently unsatisfied William found it a far cry from clinical perfection. He was especially perturbed by the horribly unsanitary practices in the operating room, including the reuse of dirty instruments, the improper preparation of the catgut needed to sew patients back together, ligatures handed to the operator from the mouth of an intern, and even nurses dragging their sleeves through the bloody surgical field.

Convinced by Dr. Joseph Lister's argument that antiseptic surgical procedures eliminated infectious germs from the operative site and afforded better results for patients, Halsted complained publicly at medical meetings about Bellevue's filthy customs. But unlike many of his colleagues who contented themselves by merely grousing, he actually did something about this problem. In 1883, he persuaded his bosses to allow him to construct a giant pavilion, a tent, with sealed flaps and an easily washed, varnished oaken floor. William's antiseptic operating theater was the first of its kind in New York City. Writing to a colleague in 1921, the year before he died, Halsted recalled the uphill battle he'd waged and eventually won: "Operations [were] performed in a large tent which I built on the grounds of Bellevue Hospital having found it impossible to carry out antiseptic precautions in the general amphitheatre of Bellevue Hospital where the numerous anti-Lister surgeons dominated and predominated."

Halsted was hardly exaggerating. Bacteriologists and doctors of this era were just beginning to appreciate the role microbes played in dreaded contagious diseases as well as their propensity to ruin the best-laid surgical plans to close an open wound or amputate a gangrenous limb. Those surgeons who did subscribe to the germ theory of disease still numbered in the minority. As a result, things remained pretty grim for those forced to submit to the surgeon's knife. At this point in medical history, there were still far too many physicians with blood and dirt on their hands trolling the wards of Bellevue, much to the disgust and alarm of the eager young bucks like William who would devote the remainder of their careers to applying the advances of bacteriology and medical science to create the life-saving methods of antiseptic surgery.

An event in the amphitheater of the Bellevue Medical College illustrates the debate between those physicians who denied the existence of disease-causing microbes and those who embraced the concept. One spring afternoon in 1882, a favorite young professor of bacteriology and pathology at Bellevue, William Henry Welch, lectured to his medical students about Robert Koch's monumental discovery of the tubercle bacillus as the cause of the white plague of tuberculosis. Welch's students ran to Bellevue's senior professor of medicine, the redoubtable and bespectacled Alfred L. Loomis, to tell him about this remarkable information. A few days later, Dr. Loomis, the author of scores of medical textbooks that had made his name, if not exactly a household word, then certainly famous among students and practitioners, ascended the lecture platform of the Bellevue Hospital amphitheater,

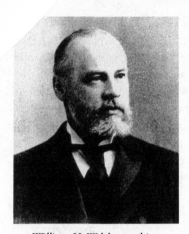

William H. Welch, age thirty, as a young professor at Bellevue Medical College, c. 1880.

looked merrily about the vast room, and declared: "People say there are bacteria in the air, but I cannot see them." Many of the medical students laughed uproariously at Loomis's witty denunciation, as students are wont to do whenever their professor makes the slightest attempt at humor. Yet when one of them later told Welch about the episode, Welch was said to have shaken his head and noted his colleague's obsolescence with an equal mixture of remorse and humor: "That's too bad. Loomis is such a nice man."

It was around this time that Welch began his long and productive friendship with Halsted. Both were junior professors in a tight-knit medical community. Welch, a frequent houseguest and dinner companion of Halsted's, grew steadily impressed with William's novel views on antisepsis, wound healing, and advancing surgical techniques. Halsted's demonstrable success was all the more fantastic in an era when postoperative hospital wards were redolent with the stink of multiplying bacteria, or what surgeons of the day misguidedly referred to as "laudable pus" and "pus of a good quality" because they thought its appearance was a sign that the body was healing itself. In reality, laudable pus was just the chemical and cellular detritus of a festering wound, one likely worsened by multiple infections.

Welch occupied his days teaching pathology and conducting bacteriological research. As a result, the bulk of his income came from the lecture admission tickets he sold to his adoring students, a once common practice in nineteenth-century medical education. Halsted, on the other hand, was already generating bountiful revenues from his surgical practice in addition to his teaching fees. Regardless of finances, they shared an intense determination to import the German research ethos into their clinical backyards and, thus, transform American medicine.

. . .

BY THE LATE FALL OF 1884, William was devoting whatever spare time he could marshal to a series of meticulous experiments using solutions of cocaine he procured from Parke, Davis and Company and water he obtained from his kitchen tap. And just as with Freud's experimental inquiries, Halsted's principal guinea pig was himself. By injecting the topmost layers of his own skin and, thence, probing deeper and deeper into muscle and nerve tissue, he carefully assembled the evidence to demonstrate how cocaine safely numbed a patient during mildly invasive procedures, such as the removal of a tooth or the closure of a skin wound with sutures, all the way to much more involved surgical operations.

One of Halsted's earliest attempts at performing major surgery with cocaine anesthesia came close to turning disastrous. In early 1885, his roommate and colleague, Thomas McBride, asked him to surgically remove the interior dental nerve in a wealthy and prominent woman suffering from trigeminal neuralgia, an inflammation of the maxillary and mandibular branches of the trigeminal nerve. Because the stabbing pain that afflicts the cheek, nose, lips, teeth, and jaw is so intense that it causes an involuntary wincing, or tic, doctors referred to the malady as tic douloureux. Halsted agreed to operate, "in a bedroom in my house." The 4 percent cocaine solution worked perfectly, but the "final snip" of Halsted's scissors nicked the internal maxillary artery. Thirty-three years later, Halsted dramatically recalled the event: "The patient's mouth filled with blood as if poured in by cupfuls. Tom McBride, whose patient she was, rushed out of the room not wishing, he told me afterwards, to be present at the death." Thanks to the surgeon's quick packing of the wound with gauze, several days of around-the-clock nursing with Halsted constantly at her bedside, and the remarkably adept clotting mechanisms of the human blood system, the woman recovered from the mishap without serious complications.

Undeterred by this setback, Halsted recruited others to help him with his pathbreaking cocaine research. Every evening, his students and assistant physicians clambered to his doorstep outfitted with pencils and notebooks, offering arms to be injected with cocaine for the purpose of figuring out where to apply the anesthetic and how much

..ld be given. Alas, not every dose of cocaine was administered ..rictly in the cause of advancing science. Increasingly, Halsted—and the others—began sneaking topical applications of the stuff onto their tongues or sniffed it into their nostrils for a quick and easy means of obliterating fatigue.

Halsted and his colleagues were quick to appreciate the sheer fun of ingesting cocaine. Theater events, dances, and even bowling matches at the University Club, a mere block away from Halsted's home, were brightened by the white powder. And like many other medicos who read of Koller's great discovery, Halsted and his associates focused only on the positive aspects of the drug as they inadvertently became drawn into its clutches, particularly after graduating from frequent oral or nasal applications to the much more direct and rapidly addicting route of injecting cocaine first into the muscular tissue of their arms and later perhaps even directly into the bloodstream.

Across the Atlantic, just as Halsted was making his unintentionally bad decision to inject cocaine, a young general practitioner struggling to build a practice in Southsea, Great Britain, became enchanted with cocaine's charms. During the long stretches between patients, the doctor occasionally experimented with the drug. On more occasions, however, he took up his fountain pen and wrote beautiful essays, stories, and even novels.

In 1887, only a few years after Koller's great announcement, the young doctor—Arthur Conan Doyle—published his first major novel, entitled *A Study in Scarlet,* in a now forgotten magazine called *Beeton's Christmas Annual.* The tale introduced the world to Sherlock Holmes, the pipe-smoking sleuth who employed a method he called "deductive reasoning," which was based on the diagnostic approach of a physician. As Conan Doyle's legion of readers would learn in subsequent episodes, Sherlock enjoyed injecting a 7 percent solution of cocaine as a means of escape after particular trying cases. Parenthetically, it is too rich to neglect to mention that one of Conan Doyle's most avid readers was Sigmund Freud. As Freud's now famous patient Sergius Pankejeff (better known as "the Wolf-Man") recalled: "Once we happened to speak of Conan Doyle and his creation, Sherlock Holmes. I had thought that Freud would have no use for this type of light reading matter, and was

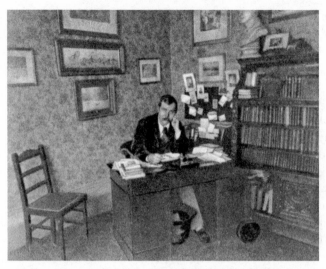

Arthur Conan Doyle, M.D.: the creator of Sherlock Holmes, 1894.

surprised to find that this was not at all the case and that Freud read this author attentively."

Three years after Sherlock Holmes's debut, in 1890, a second novel, *A Sign of the Four,* was published to great acclaim. Conan Doyle's precise description of Holmes's cocaine self-administration in this novel could just as easily be applied to Halsted's technique and mottled arm:

> Sherlock Holmes took his bottle from the corner of the mantel-piece and his hypodermic syringe from its neat morocco case. With his long, white, nervous fingers he adjusted the delicate needle, and rolled back his left shirt-cuff. For some little time his eyes rested thoughtfully upon the sinewy forearm and wrist all dotted and scarred with innumerable puncture-marks. Finally he thrust the sharp point home, pressed down the tiny piston, and sank back into the velvet-lined arm-chair with a long sigh of satisfaction.

Like the fictional detective, Halsted was instantly struck by how marvelous the drug made him feel. An injection of cocaine guaranteed freedom from all vicissitudes and slights, release from resentments and pain, and a sense of utter satisfaction so strong and compelling, exhilarating and calming that he would eventually risk or sacrifice anything just to be under its power again.

IN A MATTER OF WEEKS Halsted and his immediate circle were transformed from an elite cadre of doctors into active cocaine abusers. Tragically, some of the medical students, resident physicians, and surgeons who participated in these experiments were decimated by the drug and died early deaths. Most poignant was the fate of Halsted's close colleague, assistant, and friend Richard J. Hall. The two first met in medical school and spent time together in Vienna in 1879. Upon returning to New York, they were each appointed to the faculty of their alma mater. Present at the start of Halsted's precipitous love affair with cocaine in 1884, Hall recorded some of their earliest experiments in the *New York Medical Journal.* Unfortunately, Hall became so addicted to cocaine that he was forced to "dry out" at a sanatorium in Santa Barbara, California. In 1895, a rehabilitated Hall wrote Halsted a rambling letter boasting of a new surgical practice and explaining his long silence:

> *My dear Halsted; It is now quite a long time since I received a long letter from you and a very kind one. I am not sure that I ever answered it, for at that time I was only pulling myself together, after a long period of misery, the causes of which I do not need to describe.*

Two years later, Richard Hall died at the age of forty-four of unclear causes, though many suspect he never truly beat his demons down. William may have narrowly avoided the ultimate cocaine oblivion that took his friend at such an early age, but he hardly escaped unscathed.

CHAPTER 6

Cocaine Damnation

WHY IS COCAINE SO PLEASURABLE, so compelling, and, ultimately, so addictive?

With most substances of abuse, rapid delivery of the drug to the brain is critical. The faster the absorption, the more intense is the high. Paradoxically, the faster the absorption, the shorter is the duration of action, often inspiring the desire for more drugs. During the late nineteenth century, many cocaine fans took their drug in the form of laced teas, tonics, alcohol-based elixirs, and soft drinks. Yet the twists and turns of the stomach and intestines are simply too circuitous a path to the bloodstream and brain to yield cocaine's most explosive effects. And if there is one thing most experienced drug users seek, it is the quickest and most potent means of getting high.

Once cocaine became available in crystalline form, some, like Freud, drank it mixed in a small amount of water or dabbed on the tongue. Many others, however, began to snort or sniff a carefully ground-up dose into the nostrils, using a tiny spoonlike device or a straw-shaped object. The experienced cocaine user quickly learns the importance of grinding down the crystals with a sharp-edged instrument, such as a razor blade, into a fine powder, to avoid large pellets, which do not dissolve well and can erode or ulcerate the wet, sensitive mucus membranes that line the interior of the nose. Of greater distress to the avid cocaine user is the issue of waste: more times than not, large pieces of cocaine simply fall out at the first blow or shake of the nose. Those users who do take the time to finely chop their drug are eventually rewarded. Beneath the inner lining of the nose are thousands of tiny capillaries, which lead to larger and larger still blood vessels. The effects from such ingestions may last fifteen to thirty minutes.

A more efficient and addictive means of using cocaine is to smoke it after the drug has been chemically altered. If one smokes ordinary cocaine hydrochloride, much of the active ingredient is destroyed. To counteract this loss, in the mid-1980s drug dealers began "cooking" the cocaine in a pan laced with water and baking soda. The resulting chemical reaction frees the cocaine molecules from the attached hydrochloride salt and produces a loud popping or cracking noise—hence the drug's odd name, crack cocaine. Cocaine users soon flocked to purchase this substance from their dealers because smoking it guaranteed remarkably intense, albeit short-lived highs.

Once cocaine is chemically manipulated and smoked, psychoactive molecules are released and inhaled into tiny air sacs, called alveoli, in the inner recesses of the lungs. These are the structures where the real work of respiration takes place; molecules of life-giving oxygen are absorbed into the bloodstream and waste molecules of carbon dioxide are readied for exhalation. Surrounding the alveoli is an intricate network of blood vessels called arterioles and capillaries. In terms of surface area, these arterioles equal the square footage of a football field. As a result, the molecules of inhaled cocaine easily cross the membrane-thin layer of the alveoli and instantly enter the bloodstream, the body's equivalent of the autobahn, with a direct route to the brain.

Unlike with morphine and other opiates, relatively few cocaine addicts choose to inject the drug into their veins, although Halsted and Fleischl-Marxow may have occasionally done so. This method, alas, is dangerous, potentially painful, and highly addictive. Nevertheless, injecting cocaine rewards the addict in generating a speedy and intense high.

Whether tasted, sniffed, smoked, or injected, once inside the bloodstream, the cocaine molecules travel rapidly to other critical organs as well. Most noticeable is the drug's arrival in the heart, the central pumping and distribution system that directs the blood into the lungs in order for it to grab an allotment of nourishing oxygen before being sent to the rest of the body. Cardiac muscle is exquisitely vulnerable to cocaine's powers. Under its influence, the heart pumps harder and faster. Blood vessels will constrict, or tighten, leading to an alarming increase of blood pressure. More troubling, the drug can provoke serious disturbances in how the heart beats and may even incite a heart attack or stroke. Cocaine can also wreak havoc on the liver, spleen, and kidneys, altering those organs' functions and potentially causing serious damage.

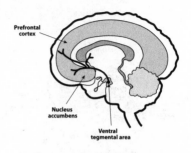

A sagittal view of the brain, showing a neuron with connections to the prefrontal cortex and its pleasure centers, the nucleus accumbens, and the ventral tegmental area.

After arriving at the brain's prefrontal cortex, cocaine travels to the ventral tegmental area (VTA), which has a direct pathway to a nearby region called the nucleus accumbens, thought to be a key pleasure center. Just about every gratifying act known to man, whether drinking a cold glass of water on a hot day, enjoying a delicious meal, feeling the warmth of the sun or the closeness of a loved one, sexual arousal and the rollicking climaxes we refer to as orgasms, the satisfaction experienced with an achievement or acquisition, or delighting in a harvest moon—essentially every experience that makes life worth living—is registered, recorded, anticipated, and mediated in this part of the brain. From this "pleasure center," these experiences are quickly translated into the recognizable signs of contentment, from a smile to a sense of well-being.

If nature set out to design an addictive drug, it could hardly do better than cocaine. This is because the drug brilliantly fools the neurons ending in the nucleus accumbens into sensing a virtual abundance of enjoyable feelings and sensations.

The predominant chemical effect of a dose of cocaine is a massive flood of receptor neurons with dopamine, the neurotransmitter that helps govern pleasure, motivation, and reward. Such synaptic flooding also occurs with two other major neurotransmitters that contribute to one's mood, serotonin and norepinephrine. Under normal circumstances, transporter proteins at the nerve endings remove these neurotransmitters from the synapse (the microscopic gap between two neurons) and recycle them back into vesicles (the transmitting neuron's storage centers). But with cocaine molecules on the scene, the trans-

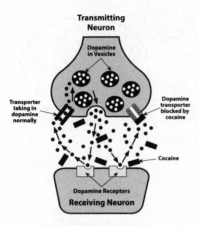

Transmitting
Neuron

Dopamine
in Vesicles

Transporter
taking in
dopamine
normally

Dopamine
transporter
blocked by
cocaine

Cocaine

Dopamine Receptors
Receiving Neuron

*The synapse between a transmitting
neuron and a receiving neuron and the
release of dopamine. The figure demonstrates normal dopamine transporter
uptake (left) and blocked dopamine
transporter uptake (right) under
the influence of cocaine.*

porter proteins are, essentially, jammed up. Consequently, the receiving neurons sense far more dopamine (as well as serotonin and norepinephrine) than usual and interpret this excess as extreme pleasure or a "rush" of euphoria. A pharmacological version of the legendary Trojan horse, cocaine essentially sneaks through the gates into the brain's finely honed reward system before seizing control.

Within a few moments of smoking, injecting, or sniffing cocaine, a sense of exhilarating delight begins. This is not the slaphappy, "I love everyone" kind of joy that transpires after a few belts of whiskey. When under the influence of cocaine, one feels supremely confident, almost electrically charged with faster thoughts, better ideas (at least in one's own mind at the time of the high), an increased speed of speaking, and a greater appreciation of such sensations as sight, sound, and touch. This energy burst also decreases the need to eat and sleep, allowing a user to stay awake all night if he consumes enough of the stuff.

And if a drug-induced sexual experience is the aim, many swear by cocaine's ability to increase desire and focus on that pursuit. Yet it is precisely in the sexual arena where one of cocaine's many perverse powers emerges. While cocaine may, indeed, catapult a person's quest for sexual stimulation and climax, the drug blocks the neurons' ability to reabsorb serotonin in the synapse. It causes vasoconstriction of the blood vessels in the penis, thus interfering with a man's ability to maintain an erection. Moreover, for both men and women, cocaine interrupts the brain's physiological processes for achieving an orgasm. Ecstatic arousal and desire are jet-propelled, but the fuel to finish the journey is defiantly lacking long before the first orbit is complete.

Cocaine, of course, also contains a brutally negative force. When the drug is metabolized and inactive in the brain, the transporter molecules begin to function again and absorb all the excess neurotransmitters in the synapse. This mop-up effort results in a shortage of these critical mood-regulating chemicals in the brain. In turn, that shortage causes the pleasure circuits to abruptly cease their orgiastic firing, a situation known all too well by experienced cocaine abusers as a "crash." Specifically, such crashes are awful, dramatic lows that occur immediately following the cocaine high; unfortunately, their effects linger far, far after the intensely pleasurable sensations are over. To make matters worse, as an individual successively fools the neurons to release, deplete, and replenish their stores of dopamine, serotonin, and norepinephrine with repeated doses of cocaine, he requires greater amounts of the drug to achieve the same levels of satisfaction, forming a perfect endless loop of addictive and destructive behavior.

In time, cocaine abuse yields significant damage not only in the brain's pleasure centers but also in the frontal cortex, the region of the brain that facilitates decision making. The extent of this neurological derangement was most starkly demonstrated during the late 1960s. Scientists gave one set of laboratory rats ample food and water, and open access to heroin; the other group was given the same food and water but the bar was serving cocaine. The heroin rats certainly became addicted to their drug, but its narcotic effects curtailed their consumption to specific times during the day. Basically, they got stoned and fell asleep, awoke, drank water and ate, and then started all over again. On the other side of the caged neighborhood, the cocaine rats did nothing but consume more cocaine. At various points some of these rats would collapse with nervous exhaustion, but once they awoke, they routinely pursued more cocaine. A month later, the heroin rats were surviving nicely, albeit addicted to narcotics; the cocaine rats were all dead.

AT THE TIME DR. HALSTED began experimenting with cocaine, he enjoyed a comfortable home life with his companion and roommate, Thomas Alexander McBride, a former medical school classmate. McBride, handsome and well-spoken, was considered quite the man about town. He maintained a prosperous carriage trade practice in addition to his duties as a clinical assistant in internal medicine at the College of Physicians and Surgeons. McBride and Halsted lived in a "luxuriously furnished" flat on Twenty-fifth Street between Madison Avenue and Fourth Avenue (now Park Avenue South) that served as the unofficial clubhouse for an expanding cadre of medical students and doctors. McBride was said to have spent "lavishly" on his roommate, but the precise contours of their domestic arrangement remain unclear. It was likely a close and loving relationship, though one that would have attracted little attention or comment in an era when discreet and separate social spheres existed for men and women, not to mention a decided aversion to publicly discussing sexuality.

In a matter of months, cocaine completely took over Halsted's life. First he missed only occasional lectures or perhaps an appointment with a colleague. Soon enough, he was referring patients to other surgeons to avoid the operating room. Although he made a somewhat confused appearance at the evening meeting of the New York Surgical Society on April 28, 1885, for most of that spring, William engaged in few, if any, clinical activities. His last recorded operations at Bellevue took place on March 23, an amputation of a laborer's leg above the knee for gangrene resulting from a crush injury and an excision of a vaginal-cutaneous sinus tract in a woman. On May 5, 1885, he ceased to be a doctor and surgeon, the path to which he had devoted the last intense decade of his life. After examining a laborer suffering from a compound fracture of the tibia, a thin, haggard, and addicted Halsted abruptly exited Bellevue Hospital to nervously hibernate and consume alarmingly large amounts of cocaine in his Manhattan town house.

Always a prolific medical correspondent with a precise literary style, the years 1885 and 1886 signaled Halsted's most fallow period as a writer. As proof, one need only consult the memorial edition of the surgeon's scientific, surgical, and academic papers, a chock-filled two volumes containing more than 150 contributions. His now famous paper on cocaine that did appear in print in 1885 was all but excised from Halsted's clothbound *Surgical Papers*. Instead, the editor lists only the paper's title and bibliographic citation, accompanied by the terse comment that it "would require such reediting as is not deemed expedient."

In fact, "Practical Comments on the Use and Abuse of Cocaine Suggested by Its Invariably Successful Employment in More Than a

Thousand Minor Surgical Operations" both advanced surgical technique and informs a retrospective diagnosis of William's condition. Many medical historians credit the article, which appeared in the September 12, 1885, issue of the *New York Medical Journal,* with introducing the world to local anesthetic by nerve blockade. The paper also demonstrated the ease with which cocaine could be injected into the skin to achieve the desired results, the means of diluting cocaine solutions to avoid toxicity and still numb the surgical area, and ways of prolonging the anesthetic effects by reducing the flow of blood to the operative site. Still, the paper is presented in a prose so disjointed, hyperactive, and overwrought that it was almost certainly written under the influence of cocaine.

> Neither indifferent as to which of how many possibilities may best explain, nor yet at a loss to comprehend, why surgeons have, and that so many, quite without discredit, could have exhibited scarcely any interest in what, as a local anæsthetic, had been supposed, if not declared, by most so very sure to prove, especially to them, attractive, still I do not think that this circumstance, or some sense of obligation to rescue fragmentary reputation for surgeons rather than the belief that an opportunity existed for assisting others to an appreciable extent, induced me, several months ago, to write on the subject in hand the greater part of a somewhat comprehensive paper, which poor health disinclined me to complete.

Even the most experienced consumer of the medical literature is forced to scratch his head when reading this seminal publication. The paper ends with the promise of more data to be published in a subsequent issue, but Halsted never wrote a "Part II."

In the summer of 1885, shortly after sending his cocaine study off to the *New York Medical Journal,* Halsted made a return trip to Vienna in search of rest and recreation. While there, he demonstrated his cocaine-injection technique for local anesthesia to his mentor Anton Wölfler and an American dentist named Thomas. Although the dentist was thrilled by the method, Wölfler declared it to be useless. Dr. Wölfler subsequently published an enthusiastic article on it in one of the daily newspapers, but without mentioning Halsted's name. To the end of his life, the surgeon recalled this slight. One person William did not record meeting with while in Vienna was Sigmund Freud.

When William returned to New York in early January 1886, his friends noticed worrisome changes in his behavior. Once modest and self-effacing, he was now abrupt, spoke incessantly, and cared little for the responses of those he was speaking with. Dr. George Brewer, a Baltimore urologist who visited Halsted around this time in search of a position at Roosevelt Hospital, complained that from early afternoon until long after it turned dark he could not get a word in edgewise. Brewer later remembered that Halsted was "very excited and talked constantly about everything under the sun from the transit of Venus to gonococci." Every time the urologist tried to beat a hasty retreat out of Halsted's house, the cocaine-fueled surgeon "would start up again."

William probably rationalized his cocaine consumption as being in the service of scientific inquiry. But long after he concluded his experiments, he abused the drug for the same reasons shared by most addicts: to simply feel better, to numb himself, to escape from the painful lows of depression, frustration, rejection, and a hundred and one other slings and arrows of life.

In late January 1886, a worried William Henry Welch took it upon himself to institute an ad hoc treatment plan to arrest Halsted's dire condition. Welch refused to accept the dogmatic pronouncements of the day dismissing alcoholics and drug addicts as hopeless, morally flawed wrecks of human beings. The pathology professor was determined to save his talented colleague from cocaine damnation. Intervening with two other concerned friends, Drs. George Munroe and Samuel Vander Poel, Welch invited Halsted into his office and offered him a potential way out of the abyss he was facing.

Welch laid all his cards on the table. He began by revealing that he knew what was going on with respect to Halsted's relentless cocaine abuse and that it needed to stop, posthaste. The solution Welch suggested was a rejuvenating sea voyage, then considered therapeutic for men of means suffering from a broad range of maladies. Convinced of the wisdom of this suggestion, Halsted joined Welch during February, March, and April of 1886 on a schooner named the *Bristol* bound for the Windward Islands in the Caribbean. Recognizing that Wil-

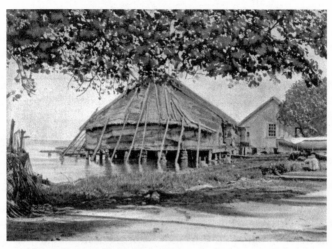

A pile dwelling where Caribbean islanders lived in the Windward Islands at the time of Halsted's restorataive ocean voyage.

liam's previous cold-turkey attempts to stop using cocaine had failed abysmally, the two physicians developed a rigorous treatment plan featuring a large supply of cocaine to be doled out by Welch while gradually cutting down William's dosage to nothing before the trip's end.

For much of the voyage down the Atlantic seaboard, things worked out rather well; but Halsted was still taking daily, albeit progressively smaller, doses of cocaine. By the time the bow pointed toward the Caribbean, he'd begun experiencing uncomfortable feelings and emotional states of the sort that bedevil any addict trying to break free of this drug. Just as the use of cocaine brings on great feelings of euphoria and exhilaration, the cocaine-starved brain complains and rebels vociferously. With smaller and less frequent doses, William's brain must have screamed to him, "Where is my drug? Feed me my tonic! If only I had some more cocaine, all would be well."

It has long been observed that cocaine abusers who abruptly stop their drug of choice do not suffer the full-blown physical symptoms seen in those who suddenly quit morphine or alcohol. Such findings formerly encouraged physicians to insist that there was no withdrawal syndrome associated with cocaine. In more recent conceptions of addiction and withdrawal, however, experts have verified a set of nasty psychological symptoms that creep in after a cocaine abuser attempts to quit, including depression, intense fatigue, unpleasant dreams, restlessness, disturbances of appetite, and even suicidal thoughts. This awful state of mind can last for many months after discontinuing use of cocaine and contributes to the high relapse rates among those seeking recovery. To be sure, the effects of withdrawing from opiates and alcohol are much more intense, physical, and acute than those involving cocaine. Yet, as Halsted surely could have testified, cocaine maintains the ability, long after it has taken its corporal leave, to communicate with the addict's brain, luring him back to partake once again, with the flimsy promise that all will be well—at least for a few moments.

Despite careful projections, Halsted could not satisfy his cocaine hunger. He grew steadily more agitated as he estimated that he would completely run out of the drug long before returning home. Late one night, miles out at sea, the cocaine-obsessed Halsted lay awake, nervously rocking in his hammock while listening to the scratching and snoring of his bunkmates. Audibly assured that they would not bear witness, he snuck out of the cabin and prowled about until he located the captain's medicine chest. It was a short time before this scion of privilege was reduced to breaking into the locked container for a much-needed dose.

A fascinating, likely embellished, and difficult to verify biography of Halsted was published in 1960. The book was written as part of a series on famous doctors and scientists for an audience of young teenagers. In it, we are told that at this point of the journey Drs. Welch and Halsted explored the island of Santa Lucia only to find a desperate doctor, a moribund patient, and an appendix doing its best to burst in the latter's abdomen. Like a fireman's horse hearing the bell, Halsted diagnosed acute appendicitis and recommended an emergency appendectomy. The island doctor vociferously disagreed, insisting that the patient's problem was the result of eating a plate of poisonous roots. William took command and insisted on beginning the operation. But first, he administered a dose of cocaine from the ship's store to both the patient and himself. The patient, of course, required the drug to avoid feeling the pain of being cut open. William, the authors claim, needed cocaine to quell his raging urges. Halsted's diagnosis turned out to be correct, and the patient enjoyed a speedy recovery from his appendectomy.

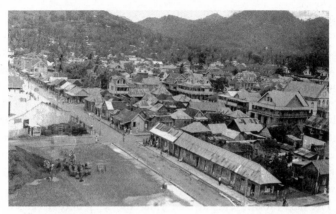

*Santa Lucia, the Windward Islands, where Halsted is said to have
performed an appendectomy during his attempt at rehabilitation
(photograph c. 1890).*

Regardless of the veracity of this tale, let alone the improbability of
operating well while under the influence, there still remained the press-
ing problem of the depleted cocaine supply Halsted needed so badly.

William consumed all of the cocaine before the ship approached
Florida, and it was then that he entered the most harrowing part of his
oceanic journey. Plagued by nightmares, exhaustion, irritability, outright suspicion of his fellow travelers, and, because he was clenching his
muscles relentlessly, aching limbs, William felt lousy. Somehow, Dr.
Welch got the cocaine-starved Halsted back to New York Harbor in
one piece in late April 1886. Before disembarking, Welch offered Halsted his best diagnosis: the surgeon needed far more intensive treatment than that afforded by a mere sea voyage; Halsted would have to
admit himself into Butler Hospital.

Butler was a well-known insane asylum in Providence, Rhode
Island, under the direction of Dr. John Woodbury Sawyer, a psychia-
trist who was having a degree of success treating morphine addicts.
This was hardly a palatable choice for the surgeon-in-exile. In William's
defense, prolonged confinement to an insane asylum was not a fate any
self-respecting or self-preserving late-nineteenth-century American
chose voluntarily.

The benevolent Welch did make sure that Halsted had a nugget of hope to take with him to Providence. Once successfully treated and released from Butler, Halsted could join him in Baltimore, where Welch was assuming command as professor and dean of the newly established Johns Hopkins University School of Medicine. Halsted quickly grasped that the invitation was a golden opportunity to make medical history. If he could only recover from his addiction, if he could only rid himself of this deadly habit, he might revolutionize the teaching and practice of surgery. Before surrendering to Welch's generous offer for recovery, however, Halsted stalled and begged for some time to think things over. Predictably, a few hours later, he was back in his town house, high on cocaine.

The next morning, Dr. Welch came knocking on Halsted's door with a list of nonnegotiable demands that began and ended with commitment to Butler Hospital. The sober pathologist and the drug-addled surgeon sat across from each other and took up their conversation where they'd left off the evening before. Halsted desperately tried to rebuff the hard evidence that cocaine was destroying his body, his social relationships, and his career. Such outlandish denials distinguish the disease of addiction from mere dabbling or recreational substance use. The addict's brain truculently conspires against common sense and

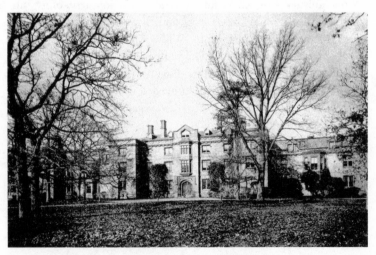

Butler Hospital, Rhode Island.

the instinct for self-preservation, urging its possessor not to quit. And it often backs up this hypnotic neurochemical spell with quarrelsome force. Quite simply, the active cocaine addict feels decent enough when the drug is coursing through his bloodstream and manipulating his central nervous system but feels downright awful when it is not.

Welch's wheedling demands somehow inspired a watershed moment in Halsted's life. A few hours later, Welch tucked him into a Pullman car leaving Grand Central Station and bound for Providence. Of all the negative thoughts running through William's troubled mind upon entering the sumptuous, marble-clad lobby of Butler Hospital, it is safe to assume that the dominant chords sounding were shame, remorse, and regret. At the registration desk, a clerk presented the surgeon with an ornate hospital register and pen. How lost and abject this proud surgeon must have felt as he timidly signed the ledger as "William Stewart" and drew a long, inky slash where "Halsted" should have been entered.

CHAPTER 7

Sigmund in Paris

N O MATTER HOW HE COGITATED on the events of 1884, Freud knew somewhere between the ventricles and atria of his heart that he had been bested by "Coca" Koller. His failure to recognize cocaine's anesthetic properties aside, a small but steady stream of respectful reviews of *Über Coca* began to trickle into print. Smelling still more academic gold to quarry, he continued to pursue his scientific investigations. His second impulse, perhaps even more powerful, was to continue abusing cocaine.

Freud proved rather adept at self-promotion. In January 1885 he convinced a reporter for the Viennese metropolitan daily *Neue Freie Presse* to write a feature story about his work on the new miracle drug. Soon after its appearance, the piece was translated and published by hundreds of American and European newspapers. This flush of fame, the equivalent of a young medical researcher today finding his work profiled on National Public Radio or in the *New York Times,* no doubt encouraged Freud to invest in five hundred reprints of the coca monograph in early 1885, which he distributed to professors and doctors who had the connections to sharpen his professional trajectory.

Around this same time, Freud published a study of cocaine's effects on the motor power of specific muscle groups and psychic reaction time in the January 31, 1885, issue of the *Wiener medizinische Wochenschrift.* He followed this up with a brief series of addenda to his *Über Coca,* which closed with a casual acknowledgment of Koller's anesthetic discovery (one he insisted that "countless others" had been working on as well). A mealymouthed Sigmund concluded that while this application was, indeed, exciting, "the present still artificially high price of the drug is an obstacle to all further experiments." A little more than a month later, in March 1885, he published a paper in the *Medizinisch-chirurgisches Centralblatt* summarizing his findings on cocaine's general effects on the human body. One of the most intriguing aspects of this paper is how Freud briefly mentions the success he had in treating acute morphine withdrawal in an unnamed addict we now know was Fleischl-Marxow, who was, by this time, no longer doing so well on cocaine: "He took about 0.40 grams of cocaine per day," the paper prematurely boasted, "and by the end of 20 days the morphine abstinence was overcome." Throughout the winter and early spring of 1885, Sigmund saw to it that all of his lectures on cocaine at prominent medical societies were abstracted and reprinted in a variety of journals.

THE BIOGRAPHIES OF FREUD and Halsted contain many odd coincidences of fate, scientific interests, and even the fact that both were rambling about the wards of the Krankenhaus in 1878 and 1879. But one of the great temporal ironies in their medical histories occurred in 1885. While Halsted was injecting himself, students, and patients with cocaine solutions, Sigmund briefly attempted to inject the drug into the trigeminal nerve of a patient with terrible facial pain. Like Halsted, Freud practiced such injections on his own arm.

He would later claim that his old boss Franz Scholz taught him how to use a hypodermic needle. Scholz had prided himself on his exemplary sterile technique in administering subcutaneous injections. It is difficult to ascertain how adept Freud was at using a needle-loaded syringe. Given his choice of medical specialty and the lack of regular opportunities to practice injection techniques, however, it is safe to wager he was less than proficient.

Tracing the lithe trigeminal nerve as it traverses a person's face, the ropy ulnar nerve as it slithers along the path of the arm, or a spongy blood-filled vein bulging beneath the skin, let alone isolating those structures long enough to accurately insert a needle, requires real skill. Halsted clearly possessed that ability, and his deft injections led to the advent of local anesthesia, one of the greatest gifts to modern surgery and dentistry. Both men were unabashed medical geniuses, but Freud would never be able to claim the manual dexterity of a surgical virtuoso like Halsted. In fact, Sigmund garnered lackluster results with the cocaine injections and soon abandoned the method.

Freud's clumsiness may well have saved him from Halsted's landslide fate. The surgeon's reliance on rehearsing this technique on himself provided a faster, more intense high but also increased his tolerance and desire, if not outright compulsion, for more of it. Halsted's path from scientific investigator to full-blown addict required only a few months; Freud's cocaine abuse, which centered on the application of the drug into his mouth or nasal passages, continued for years in a somewhat more measured manner.

Regardless of the route of entry, in 1885 and 1886 Freud was self-medicating with greater and more frequent doses of cocaine. On too many days and nights, at social occasions and alone in his quarters, when the pain of being Sigmund was simply too great to bear, he availed himself of some of the "magical drug." At other times, as while writing to his beloved Martha, cocaine served as an aphrodisiac, unleashing flowery and uninhibited words of love.

IN MARCH 1885, while waiting to be appointed *Privatdozent* at the Vienna General Hospital, Sigmund applied for and received the University of Vienna's prestigious Jubilee Fund travel grant. Awarded annually to the training doctor deemed to be most worthy of additional medical study in another country, it came with a stipend of 600 gulden and the stipulation that half was given to the winner before embarking, with the balance to be paid upon his return and presentation of a formal report to the medical school. Although this arrangement meant Sigmund would have to be extremely miserly with his expenditures, he made immediate plans to leave for Paris to study neurology under Jean-Martin Charcot, the world-famous neurologist, pathologist, and clinician. A leading light of the Paris clinical school, Dr. Charcot held court at the Salpêtrière Hospital, on the Left Bank of the river Seine. Scheduled to begin his fellowship in the fall, Sigmund first took a brief summer visit to Martha's country home in Wandsbeck, near Hamburg. After a teary farewell, he was off for France.

Freud's initial days in Paris were lonely and trying. In one early October 1885 letter to Martha, he records every expense, from stationery to matches, in view of the tight budget forcing him to squeeze every centime to its maximum value. Freud managed on 300 francs (or $60) a month for meals, room, and books. He dutifully sent home any extra monies to his mother, excepting the one month he splurged on purchasing a complete set of the journal *Charcot's Archives* for 80 francs. His hotel accommodations at the Hôtel de la Paix in the Latin Quarter were cheap, 55 francs a month, but woefully dingy. His second address, Hôtel du Brésil on the Rue de Goff, was a far better bargain at 155 francs a month for both room and board. On one occasion, Dr. Freud of the famously filthy Krankenhaus was disgusted to discover that the curtains surrounding his hotel bed were green and menacing. Ever the scientific investigator, before retiring that night, he made a trip to the local chemist and brought back a parcel of chemical reagents to test his room for arsenic. The inquiry, fortunately, proved to be negative.

As Sigmund began to explore the City of Lights, he found it to be "magnificent and charming," a delightful place of "magic." Freud reveled in the beauties of the winding Seine. He visited the Louvre Museum's Egyptian and Assyrian collections and ogled the Venus de Milo. So enchanted was he by the grand museum's ancient collections that he neglected to wander into the famed picture galleries. On many nights, he climbed the twisting stairs of Paris's theaters, where he made do with "shameful pigeon-hole loges." These were the only seats he could afford but well worth it for the chance to watch the legendary Sarah Bernhardt in Victorien Sardou's *Théodora*. Upon returning from her performance, Sigmund raved about the actress to Martha: "But how that Sarah plays! After the first words of her vibrant lovely voice I felt I had known her for years. . . . I believed at once everything she said." Sigmund also attended productions of Hugo's *Hernani*, Sophocles' *Oedipus Rex*, Beaumarchais's *Le Mariage de Figaro,* and Molière's *Tartuffe*. Beyond Freud's love of the stage, there was a practical reason for his frequent theater attendance: the performances served as valuable French lessons.

Some afternoons, Sigmund walked through the grim grounds of the Père-Lachaise Cemetery to pay homage to a large number of recumbent but great French literary, medical, scientific, and artistic lights. On others, he smelled the flowers and greenery of the glorious Tuileries Gardens, negotiated the traffic of the Champs-Élysées, gazed at the "real

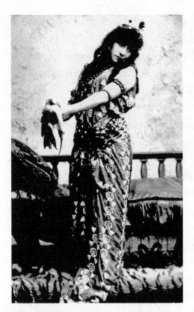

"The Divine Sarah": Sarah Bernhardt in 1905, at age sixty-one, in Victor Hugo's romantic drama Angelo. *Bernhardt was one of Freud's favorite actresses; as a postgraduate fellow in Paris in 1886, he saw her perform.*

obelisk from Luxor" in the Place de la Concorde, and sat on hard pews in the Cathédrale Notre-Dame. Less attractive were the Parisians, whom Sigmund found to be "possessed of a thousand demons . . . they are people given to psychical epidemics, historical mass convulsions, and they haven't changed since Victor Hugo wrote *Notre-Dame.* To understand Paris," he wrote Martha, "this is the novel you must read; although it is fiction, one is convinced of its truth."

THE SALPÊTRIÈRE WAS one of the largest hospitals in all Europe. As its name implies, it was originally a gunpowder and saltpeter factory but was converted, by order of Louis XIV in 1656, into a giant warehouse for Paris's most rejected yet still living flesh and bones. At the dawn of the French Revolution, the hospital had a capacity of more than ten thousand patients and at least three hundred prisoners, including some of the city's most defiled prostitutes. Home to a quivering, teeming mob of the mentally impaired, epileptic, insane, and simply destitute, it was the largest madhouse in the world. But on May 24, 1793, a medical revolution transpired there when the Salpêtrière's physician-in-chief, Philippe Pinel, descended into the hospital's subbasement ward of poorly lit and badly ventilated cells. In one of these dank hospital wards, Pinel ceremoniously liberated forty-nine insane patients from the chains holding them down, thus inaugurating an era of humanism toward the mentally ill that has continued in fits and starts for more than two centuries.

The smell that afternoon in 1793 must have been overpowering to the well-bred doctors and students making their historic rounds: rotting feces, fetid urine, and nauseating vomit spilled onto the floor from buckets serving as makeshift toilets; feculent sludge oozed from walls built too close to the city's sewers, which ran at the same subterranean level. All of these nasal assaults were combined with the sweaty and foul emanations of unwashed patients locked up for years on end. In an era when many considered the cause of ill health to be inhaling miasma and vitiated effluvia—or tainted air—it was little wonder that the doctors attending these patients covered their mouths and noses with scented handkerchiefs, in a misguided effort at self-protection. Other than the physicians, nurses, orderlies, students, and the multitude of inmates, the only other living beings down there were the cockroaches, fleas, and a herd of ferocious rats, which tortured the incarcerated on a regular basis. Dr. Pinel's removal of the iron restraints binding these unfortunates must have been very welcome indeed, and from every account of the event, all of the patients responded favorably.

Less than a century later, on the morning of October 20, 1885, Sigmund Freud first entered the Salpêtrière. Situated on seventy-four acres and bounded by a grid of cobblestoned streets, its forty-five buildings housed more than six thousand patients. The complex's grandest suites, wards, clinics, and amphitheaters were reserved for Dr. Jean-Martin Charcot. At its center and replacing the manacles and chains Pinel had

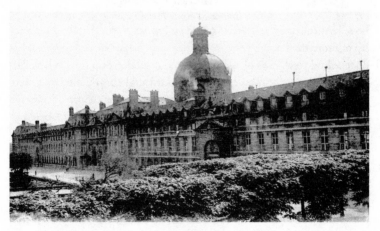

The Salpêtrière Hospital of Paris, where Freud studied under Charcot.

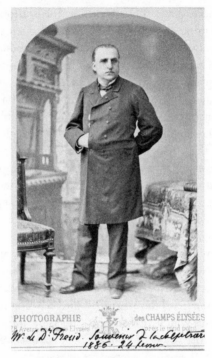

"Souvenir of the Salpêtrière, 1886.
24 February": Jean-Martin Charcot
inscribed this photograph as a farewell
of sorts commemorating Freud's taking
leave of Paris for Vienna.

once found were rows of polished-wood display cabinets with beveled-glass fronts, their shelves holding cylindrical glass jars; the latter were filled with formaldehyde and the brains and spinal cords of patients who'd failed to be discharged alive. Each jar was pristinely labeled in tiny French script, giving the precise pathological details of the individual's case. This macabre but impressive hallway—essentially a museum of neurology and insanity—led directly into Dr. Jean-Martin Charcot's consultation room.

Neurology, as a clinical specialty, was in its infancy when Dr. Charcot entered the field. The complex set of diseases met its match in a mind laserlike in focus and as wide as a canyon in terms of what the great physician collected, analyzed, and processed. Charcot was particularly gifted at synthesizing a patient's signs, symptoms, and medical history and then correlating them to the brain lesions and anomalies he'd found at the autopsy table. His major discoveries included the first definitive descriptions of multiple sclerosis, amyotrophic lateral sclerosis (often referred to as Lou Gehrig's disease, after the famous New York Yankee first baseman who was diagnosed with it in 1939), and a group of the most common inherited degenerative neurological disorders that still bears his (and his colleagues') name, Charcot-Marie-Tooth disease.

A mesmerizing speaker, Charcot illustrated his formal tutorials with vivid chalk diagrams he drew on the blackboard while lecturing, never losing his train of thought or misplacing an anatomical structure. A technophile long before the term was coined, he employed the latest lantern slides, lighting techniques, photographs, and clay models. Like many an excellent neurologist, he was a superb mimic of his patients' symptoms. Each morning, Charcot masterfully demonstrated to his students the limping gait of a polio victim, the storklike walk of someone with end-stage syphilis, the slurred speech of a stroke victim, or the unresponsive face of a person with Parkinson's disease. Such techniques were neither a form of ridicule nor a means of entertainment. Instead, they were critical tools in teaching nascent doctors to better recognize these diagnostic features in their own patients.

Freud arrived at Charcot's neurology clinic on the morning of October 20, 1885, and promptly paid a deposit of 3 francs for a key to the laboratory closet and an apron. Soon after, he found Charcot's *chef du clinique,* Dr. Pierre Marie, examining outpatients in front of a captive audience of interns and physicians, many of whom came from distant locales and all of whom leaned off their seats with such absentminded intensity that only a few inches of buttocks kept them from falling onto the floor. A valued collaborator of Charcot's and a skillful neurologist in his own right, Dr. Marie made his name in 1886 by identifying the pituitary gland tumors that cause acromegaly, a rare disorder in which the brain produces too much growth hormone, leading to enlargement of the hands, feet, and facial features, as well as damage to the heart, eyes, and other organs.

Precisely when the clinic's big wooden clock struck ten, Dr. Marie brought his comments to a rapid close and deferentially stepped aside. Before the second hand had a chance to mark the passage of a single minute, Charcot made his dramatic entrance from a side door. Without looking at his notes, the professor thrust himself into pontificating on a puzzling case with the confidence of a virtuoso playing a Mozart piano concerto. What developed was an intricate rondo of competing stories, one containing the mystery within the patient and the second the physician's compulsion to unravel that secret. But there was never a doubt as to who was in command and playing the role of featured soloist.

Afterward, Sigmund shyly approached Drs. Charcot and Marie. Summoning up as much courage as he could muster, he presented his impressive credentials and letters of reference to Marie, who quickly read them and handed them to Charcot for the senior professor's review. After a pregnant pause, the clinical lion warmly welcomed Freud by exclaiming, *"Charmé de vous voir."* He then graciously proceeded to advise the young physician about how to make his working arrangements with the *chef du clinique* and showed Freud around the impressive laboratory and wards. To Sigmund's great delight, he was accepted into the Salpêtrière "without further ado."

The bonhomie of Charcot's clinic must have been remarkably freeing for the tightly wound and repressed Sigmund. On a daily basis, he was exposed to some of the finest clinicians and pathologists alive. Instead of feeling snubbed because of his Jewish-outsider status, as in Vienna, Sigmund was welcomed with joyous salutations. Added to this freedom was the French clinicians' willingness to think outside the box of conventional wisdom and explore such controversial methods as hypnotism and electrotherapy in the treatment of nervous disorders.

The next night, after returning to his hotel room satiated by a hearty dinner with some wine that was "very cheap, a deep red, and otherwise tolerable," Sigmund wrote Martha a long letter. He described Charcot as "a tall man of fifty-eight, wearing a top hat, with dark, strangely soft eyes (or rather, one is, the other is expressionless and has an inward cast), long wisps of hair stuck behind his ears, clean shaven, very expressive features with full protruding lips—in short, like a worldly priest from whom one expects much wit and an appreciation of good living."

In an excellent example of the literary abilities that would one day make him world-famous, Sigmund recorded all of Charcot's mannerisms and actions as he examined patients that morning. The young physician was bedazzled by Charcot's brilliant diagnostic powers "and the lively interest he took in everything, so unlike what we are accustomed to from our great men with their veneer of distinguished superficiality." Freud, of course, was always in search of father figures like Brücke, Nothnagel, and Meynert to elevate his spirit and his professional standing. As Martha read Sigmund's latest dispatch from Paris in her cosseted bedroom in Hamburg, it was clear that Freud had discovered his next hero.

During the following weeks, Sigmund's emotional geyser continued to erupt. On November 24, he wrote Martha:

> *I am really very comfortably installed now and I think I am changing a great deal. I will tell you in detail what is affecting me. Charcot, who is one of the greatest of physicians and a man whose common sense borders on genius, is simply wrecking all my aims and opinions. I sometimes come out of his lectures as from out of Nôtre Dame, with an entirely new idea about perfection. But he exhausts me; when I come away from him I no longer have any desire to work at my own silly things; it is three whole days since I have done any work, and I have no feelings of guilt. My brain is sated as after an evening in the theater. Whether the seed will ever bring forth fruit, I don't know; but what I do know is that no other human being has ever affected me in the same way.*

At the same time that Sigmund's thoughts were expanding with inspiring neurological insights, his brain and body were becoming increasingly accustomed to his favorite chemical substance. He'd likely have brought a supply of cocaine with him from Vienna, but even if he ran out, there were plenty of chemists in Paris glad to sell him more. And, in a pinch, a tasty bottle of Vin Mariani could be purchased and quickly consumed.

Between January and February 1886, Freud was invited to a series of six balls, dinners, and "at homes" at Dr. and Madame Charcot's palatial residence at 217 Boulevard St. Germaine. On January 18, Sigmund

excitedly wrote Martha about an invitation to the neurologist's home
the following evening. Sigmund anticipated his nervousness and told
Martha how he planned to pharmacologically alter it:

> [Charcot] *invited me (as well as Ricchetti) to come to his house
> tomorrow evening after dinner: "Il y aura du monde." You can
> probably imagine my apprehension mixed with curiosity and
> satisfaction. White tie and gloves, even a fresh shirt, a careful
> brushing of my last remaining hair, and so on. A little cocaine,
> to untie my tongue. It is quite all right of course for this news to
> be widely distributed in Hamburg and Vienna, even with
> exaggerations such as that he kissed me on the forehead (à la
> Liszt). As you see, I am not doing at all badly.*

In preparation for Charcot's formal soiree, Sigmund had his hair set
and his "rather wild beard" trimmed by a barber "in the French style."
To complete the picture, he donned evening dress, a custom with
which he was not yet comfortable despite having spent a huge sum for
a brand-new tailcoat. In fact, Sigmund had a devil of a time attempting
to tie the white bow tie he had just purchased. After several botched
tries, he was reduced to putting on a ready-tied black one he had
brought with him from Hamburg. Later, he learned that Charcot, too,
could not tie his own bow tie and had had to ask for his wife's help earlier that evening.

The starry-eyed Freud must have found his first visit to chez Charcot, on January 19, 1886, breathtaking. At one point in the evening, an
envious Freud snooped about Charcot's study. It was, he later told
Martha, a "room worthy of the magic palace he dwells in," divided into
two sections: "the larger one devoted to science, the other to comfort
[with] two slight projections from the wall [to] mark them off." Sigmund swooned at the sight of Charcot's elaborate bookcases stretching
from the floor to the house's second level, "each with steps to reach the
upper one," the stained-glass windows overlooking a leafy green garden, an "enormous long table covered with periodicals and odd books,"
Charcot's writing table, "quite flat and covered with manuscripts and
books," an ornate fireplace, "closets containing Indian and Chinese
antiques," and walls "covered with Gobelins and pictures."

All of Sigmund's insecurities screamed at him to self-fortify with cocaine. Whether out of sight in his hotel room, before walking up to the Charcots' front door, or during the party itself, Sigmund consumed more. As soon as the drug took effect, his pulse began to bound. He sweated profusely, a reflection of cocaine's elevating effect on internal body temperature. And because cocaine numbs whatever human tissue it touches (the very quality Sigmund had missed but had brought Carl Koller international acclaim), his mouth was dry and fuzzy and his speech was slurred. No amount of swishing his tongue against his teeth and lips or swigs of wine seemed to resolve this oral desiccation. All these signs conspired to reveal that he was under the influence and gave Sigmund good reason to worry about the impression was making. Yet despite having so much at stake, Freud convinced himself that cocaine enhanced his performance at these nerve-racking parties, even as the objective evidence suggested otherwise.

One night in early February, before he went for a return engagement at the Charcot home, he wrote a cocaine-influenced but remarkably self-analytic note to Martha:

> *The bit of cocaine I have just taken is making me talkative, my little woman. I will go on writing and comment on your criticism of my wretched self. . . . I believe people see something alien in me and the real reason is that in my youth I was never young and now that I am entering the age of maturity I cannot mature properly. There was a time when I was all ambition and eager to learn, when day after day I felt aggrieved that nature had not, in one of her benevolent moods, stamped on my face with that mark of genius which now and again she bestows on men. Now for a long time I have known I am not a genius and cannot understand how I ever could have wanted to be one. I am not even very gifted; my whole capacity for work probably springs from my character and from the absence of outstanding intellectual weaknesses. But I know that this combination is very conducive to slow success, and that given favorable conditions, I could achieve more than Nothnagel, to whom I consider myself superior, and might possibly reach the level of Charcot. By which I don't mean to say that I will get as far as that, for these favorable conditions no longer come my way, and I don't*

possess the genius, the power, to bring them about. Oh, how I run
on! . . . You know what Breuer told me one evening? I was so moved
by what he said that in return I disclosed to him the secret of our
engagement. He told me he had discovered that hidden under the
surface of timidity there lay in me an extremely daring and fearless
human being. I had always thought so, but never dared tell anyone.
I have always thought I inherited all the defiance and all the
passions with which our ancestors defended their Temple and could
gladly sacrifice my life for one great moment in history. And at the
same time I always felt so helpless and incapable of expressing these
ardent passions even by a word or a poem. So I have always
restrained myself, and it is this, I think, which people must see
in me.

Here I am making silly confessions to you, my sweet darling, and
really without any reason whatever unless it is the cocaine that
makes me talk so much.

As Sigmund tells Martha about the "defiance and all the passions
with which our ancestors defended their Temple," he suggests a heroic
image of the Jew breaking out of the mortification and repression that
was Vienna. Warmed by the glow of intellectual fraternity permeating
Dr. Charcot's salon, Freud began to embrace a mind-set in defiance of
the norm; it was a mentality that celebrated his outsider status in the
rigid medical profession and yet still clung to the righteous anger that
ignited his brilliance. Equally fascinating, Sigmund freely declares his
most repressed thoughts, ideas that he "always thought" but had "never
dared tell anyone."

In the short term, of course, cocaine inspires loquaciousness. In
many, the drug instantly releases a torrent of repressed thoughts, ideas,
or feelings that formerly enjoyed sanctuary. In one sense, Sigmund's
cocaine abuse represents a pharmacologically induced, perverse object
lesson about the power of uninhibited expression for gaining access to
deeper, unconscious levels of psychological meaning. As Freud was to
learn in the coming years, however, the drug-free techniques of talk
therapy and free association contain far fewer dangerous side effects
than those encountered with regular cocaine consumption.

There is also the notorious "crash" of moods that follows cocaine
ingestion, and Freud demonstrates this depressive experience in the

reprise of his letter to Martha that night. Upon returning from Charcot's party that evening, Sigmund wrote:

> *Thank God, it's over and I can tell you at once how right I was.*
> *It was so boring I nearly burst; only the bit of cocaine prevented me*
> *from doing so. Just think: this time forty to fifty people, of whom I*
> *knew three or four. No one was introduced to anyone, everyone was*
> *left to do what he liked. Needless to say, I had nothing to do: I don't*
> *think the others enjoyed themselves any better, but at least they could*
> *talk. My French was even worse than usual. No one paid attention*
> *to me, or could pay attention to me, which was quite all right and*
> *I was prepared for it.*

It is also telling that he does not reveal to Martha the precise amount of cocaine he was ingesting. In fact, throughout his notes during this period, Freud minimizes the amount and frequency of his cocaine dosage, using such terms as "a little cocaine" or a "bit of cocaine," a tactic many substance abusers employ to avoid the disapproval or intervention of others.

As HIS FELLOWSHIP IN PARIS drew near a close, Freud finally relaxed in the presence of his great teacher and explored a few cases on his own. He was still wily enough to watch the interactions of the other young, ambitious doctors who crowded Charcot's clinic and whose competitive maneuvering was an essential aspect of the academic medical merry-go-round.

On February 9, a Viennese gentleman whom Freud described as "a truly dreadful fellow" arrived at the Salpêtrière. The doctor was trained in both neuropathology and hydrotherapy, the latter being a once-popular sect of medicine that proposed cures through warm baths in water sources rich in natural salts. Armed with a flattering letter of introduction from his mentor Wilhelm Winternitz, the director of a prominent hydropathic clinic in Kaltenleutgeben, near Vienna, the newcomer told Sigmund that it was only a matter of time before he was embraced by Dr. Charcot and advanced to the head of the class. He made "all kinds of condescending remarks," Sigmund reported to Martha, "which I took in my stride, confident of imminent revenge."

Imagine Freud's glee when Charcot read the applicant's dossier and responded, like a café waiter, "*À votre service, Monsieur.*" Dr. Charcot quickly palmed the newcomer off onto Sigmund, adding sweetly, "Do you know Monsieur Freud?" Reflexively, both Austrian physicians clicked their boots together and lowered their heads in deference to the other, "he rather taken aback," Sigmund explained to Martha, "I silently pleased."

A few days later, another foreigner arrived at the hospital. Sigmund described him to Martha as "a definitely Germanic type and yet somehow different." As the students and doctors strolled over to the eye clinic, however, it became obvious that wherever he came from, the guest was no neophyte. There, the foreign physician conducted several examinations and offered his diagnoses with considerable authority and expertise. When he presented his card to the attending ophthalmologist, the latter responded with great deference and begged him to grace the clinic again the following morning. The visitor's name was Hermann Jakob Knapp; New York City's most prominent ophthalmologist, he was an early proponent of cocaine anesthesia in the United States and a colleague of William Halsted's.

The ambitious hydrotherapist, sensing a medical dignitary with whom he could network, sidled up to Dr. Knapp. "I heard you speaking German [and] I'd like to introduce myself," he interjected while handing Knapp one of his richly engraved calling cards. Knapp graciously replied, "I am a German, but I emigrated to America long ago." Freud, desperately wanting to be part of the conversation, fumbled through his coat to locate one of his own cards. Upon discovery of a particularly rumpled one, he was embarrassed to note that it stated only his name but neither his address nor his hospital affiliation. Knapp glanced at the card Sigmund timidly offered him and enthusiastically asked, "Could you be Dr. Freud from Vienna? I've known your name for a long time, from your publications, especially the one on cocaine."

The Viennese hydrotherapist condescendingly queried Freud, "Have you also written about cocaine?" Not waiting for Sigmund to answer, Knapp interjected, "Of course he has, it was he who started it all." Sigmund told Martha, "I greeted [Knapp] accordingly and my *bête noire* stood there looking rather sheepish, first of all because he had failed to recognize the man, and second because he had again managed to make a fool of himself."

Young physicians, eager to get a leg up on their careers, spend inordinate amounts of time actively seeking the attention of their superiors. After all, one never knows when a senior man can help out a junior one. It is not rare during these reindeer games that the more callow let their desire to win acknowledgment overcome their intellectual prowess. The result is, invariably, an exhibition of bluff as the youngster overstates his medical skills and knowledge. The only joy for those forced to silently endure this process of one-upmanship is the rare occasion when the charlatan is found out by the possessor of the very hindquarters about to be kissed. For Sigmund, this was one of those wonderful moments.

ON FEBRUARY 23, 1886, Freud left the Salpêtrière and Paris. He first spent a few weeks studying childhood neurological diseases under the great German Jewish pediatrician and later director of the Kaiser and Kaiserin Friedrich Kinderkrankenhaus, Adolf Baginsky. Soon after, he returned to Vienna to commence his private practice. At this point in his life, Freud would not be diagnosed as a cocaine addict according to modern medical definitions. Today, doctors imbue the terms "abuse" and "addiction" with separate meanings. "Substance abuse" implies use with adverse consequences, while "addiction" is defined by a loss of control and impairment of one's mental faculties with continued use. Freud, it appears, was able to maintain some semblance of control over the timing and dosage of his clandestine cocaine consumption as he continued his medical studies. Nevertheless, by this point he was chronically abusing the drug and exhibiting signs of dependency.

Sigmund never saw his inspirational teacher again, but he revered Charcot for the remainder of his life. On Freud's last morning in the Salpêtrière Hospital neurology clinic, Charcot fondly bade him adieu. During their time together, the French neurologist had guided Sigmund toward studying hysteria, a strange and vexing disorder that defied physical and psychological boundaries. The sage teacher was also careful to warn his pupil, "Theory is all very well, but that does not prevent facts from existing." Both this research interest and the advice were about to change the course of Freud's life.

CHAPTER 8

Rehabilitating Halsted

MODERN PSYCHIATRY WAS IN an embryonic state when Halsted admitted himself to Butler Hospital for the Insane. The hospital was founded in 1844 thanks to a large bequest from the Rhode Island industrialist Cyrus Butler and additional funds from the millionaire merchant, philanthropist, and benefactor of an eponymous university, Nicholas Brown Jr. In the decades that followed, the facility garnered an excellent reputation in treating the mentally troubled from America's finest families but also, with the help of subsidies from the state's treasury, many impoverished mentally ill Rhode Islanders.

Situated a distance away from the bustle and stresses of downtown Providence, Butler Hospital's buildings, rolling hills, ravines, trees, shrubs, and manicured gardens were designed to create a calming campus for psychic healing. Its therapeutic philosophy was centered on removing a mentally ill person from the social environment that appeared to cause his or her problems. Such enforced separation, the hospital staff believed, helped restore the troubled individual to sanity.

The care of the mentally ill during this period often veered toward the cruel and punitive. Moral judgments abounded. Many doctors practiced harsh and even painful clinical methods that had remained unchanged for centuries. More broadly, Americans considered the insane to be a potential menace to society and mandated their warehousing in walled-off enclaves.

Most asylums in the United States did not enjoy Butler's lavish financial resources, and some struggled to put food on the table and doctors and nurses in the corridors. Such institutions were funded by sporadic contributions from the local communities that built them and

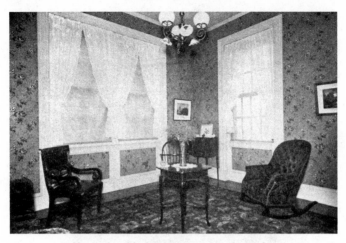

Butler Hospital bedroom, c. 1886, similar to the one
Halsted stayed in as a patient.

occasional appropriations from state and municipal governments not known for their largesse in caring for the mentally ill. Short-staffed, often filthy, and overcrowded, many asylums were regarded as "snake pits" well into the twentieth century.

Butler, to be sure, was very much an insane asylum of nineteenth-century sensibilities. But it was hardly Bedlam, the notorious London madhouse once considered so dangerous that the eighteenth-century physician William Buchan described it as "more likely to make a wise man mad than to restore a madman to his senses." By all accounts, the Butler Hospital's staff and trustees labored to understand the disruptive force insanity and addiction imposed on their patients, and they devoted their working lives and fortunes to ameliorating such conditions. Hence, it is not surprising that their superlative work came to the attention of William Welch, who kept abreast of everything that was going on in clinical medicine. Without question, Butler Hospital was one of the best of its kind in the United States during the 1880s.

WHEN HALSTED FIRST ARRIVED at Butler, he was unlikely to have taken much notice of the institution's sumptuous grounds and residence halls. His nerves were jangled and his mood depressed by

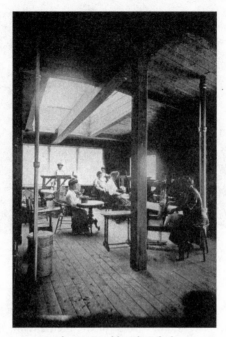

Butler Hospital handicraft class.

chronic cocaine abuse. He was also struggling with the realization that he had damaged his health and all but destroyed his career.

There were, of course, no effective medications for either mental illness or addiction in the 1880s. Even at the world's major medical centers, where cutting-edge medicine was being sharpened each day with new discoveries and treatments, many American physicians considered mental illness to be an unfathomable spiritual, social, and physical imbalance. According to the Hippocratic concepts of humoralism, each person, and the organs residing within him, had their own composition, or *krasis* (mixture or temperament). Medical doctrine held that while there was a limited range of variation for such individuality, similar patterns of disease or disequilibrium appeared in many people. Achieving equilibrium in one's thoughts, actions, demeanor, physical health, mental health, work, leisure, sleep cycle, emotions, environment, relationships, and diet was the quintessential therapeutic goal of physicians and patients alike.

In the 1880s, medical professionals specializing in mental illness typically referred to themselves as "alienists." This name has its roots in how insanity was understood in nineteenth-century American society. So "alienated" and separated from human society were insane individuals, so disjointed and unreal were their thoughts, feelings, and experiences, that only a trained specialist could restore their disordered world and bring them back safely to the realm of the sane and rational. One such practitioner was the creative and compassionate medical superintendent of Butler Hospital, Dr. John Woodbury Sawyer. Fortunately for Halsted, and unlike most asylum superintendents then working in the United States, Sawyer also had an abiding interest in facilitating the recovery of alcoholics and opium addicts.

It is difficult, if not impossible, to re-create the precise treatment plan for a psychiatric patient from a distance of more than a hundred years. To begin, such records are often kept confidential, for all the obvious reasons. (This protection has only grown stronger in recent years with the passage of federal patient privacy acts.) More problematic is the current practice by some hospitals of destroying decades-old patient records and charts. Medical centers are prone to enacting such plans because of the exorbitant fees for storing them. One shudders when contemplating the priceless loss this burgeoning practice exacts upon the historical record. That said, the *Annual Reports of the Trustees and Superintendents of the Butler Hospital for the Insane* do exist, and from these yellowed and brittle pages we are able to garner a sense of the institution Halsted entered and, eventually, left.

In 1886, when William was admitted to Butler, there were 186 patients, 82 men and 104 women, already residing there in altered states of mind. During the course of that year, another 83 patients were admitted (37 men and 46 women; one man and one woman required two stays during the same year). On a positive note, 103 patients were safely discharged that year to resume their daily lives. Thirty-six patients were thought to have been insane for less than three months; 23, for less than a year; 7, between one and two years; and 16, for more than two years. Thirty-one of the patients were married, 44 single, and 8 widowed; many were from New England, but 3 patients came from other states. Thirteen unfortunate souls never left the place and, instead, died from causes ranging from tuberculosis, heart disease, and stroke to exhaustion following acute mania and epilepsy. Three patients were not considered insane and were, instead, specifically admitted for addiction problems. One was William Halsted.

The hospital's annual report to the trustees for the fiscal year 1886–87 described in great detail the metrics and conditions of Butler's insane patients. Predictably, in an era when substance abuse problems remained shrouded in secrecy, the report includes only a mere sentence about depicting the treatment of that year's patients with addiction problems: "It has seemed to me best, also, in order that the statistics of insanity may be more accurate, to discharge those who have been treated for the opium and alcohol habits as 'not insane' rather than as 'recovered.' "

Nineteenth-century American alienists contended that severe mental illness was a "great leveler" among the rich, poor, educated, and illiterate, making them all suitable and congenial housemates. Yet in a culture rife with rigid social standings and distinctions, such egalitarian thoughts rarely worked out in practice. The Butler medical staff, for example, worked intensively to "quarantine" the "hopelessly demented" (read: impoverished ill) from the wealthier patients as a means of protecting the latter against the "depressing and unfavorable influence" of the former. And while the hospital certainly admitted the poor and insane of Rhode Island, the majority of its patients came from the upper classes.

The desire (and financial need) to attract paying patients was the major impetus behind the Butler doctors' intense lobbying for better and more luxurious facilities. In January 1888, for example, the medical superintendent unfurled an ambitious plan for improving the hospital's physical plant that required a budget totaling over $80,000 (approximately $1.8 million in 2010). A year later, Butler Hospital boasted one of the most modern and spacious facilities of its kind along the eastern seaboard:

> Those who study these plans carefully, will see that there are rooms in suit[e], connected with which are all the conveniences and comforts which can be found in a first-class private house or hotel; and that beside a better classification of patients, afforded by a larger number of wards, there is found, also, the means of

separation or isolation, so very important in the treatment of certain forms of mental disease; and the conveniences so needful to many patients accustomed to and able to pay for every comfort—persons whose mental balance is disturbed, without the loss of their tastes, or of desire for some of the companionships and even elegancies of life to which they have been accustomed.

COCAINE ABUSE WAS AN ENTIRELY NEW phenomenon when William entered Butler. And while it is always treacherous for a historian to label a particular event or individual as the first of its kind, it seems safe to assert that Halsted was, at least, a charter member of the earliest cohort of cocaine addicts to come to the attention of medical professionals in the United States.

As more and more people indulged in the chemically processed white powder hailing from South America, a growing number of doctors began reporting on the hazards of cocaine. Like many of today's "new" medicinal agents that have ultimately proved dangerous, cocaine followed a specific and predictable track: doctors, scientists, and pharmaceutical companies first develop a new drug, then extol and mass-market its virtues and wonders. As a result, patients begin to clamor for it. In the worst scenarios, reports of adverse side effects or complications proliferate, accompanied by heated assertions to the contrary from doctors and patients refusing to acknowledge such risks. Typically, these pharmacological morality plays end with the drug relegated to the medical equivalent of the proverbial doghouse.

Some of the earliest reports on cocaine's dangers emerged in direct response to Sigmund Freud's glowing advocacy of the drug as a treatment for morphine addiction. Over the summer of 1884, the editors of the *St. Louis Medical and Surgical Journal* commissioned a brief translation of Freud's cocaine monograph for their December issue. To protect himself from some of the charges he was hearing at medical meetings, Freud asked a still coherent Fleischl-Marxow to append a brief note describing his success with cocaine in treating his morphine addiction. Fleischl-Marxow's addendum neglected to mention how much cocaine and morphine he was consuming at the time and erroneously con-

The St. Louis Medical and Surgical
Journal *December 1884 issue in which
Freud argues that cocaine is not
addictive or dangerous.*

cluded that abusing the two drugs simultaneously was "antithetical."
The morphine- and-cocaine-addicted doctor went as far as to add that
because of cocaine "inebriate asylums can be dispensed with."

Among the most powerful salvos against cocaine was one from the
highly respected Viennese neurologist Heinrich Obersteiner, a friend
and colleague of both Sigmund's and Fleischl-Marxow's. On January 11, 1886, Obersteiner reported that "since the use of cocaine had
become frequent, several cases of cocaine intoxication had occurred;
their status is similar to the alcohol delirium and especially characterized by the hallucination of tiny animals crawling over the patient's
skin," the very symptom Fleischl-Marxow experienced. A few months
later, in May, Johann A. A. Erlenmeyer, a German physician, an expert
on morphinism, and a vociferous critic of Freud's work, published a
paper declaring cocaine to be a scourge upon mankind because it was so
dangerous, poisonous, and a definite cause of addiction. Sounding an
alarm specifically meant for Freud and his supporters, Erlenmeyer

wrote, "Today, I count myself fortunate for not having found it possible to recommend the use of cocaine in the morphine withdrawal cure."

That same year, in the United States, Dr. E. W. Holmes, once a strong proponent of using cocaine for treating hay fever, fatigue, and exhaustion, warned readers of the *Therapeutic Gazette* that the drug could be habit-forming and that the doctor self-prescribing cocaine was the equivalent of the lawyer representing himself in court: each had a fool for a patient or client.

In the months that followed, Freud continued to fight back in print, contesting claims that cocaine was addictive. But by July 1887, with Fleischl-Marxow's decline in full force, he employed an ever-shifting set of rationalizations in a paper on the craving for and fear of cocaine. Although Freud admitted that cocaine might not be the wisest course of therapy for those already addicted to morphine, he continued to assert that the drug was entirely safe for recreational users like himself. He also distinguished between injecting cocaine and ingesting it into the mouth or nose:

> All reports of addiction to cocaine and deterioration resulting from it refer to morphine addicts, persons who, already in the grip of one demon[,] are so weak in will power, so susceptible, that they would misuse, and indeed have misused, any stimulant held out to them. Cocaine had claimed no other, no victim of its own. I have had broad experience with the regular use of cocaine over long periods of time by persons who were not morphine addicts and have taken the drug myself for some months without perceiving or experiencing any condition similar to morphinism or any desire for continued use of cocaine. On the contrary, there occurred more frequently than I should have liked, an aversion to the drug, which was sufficient cause for curtailing its use. . . . I consider it advisable to abandon so far as possible subcutaneous injections of cocaine in the treatment of internal and nervous disorders.

Unfortunately for Fleischl-Marxow, Halsted, and their peers who became addicted to cocaine between 1884 and 1886, such academic debates did little to stem the rising tide of cocaine use. In fact, it took several more years before the medical profession in Europe and North

America gained a greater appreciation for cocaine's rapaciously addictive dangers.

What particularly startled those first doctors treating the earliest cocaine addicts were the rapid, degenerative changes in physical appearance and personality, especially when these patients were compared to those addicted to opium or morphine. The latter tended to simply nod off alone in their rooms when under the influence and often kept up their clandestine substance abuse for years before falling to pieces or being discovered by family members or coworkers; their color may have been pale and their bowel habits halting, but they nevertheless functioned. Active daily cocaine users, on the other hand, became haggard and haunted in a matter of weeks to months. Their mannerisms were jittery and nervous. They could barely sit still and often walked aimlessly. Incapable of participating in meaningful conversations, they spoke nonstop with little regard for their listeners, let alone control of word choice and sentence structure.

In 1888, Charles Bunting, a physician who treated many alcoholics and addicts, reported how within months one patient was transformed "into an emaciated, hollow-eyed, bilious-faced, flat-chested, helpless limp of humanity—a very caricature of manhood, with a look like a hunted beast, the shrunken frame trembling." Similarly, in 1891, a California physician named H. G. Brainerd described the speed with which such striking changes occurred: "Within a few months . . . the character of the cocaine habitué is changed, and he becomes unfitted for business."

An American physician named J. W. Springthorpe, who accidentally became a cocaine addict around the same time as Halsted, published a tortured memoir titled "The Confessions of a Cocainist" in 1897. Springthorpe poignantly recalled that "every part of the body seems to cry out for a new syringe . . . one syringe self-injected is absolutely sure to produce the fascinating desire for a second."

Only twelve months later, in 1898, C. C. Stockard of Atlanta portrayed the intense paranoia his cocaine-abusing patients exhibited after several days of use. For example, one of his morphinism patients ingested a rather large amount of cocaine to counteract the unadulterated agony of opium withdrawal. The resulting signs and symptoms Stockard describes perfectly capture the paranoiac hell of acute cocaine intoxication. The patient was convinced, he writes, that the people in the house were watching his actions and were talking about him and planning against him. The sparrows singing in the street were talking about him, the ticking clock was a telegraph machine of some sort, through which people were communicating about and plotting against him.

That same year, Dr. T. D. Crothers unequivocally stated that "cocaine is probably the most agreeable of all narcotics, therefore the most dangerous and alluring." Crothers also observed that the majority of the cocaine abusers he treated were professional men over the age of thirty who had already used alcohol and opium recreationally before turning to cocaine as a stimulant after a hard day's work. Not coincidentally, more than 60 percent of the cocaine abusers in Dr. Crothers's study were members of the medical profession.

MOST AMERICANS OF THIS ERA considered substance abuse to be a vice, an evil habit that could be conquered by seeking out a new environment, building up a sound physical constitution and one's willpower, and, depending on one's religious beliefs, praying for divine intervention. It was a moral or character defect and only those favored (and forgiven) by God had any chance at success. A subtext to this thinking was a tendency to blame alcoholics and addicts for creating their own problems.

With respect to cocaine, many physicians, including Freud, continued to argue that the drug was not addictive itself; rather, the person who took it to excess suffered from a personality or set of characteristics that put him or her at risk for abuse. This argument, often summarized by the label of the "addictive personality," continues to resonate in the twenty-first century, although many critics decry it as a means of stigmatization. Like many clichés, this one has some elements of truth; certain types of people are more likely than others to become addicts, such as those who enjoy taking risks or have emotional difficulty enduring painful stimuli and delaying gratification. But it is also important to note that, at present, more than half of all adults diagnosed with substance abuse problems simultaneously suffer from one or more mental health problems, such as depression, mood disorders, or attention deficit disorder. Furthermore, evidence is being uncovered each day demonstrating the genetic basis of addiction and of a host of other mental illnesses. One doubts that these epidemiological trends were that much different in the late nineteenth century, even if the diagnostic categories existed under different names and rubrics. All of these personality factors, genetic attributes, and mental health disabilities can play significant roles in an individual's decision to self-medicate his problems away with a drink, a joint, a syringe, or a line of mind-altering substance. Nevertheless, the notion of the addictive personality persists and thrives in the popular imagination.

FROM MAY TO NOVEMBER 1886, Halsted surrendered to his alienists' rigid prescriptions of seclusion, fresh air, exercise, healthy diet, and daily counseling sessions in order to achieve a gradual but determined withdrawal from cocaine. It would be anachronistic to call William's treatment "talk therapy" in the Freudian sense. But Dr. Sawyer's modus operandi for treating addicts and alcoholics was to gently converse with them, build up their self-confidence, suggest sober frames of reference for living the rest of their lives without the offending substance, and imbue them with an understanding of what would happen if they continued to abuse drugs. Dr. Sawyer wisely wasted no time berating Halsted for his failings or lack of self-control. Instead, he and his superb staff spent the next six months convincing William that the most productive part of his life and career was about to begin, provided he could get a handle on his illness.

Most mornings, William ambled through the bucolic grounds of the hospital and spent time weeding the hospital's fragrant flower garden and vegetable farm. He also attended weekly stereopticon lectures and, less frequently, Sunday church services. On many afternoons, he took the sun in the hospital's conservatory, went horseback riding, and made visits to the well-stocked library to peruse the latest edition of the *Graphic* and other popular magazines of the era. Because of his social station and financial resources, it is highly doubtful that Halsted spent much time interacting with the asylum's severely alienated inmates. In fact, William resided in a nicely decorated room in a building separated from the locked asylum wards by a lengthy corridor designed to muffle the sounds of the screaming patients at night.

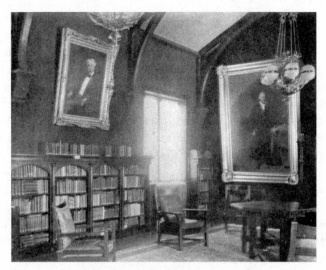

The Butler Hospital library, c. 1890.

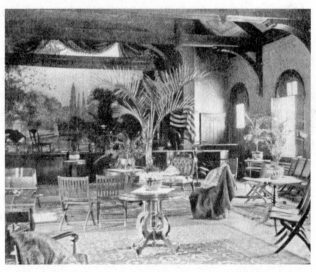

Butler Hospital musicale for patients in Isaac Ray Hall, c. 1887.

Extreme agitation and unrelenting insomnia constituted William's most troubling symptoms. So powerful were these unpleasant reactions that they were untouched by either soothing hot towels or sedative doses of chloral hydrate and bromides. William simply needed something stronger to counteract the emotionally draining symptoms of quitting cocaine. Disastrously for Halsted, the doctors at Butler succumbed to an urge that the profession has been victim to since well before the invention of the prescription pad. If one drug does not work, doctors are trained to substitute another, or simply combine a few new drugs. We have already seen how Sigmund applied such a therapeutic construct on his friend Fleischl-Marxow in Vienna.

The intense withdrawal symptoms from morphine and alcohol compelled doctors of this era not just to stand there but to do something. For example, the withdrawing alcoholic who experienced intense hallucinations, or delirium tremens, and seizures was often calmed with doses of morphine; morphine addicts enduring painful narcotic withdrawals were given a few shots of whiskey or, better still, several strong hot toddies. Not surprisingly, William's paranoia and agitation inspired his alienists to pull out a syringe filled with morphine and inject its soothing balm into his arm.

Halsted's doctors lacked a complete understanding of the dangers of their treatments. The psychiatrists at Butler Hospital were as kind, competent, and professional as any to be found in the world. But their reliance on the liberal use of morphine caused additional addictive problems for Halsted that lasted for the remainder of his life.

Halsted made excellent progress in eschewing cocaine during his six-month stay at Butler, no doubt thanks to the emotional support he was getting from his doctors, the lack of access to cocaine, and the calming effects of his daily morphine injections. But before he was able to venture out of Butler's safe haven to reclaim his surgical instruments, he endured two more traumatic events.

On August 31, 1886, Halsted's beloved roommate, Thomas McBride, was fatally struck down by an attack of Bright's disease (as kidney failure was then known). The forty-year-old McBride was sailing home on the North German Lloyd's steamship *Aller*, after a buoyant and activity-filled European jaunt, when he died; he was quickly buried at sea. Some have speculated that cocaine, and perhaps morphine, contributed to McBride's early demise; others have waxed poetic on what this talented young physician might have accomplished had he lived longer. Less debatable was the enormous impact McBride's death must have had on William when he was at his most psychologically vulnerable.

Another emotional blow struck near the end of 1886, when Dr. Sawyer became severely ill with what was likely a severe streptococcal throat infection. One apocryphal account of their final lucid visit describes Dr. Sawyer urging William not to be discouraged by his addiction. "I've seen enough of drugs," Dr. Sawyer reputedly said, "to know that it is not an easy thing to break off. Many more fail than succeed. In your case you are, at this moment, succeeding. Don't let anything stop you from trying. You are young—is it thirty-four? Our profession needs you. Think of it that way and don't let modesty interfere."

Whether his alienist told him this or not, it is clear that Halsted did summon the strength to tame his voracious beast of a disease. He actually got better, if not completely cured. Each day's abstinence fortified his desire to rejoin the world at large. Like an unemployed actor hungering for a theater filled with adoring fans, Halsted desperately wanted to return to the operating room and, thereby, change the course of medicine. Such a magnificent destiny, however, was only accomplishable if he could stay healthy enough to seize it. By late November 1886, the medical staff at Butler agreed that he was well enough to leave the asylum, provided he submit to living under the watchful eye of his friend and benefactor William Henry Welch.

TRUE TO HIS PROMISE, Welch took Halsted two hundred miles south of New York City and his cocaine-abusing cronies, to the homier Baltimore. There, Welch was charged by a group of energetic trustees and a magnificent endowment of $7 million (or more than $132 million in 2010 dollars) to design and populate what became the most important center of healing, education, and research of its day, one that would eventually rival, if not completely dominate Vienna, Berlin, Leipzig, Paris, London, and all of North America.

It was to be named the Johns Hopkins Hospital and Medical School, after the wealthy but dyspeptic bachelor and Quaker merchant

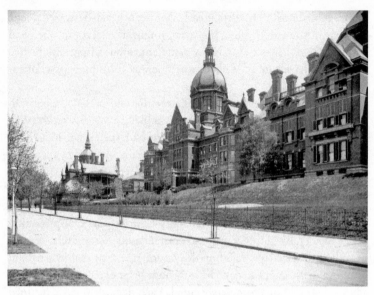

The Johns Hopkins Hospital, early 1900s.

who forked over the funds for the enterprise. When Mr. Hopkins died, in 1873, his last will and testament explicitly called for the creation of a first-rate medical school and hospital as an integral part of a fully endowed research university. By 1887, the university had been up and running for twelve years, but the hospital and medical school were still being pondered and planned. Given Welch's appreciation for all things *deutsche,* it is not surprising that he organized the medical school along the German model of research institutes and laboratories. The school was to be physically and intellectually connected to a magnificent hospital that not only served Baltimore's destitute, as directed by Mr. Hopkins's will, but also attracted ailing people from around the world as its doctors developed new ways to treat, cure, and prevent disease.

The medical campus's collection of buildings constructed of ferrous-red brick and West Virginia sandstone was designed by John Shaw Billings. A physician and surgeon, Billings served as officer in charge of the surgeon general's library from 1865 to 1895 and initiated two major indexes of the world's burgeoning medical literature, *Index Medicus* (1879) and the *Index Catalogue of the Surgeon General's Office*

(1880). In 1896, after a distinguished career with the United States federal government, he was named the first director of the stately New York Public Library on Fifth Avenue and Forty-second Street.

For Johns Hopkins, Dr. Billings created a space of healing and discovery that was efficient and inspiring, practical and grand, topped by a magnificent slate-clad, copper-ribbed dome that could be seen from virtually every point of Baltimore and, on a clear day, from the head of Chesapeake Bay. Underneath its spire were well-appointed rooms for private patients, comfortable quarters for the resident medical staff, pristine operating rooms, spacious teaching amphitheaters, laboratories, workshops, and endless wards separated into pavilions in order to keep the spread of infection among the patients to a minimum.

Although Welch possessed the loudest voice in selecting those who would participate in his greatest medical experiment, he still required the final approval of the university's board of trustees. The mutton-chopped, frock-coated men who sat on this board were a powerful group of Baltimore businessmen who understood the need to create something entirely different and modern but were also bound, by custom and legal precedent, to protect the massive investment their late colleague had entrusted to their care.

When Halsted arrived in Baltimore in December 1886, the medical campus was still a morass of muddy streets, wooden and iron scaffolding, and piles of bricks. The hospital would not formally open its doors until the spring of 1889, and the medical school did not embark on its teaching mission until 1893. Suitably impressed by Halsted's facility with the scalpel and his potential to reinvent the science of surgery, Welch hoped to appoint his protégé as the first professor of surgery at Johns Hopkins. But Welch was nothing if not politically savvy; he understood that in academia, as in so many other professional pursuits, timing was everything. Ever the benevolent puller of strings and manipulator of lives, Welch initiated William's clinical reentry with the rather tenuous designation of "special graduate student" in his pathological laboratory. There, the surgeon could accrue additional time recuperating from what was euphemistically referred to as "health problems."

Welch was interested in supporting Halsted for many reasons. Foremost, Professor Welch loved helping young men. A lifelong bachelor who resided in a series of boardinghouses, Welch spent most evenings in the company of other successful men at the stuffy and tobacco-stained dining clubs then so popular in New York and Baltimore. In these richly paneled rooms as well as the amphitheaters and classrooms of Johns Hopkins, Welch's eye was always caught, and sometimes bedazzled, by the promise of ambitious, younger physicians eager to climb the greasy pole of academic medicine.

In recent years, many medical historians have speculated about Dr. Welch's sexuality. His students, far less sophisticated, coined a few lines of doggerel verse hinting at the mysterious proclivities of the teacher they warmly nicknamed "Popsy" Welch:

> Nobody knows where Popsy eats,
> Nobody know where Popsy sleeps,
> Nobody knows whom Popsy keeps,
> But Popsy.

From the distance of nearly a century, Welch remains an enigma of personality and appeal. Many of his rank-and-file medical students derided him as an aloof and indifferent lecturer. His family wondered about his solitary summer vacations to ocean resorts where he pursued

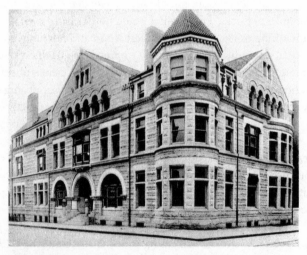

The Maryland Club, where Halsted and Welch dined nightly, c. 1890s.

sweets of all kinds, long naps on the beach, and wild rides at amusement parks. And not a few colleagues commented on how he spent the overwhelming majority of his time in the company of his young laboratory men, who remained loyal to their chief until their dying days. The historical documentation necessary to answer the questions posed by the "Popsy poem," however, has been definitively removed from the table. Welch's highly developed sense of privacy extended to what he saved for the archives and posterity.

Regardless of inspiring impulses, Welch had an unerring eye. For the next four decades, the crème de la crème of American medical and public health schools, foundations, and research institutes all came from the successive litters of students he lovingly referred to as "Welch's Rabbits." Of all these professorial and, perhaps, closer relationships, Welch immediately grasped that William Halsted was one of his greatest discoveries.

Welch assumed the role of William's protector and arranged for the surgeon to reside in his suite of two furnished rooms on the third floor of a boardinghouse at 20 Cathedral Street that he rented for $35 a month. There, about a mile away from the hospital, Mrs. Thomas Simmons, a Civil War widow and landlady in rather reduced circumstances, and her unmarried daughter doted on the two gentlemen bachelors. Having little choice in the matter and worried by the constant threat of returning to his wildly addictive ways, Halsted readily agreed to his prescribed living arrangements. One of Welch's many custodial tasks was to closely monitor the surgeon's cash flow to make sure he did not have enough money to purchase cocaine. On most evenings as they dined together at the venerable Maryland Club, before they retired for the night, and again in the morning, as they readied for another day of work, Welch patiently coached Halsted on how to earn the trustees' respect and endeavored to boost his shaky confidence.

BALTIMORE WAS SMALL IN SCALE and acreage and southern in temperature and temperament. Welch and Halsted lived in the "better" part of town, which included several prominent neighborhoods along Charles, St. Paul, and Cathedral streets, extending to and beyond Millionaire's Row, on Mount Vernon Place. Elegant brownstones, limestone mansions, and red-brick row houses with marble stoops fronted tree-lined, cobblestoned pavements. If you were wealthy and white, Baltimore was a most amiable town, communal by nature, busy with social events, and, as the pathologist W. G. MacCallum described it, "a delightful, friendly place to live and one was happy."

Traveling closer to the hilly neighborhood where the Johns Hopkins Hospital was situated, however, one encountered shabbier homes, unsavory tenements, a teeming mass of immigrants from Italy and Eastern Europe, African Americans, Irish Americans, and other charter members of the American urban poor. The streets reeked of manure and human refuse. Baltimore did not offer the "modern conveniences" of indoor plumbing and adequate sewage systems for all its residents until well into the twentieth century, a status that went a long way toward explaining why the "Charm City" once had the highest rate of typhoid fever in the United States.

Early each morning, a horse-driven carriage took Halsted from his leafy neighborhood to a squat, red-brick building situated behind the developing skeleton that would ultimately become the hospital. In sub-

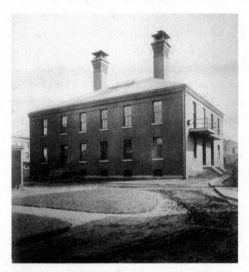

The Old Pathological Building at Johns Hopkins,
c. 1886; Halsted's laboratory was on the
second floor.

sequent years, this structure came to be called the "Old Pathological Laboratory," and it was where Halsted toiled at some of his most important experiments. As he made his way to East Baltimore, his nervously twitching eyes elicited far less attention from the pedestrians he passed than did his formal dress. He adorned his muscular frame with bespoke suits made from the finest woolens on London's Savile Row, hand-sewn linen shirts and silk neckties from Charvet, impeccably crafted leather shoes from Paris's best cobblers, and, as MacCallum described it, "a glistening high silk hat when no one else wore one . . . not done in any air but only because it was his habit."

Upon arrival to the Old Pathological, William bounded up the stairs and thrust open the door to his poorly ventilated laboratory. After hanging his hat and coat on the pegs behind his door, he focused on his scientific tasks with intensity and purpose. These long days satisfied both his obsession for surgical perfection and the design of his recovery program. Hardly a debtor or a criminal like the original "addicts" of ancient Rome, William, nevertheless, was acutely aware of his bondage to cocaine.

Abstinence is a monumental challenge for any addict, even for one as motivated and disciplined as Halsted. Heroin addicts have an odd slang term called "jonesing," which refers to the strong cravings one experiences even after quitting the drug. The addicted brain, after all, has an excellent memory for the substances it has learned to love. With time, treatment, and patience, the urges tend to subside or, at least, the successfully recovering addict is taught how to tame them and take the necessary steps not to act upon them. Such seductive and destructive thoughts, which can crop up at any time in a recovering addict's life, are among the many reasons so many well-intentioned addicts relapse. To allay his potent waves of addictive desire, Halsted remained fixed to his workbench, and it was not uncommon to see the gaslights burning in his laboratory well into the next day's early morning hours. Resolved to repay Welch for his support and reclaim his position in the medical profession, William confined himself to perfecting surgery.

Halsted found himself among the extremely good company of young, obsessive, eager scientists determined to make their own healing discoveries. His laboratory, which he shared with the brilliant anatomist Franklin P. Mall, was in the southeast corner of the building, directly across the hall from Dr. Welch's southwest corner office. Elsewhere on the second floor were William T. Councilman, Welch's associate pathologist, who in 1892 was appointed the Shattuck professor of pathological anatomy at Harvard Medical School; George Sternberg, who wrote the first major American textbook of bacteriology and eventually rose to become the surgeon general of the U.S. Army; Maude Abbott, a pathologist who pioneered the field of congenital heart defects; Christian A. Herter, a pathologist, biochemist, neurologist, and pharmacologist who in 1905 would cofound the prestigious *Journal of Biological Chemistry;* Walter Reed, who became internationally famous in 1900 for his elucidation of the role mosquitoes play in spreading yellow fever; and many other budding leaders in the fields of bacteriology and pathology.

Unlike during his hurried clinical days and nights in New York, Halsted now had the dedicated time, as professors like to say, to think the great thoughts. Restricting himself to dogs, which he treated with all the attention and care he'd once offered to his human patients, Halsted explored their intestines. Working with Franklin Mall, he operated on these canines employing a number of different suture, or stitching, techniques. This was no mere exercise in idle sewing. To operate successfully

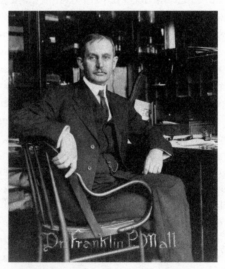

*Franklin P. Mall, professor of anatomy and
colleague of Halsted's at Johns Hopkins, 1893.*

on a patient's guts, the surgeon had to know which layer of the intestines would hold the stitch the best and not come apart once he completed the procedure and closed the incision. Anything less might invite a bout of peritonitis, the spilling of fecal material and the bacteria it carries into the abdomen; this disastrous surgical complication often resulted in the painful death of the unfortunate patient incorrectly put back together. These detailed and exacting studies demonstrated Halsted's creativity, acute observational skills, and intense patience as he searched for new ways to extend the surgeon's reach. Eventually, he concluded that the critical place to rejoin severed ends of the intestines was the submucosal layer, a monumental discovery that allowed surgeons to safely invade the gastrointestinal tract and emerge victorious.

THERE EXISTS A CAPTIVATING ACCOUNT about a winter afternoon in 1889 when Dr. Welch invited the sweaty, bloodstained surgeon into his office. At the meeting, perhaps over a cup of tea, Welch repeated how he was engineering the appointments of the professors both of medicine and of gynecology at the soon-to-be-opened medical school. But, he confided to Halsted, neither he nor the trustees had yet designated a professor of surgery for Johns Hopkins. That person, Welch said as he leaned over his desk, was to be William Stewart Halsted. Once the toast of New York's elite medical circles and now merely a dog surgeon, William protested that such a prestigious appointment could never be his. Without knowing the specific details of his illness, many had heard about Halsted's abandonment of a patient on the examining table four years earlier. William's crime, in the eyes of many, was the unforgivable moral equivalent of a sea captain abandoning his sinking ship.

The always confident Welch dismissed Halsted's objections with a principle that remains a cornerstone of drug rehabilitation: a recovering addict needs to learn to trust himself and his ability to resolutely say no when cravings hit him. That hardly meant Halsted had to go it alone, Welch added in his plummy voice. William could always come to him for guidance and, if need be, figurative hand-holding. Confidence, good faith, and hard work, Welch insisted, would help William conquer his addiction and deliver his healing gifts to all humankind.

At the end of this discussion came one of many details that strain credibility: Welch handed Halsted a small vial containing cocaine—a measure physicians today would hardly contemplate, let alone act upon. Welch instructed William to carry the vial at all times but never to break into it; to delay the opening of the vessel for another day; to, in essence, gain experience in saying no to his addiction. Once he achieved mastery over his cocaine cravings, Welch predicted, William's confidence—a critical personality trait for anyone who earns his living cutting people open while the motor is still running—would return. And it was then, the pathologist gently said as he placed his ample hand on one of the surgeon's shaking shoulders, that the hospital trustees would appoint him surgeon-in-chief over the most important surgical empire ever created on American shores.

Even if we discount many of the details and assertions of such a tale, it is certain that there were many painful conversations between Welch and William about the destructive force of cocaine. The precise details of those conversations are, sadly, lost, making it impossible to measure their effect and consequences. Predictably, William's cocaine addiction proved to be the stronger combatant. In keeping with the remitting, relapsing, and chronic nature of his illness, Halsted would never maintain total abstinence, even under the watchful eye of his mentor. In April 1887, for example, William confessed to Welch that his problem had returned with a vengeance. It is unknown how William acquired a supply of cocaine—but this was not a terribly difficult task for a physician with such easy access to the drug in his surgical laboratory or at any local pharmacy. Regardless, Halsted did relapse around this time and was quickly hustled back to Butler Hospital, in Rhode Island, for more intensive therapy. There he remained, along with 3 other addicts and 171 mentally ill patients, for nine months of therapeutic seclusion and morphine. He was discharged on December 31, 1887.

When he returned to Baltimore in January 1888, he appeared much stronger and was eager to return to his laboratory. Halsted immersed himself in a series of important experiments on wound healing, antisepsis, and the surgical treatment of thyroid gland disease, breast cancer, and several other serious maladies. By most accounts, he was abstaining from cocaine. Yet all who knew him well fretted over how much he had changed from his boisterous and bold days as an operator in New York. With his now cloistered life as a surgical scholar, he seemed older, more guarded, remote, and cautious in his demeanor and actions, less friendly with others, even downright caustic and rude. The once-sociable Halsted now took great pains to avoid close relationships with anyone save Welch, a difficult feat when working in the company of dozens of lonely, twenty-five- to thirty-five-year-old men whose lives were bounded by the walls of the hospital and laboratory.

Already the recipient of several second chances, Dr. Halsted could not afford another encounter with cocaine. Every morning he awoke to the realization that relapse meant shameful discovery, readmission to Butler Hospital, and a career that even the redoubtable William Henry Welch could not resurrect. The intense pressure to succeed must have come at a huge emotional price for William Halsted. On many days, and not a few evenings, fighting to establish his hard-won sobriety, the increasingly isolated surgeon walked around the grounds and corridors of Johns Hopkins as if he was a condemned man. His body smarted from the long hours of leaning over the anesthetized dogs on his operating table. His posture sagged as if he were Atlas carrying the weight of the world on his shoulders. And always on his mind was the fear of cocaine's absolute power to ruin everything—his health, his reputation, his career, and, as it turned out, the future of modern surgery itself.

CHAPTER 9

The Interpretation of Dreams

O N APRIL 25, 1886—Easter Sunday—the Vienna *Neue Freie Presse* ran a small news announcement that likely received little attention. In an agate font, the squib heralded, "Herr Dr. Sigmund Freud, Docent for Nervous Diseases at the University, has returned from his study trip to Paris and Berlin and has consulting hours at [District] I, Rathhausstrasse No. 7, from 1 to 2:30." Freud announced to his corner of the world that he was no longer a mere physician-in-training; he had officially cast his hat into the ring of the Viennese medical profession.

Such a declaration demanded that he raise a steady stream of clinical revenue, a task that he initially found to be quite difficult. The shabby appearance of his frayed frock coat revealed that he was subsisting on the fringe, scrimping so much to make ends meet that often he could not afford cab fare for his obligatory house calls. Still, that September, Sigmund threw all caution to the wind and finally married Martha Bernays; a few months after the nuptials, the Freuds were expecting their first child, whom they would name Mathilde, after Josef Breuer's wife.

Toward the end of his life, Sigmund wrote, "In the time span of 1886 to 1891, I did little scientific work and published almost nothing. I was occupied in finding my way in my new profession and in securing material subsistence for myself and my rapidly growing family." He was being either modest or forgetful. Among his publications during this era were some illuminating investigations on aphasia (an inability to speak because of damage to the language centers of the brain) and infantile cerebral palsy, the latter based on his thrice-weekly pediatric neurology clinics at the Erstes Öffentliches Kinder-Krankeninstitut, (the Vienna First Public Institute for Sick Children).

More important, this period marks when Freud shifted from the anatomic-, structural-, and lesion-focused research of his medical training to the introspective, analytic inquiries that would make his name. And because of the trailblazing but introspective questions he chose to ask, he became, by necessity, his primary analytical subject. Indeed, these were the years when Freud began pondering what would become his signature ideas on neuroses, sexual conflicts, and the "talking cure," with the express goal of mitigating the psychological foibles that drive many of us slightly mad.

IN FREUD'S LETTERS OF THIS PERIOD, the major chord struck is of the great effort required to establish his private practice. On too many mornings, he awoke to too many open slots in his appointment book and too much red ink in his bank ledger. Such precarious finances forced Sigmund to obsequiously court established physicians who might send well-to-do, mentally disturbed patients his way. At the same time, however, the ambitious Dr. Freud remained on the lookout for a stunning medical discovery.

Specializing in the nascent arena of debilitating neuroses, Freud employed newfangled and, in Viennese medical circles, poorly regarded "French techniques" such as hypnosis and electrotherapy. Several Krankenhaus physicians heatedly criticized these unorthodox methods as quackery, eventually forcing him to abandon them for fear of gaining a reputation as shatter-pated.

Day after day, Freud pandered for new patients while Martha worried about paying the stack of bills sent by their grocer, their butcher, and the tradesmen who serviced their brand-new, fashionable flat off the Ring at Maria Theresienstrasse 8. The flat leased for 1,600 gulden a month, but this actually represented a bargain in that the apartment building had been erected on the former site of the famous Ring Theater, which had burned to the ground on December 8, 1881, killing hundreds of people, and was considered by many superstitious Viennese to be an unlucky location.

The young physician kept strict accounts of all monies received

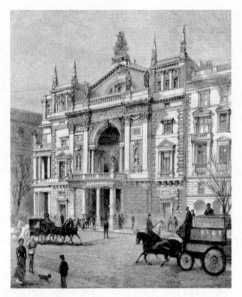

The Ring Theater, which burned to the ground in
1881; built on its site a few years later was the
apartment house where the Freuds first lived.

from his thin list of patients. Each evening, he turned over to Martha
every check and cash payment for safekeeping in a strongbox. The following morning, depending on their requirements, Freud withdrew a
precise amount of money, including about 10 cents for his daily allotment of cigars. As the new day progressed, he labored to replenish the
strongbox before nightfall. There were many days when he was not successful at this task, a reality that forced Sigmund and Martha to all but
ignore the gaiety of Vienna's legendary cultural life and to postpone the
purchase of furniture, let alone an elegant gold snake bracelet for her, a
common gift university-affiliated physicians gave their wives to distinguish them from the spouses of less-accomplished doctors. After the
arrival of their daughter Mathilde, the Freuds stretched Sigmund's
dribbling income even further. As the cultural historian Frederic Morton bluntly put it, "every kreutzer counted."

   Despite his pecuniary travails, Freud still managed to scrape together
the gulden to purchase cocaine. One way of raising cash involved his
pen: translating Charcot's French medical texts into German and—

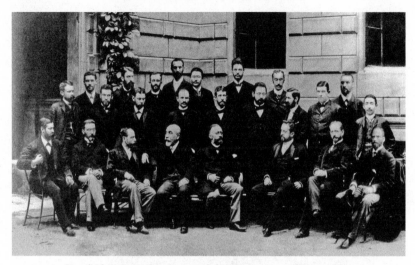

Freud (first row, left corner) and the Vienna First Public Institute for Sick Children staff, c. 1893.

perhaps the lowest rung of academic hell—writing unsigned articles for a medical dictionary. He performed this work late at night, when he would have been better served by a decent night's sleep. Aside from the money and what it might have been used to purchase, there was one virtue to his contract medical writing: the time spent thinking about and explaining complex concepts in neurology and psychology was an important early step in his becoming a masterful writer.

Freud's demeanor oscillated up and down, depending on the day and his social encounters. Lonely and alienated from many of his medical colleagues, he began to take out his frustrations on his wife in a most upsetting and irritable manner. In face-to-face conversations and in the occasional sheepish letter, a guilty Sigmund apologized to Martha for being "violent and passionate, with all sorts of devils . . . [that] rumble about me inside or else are released against you, you dear one." Sigmund's professional insecurity and his long but not always productive work hours, combined with the psychic costs of cocaine abuse, encouraged a melancholic state of mind. He frequently described his mood during these years as "dead tired" and complained to friends that he felt as if he were being devoured by a cancer.

Sigmund also appears to have engaged in reckless behavior, sexual

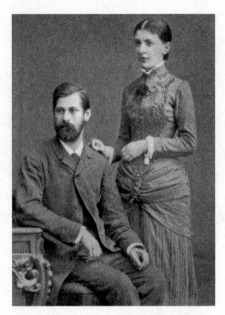

*Freud, age twenty-nine, and Martha
Bernays, age twenty-four, at Wandsbeck, near
Hamburg, in 1885, during their protracted,
four-year engagement. Freud wrote her on
January 6, 1886, "Such perseverance as we
have shown should melt a heart of stone, and
you will see that when we marry the whole
family will wish us luck."*

indiscretion, and a deceptively double life during these years. Long
debated by Freudians is the question of whether he had a clandestine
physical relationship with his sister-in-law Minna Bernays. At almost
the same moment he was courting and falling in love with Martha, in
April 1882, he was smitten with her younger, bright, and sarcastic sister.
For many years, Sigmund wrote Minna warm, loving letters, and they
appear to have enjoyed a rich and deep platonic relationship; indeed,
Sigmund freely discussed his intellectual life with Minna on a level he
never did with Martha. In 1896, a year after Sigmund and Martha
elected to become sexually abstinent after the birth of their sixth child,
Minna came to live with them in Vienna and stayed for the next forty-
two years.

According to Carl Jung, who visited the Freud family in early March 1907, Minna asked to speak with him. "She was very much bothered by her relationship with Freud and felt guilty about it," Jung recalled decades later, in 1969. "From her I learned that Freud was in love with her and that their relationship was indeed very intimate." During their 1909 trip to Clark University in Worchester, Massachusetts, Freud told Jung of "some dreams that bothered him very much. The dreams were about the triangle—Freud, his wife, and wife's younger sister." When Jung pressed him for some more personal details, Freud—who was unaware of the conversation Jung

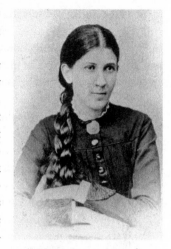

Minna Bernays, Freud's sister-in-law, at about the age of twenty-five, c. 1890.

had had earlier with Minna—abruptly stopped. "He looked at me with bitterness and said, 'I could tell you more but I cannot risk my authority!'" Many historians initially dismissed this account because of the subsequent ugly turn of Jung and Freud's relationship.

In 2006, however, a German sociologist uncovered a leatherbound register from the Schweizerhaus, an inn in Maloja, Switzerland. It documents Minna and Sigmund's three-day stay there in mid- to late August 1898. With the practiced duplicity of an accomplished substance abuser, Sigmund registered for room 11 in his spiky handwriting: *"Dr. Sigm Freud u frau."* Although Freud kept this affair of the heart, like his cocaine abuse, a guarded secret, the newly discovered hotel register has convinced many doubters that there was, in fact, a physical relationship. No matter what transpired during those summer nights in that double room in the Swiss Alps, or elsewhere, it would have invited certain scandal if discovered at the time.

INTELLECTUALLY, FREUD REMAINED EXCITED by what he learned from Jean-Martin Charcot, even if the master was not nearly as revered in Vienna as in Paris. Sigmund was particularly captivated by the Frenchman's observation that "anatomy has finished its work and the theory of organic disease might be called complete; now the time of the neuroses had come." None of the listings in the long catalog of psychological quirks met this requirement better than hysteria, an entity that baffled mental health experts and laypersons alike.

The diagnosis of hysteria has long since been deleted from the American Psychiatric Association's authoritative *Diagnostic and Statistical Manual of Mental Disorders.* Today the term is typically used in the vernacular to cast aspersions on a person's over-the-top responses to daily vicissitudes. Yet such pith diminishes the clinical importance the word once held, especially during the nineteenth century. The term's derivation from the Greek root for "uterus" indicates that many doctors of centuries past erroneously considered aberrant behaviors exhibited by women to have originated within their sexual organs. The removal of a uterus is still referred to as a hysterectomy. Before the advent of modern gynecology, this surgical procedure was considered a definitive means of curing a woman of her hysteria. Regardless of its exact cause, hysteria was strange, dramatic, and disturbing. As *The Oxford Companion to Medicine* succinctly notes, its victims suffered from intense "sensory and motor dysfunction, such as a loss of sensation over parts of the body, temporary blindness, paralysis of the limbs, loss or impairment of speech or hearing, convulsions, lack of concern over one's body and health, and often worse."

Although Freud had seen his share of hysterics in Vienna, his interest in them certainly intensified while he was studying with Charcot. Few prominent Viennese neurologists or internists considered the "female problem" of hysteria to be worthy of their time, let alone clinical consideration. But in Paris, Dr. Charcot initiated a revolutionary turn by proposing that hysteria affected both women and men and was caused by either a heretofore unidentified, underlying, inheritable organic lesion or a chemical imbalance that required a triggering traumatic or emotional event to come to the surface.

Every Tuesday, Professor Charcot demonstrated a long parade of hysterical women, and occasionally some men, in varying states of undress and sexually charged, semiparalyzed poses. These poor souls writhed and moaned, simultaneously titillating and revolting a crowded auditorium of curious students. The French neurologist also

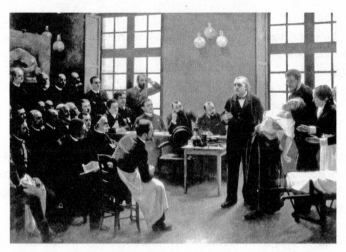

A Clinical Lesson with Doctor Charcot at the Salpêtrière Hospital, 1887. *Painting by Pierre André Brouillet. The patient being demonstrated to the audience is suffering from hysteria. Freud hung a copy of this painting in his consulting room.*

wrote dozens of dispatches on the subject in his famous journal, *Charcot's Archives,* which was avidly followed by doctors around the world. Millions more throughout Europe and North America read about and saw carefully staged photographs of Charcot's hysterical patients in the popular press. With all this attention, it is hardly surprising that Freud and many other physicians of his generation clamored to find and treat such intriguing patients. And lo and behold, as is seen with most newly proposed, collected, and celebrated medical diagnoses, these doctors promptly discovered their own cases. Almost overnight, hysteria became a respectable disease. Throughout Europe, wealthy, well-born, depressed, nervous wrecks of men and women, disassociated from their surroundings and contorted into strange body positions and facial expressions, crowded neurology and psychiatric clinics, begging for help.

In time Charcot grew frustrated with diagnosing hysteria, because he could not identify a precise physical abnormality underlying it. As Freud reminisced in his 1925 autobiography, "It was easy to see that in reality he took no special interest in penetrating more deeply into the psychology of the neuroses. When all is said and done, it was from pathological anatomy that his work had started." Still, it is important to recall that one morning in late 1885 or early 1886, the Frenchman suggested to Freud that the cases of hysteria they were examining together had not a little to do with sex: *"C'est toujours la chose génitale, toujours . . . toujours . . . toujours."*

IN THE INTERCONNECTED WORLD of Viennese medicine, Freud grew close to Josef Breuer, a superbly trained Jewish internist and physiologist who was fourteen years older than Freud and once treated their mutual friend Fleischl-Marxow. Sigmund admired Breuer for his exquisite bedside manner, his ability to ferret out the most obscure of diagnoses, and his successful private practice, which numbered many of the Vienna Medical School's most prominent physicians as patients. Breuer saw Sigmund as a precociously bright younger brother and medical protégé. He and his wife virtually adopted Freud, frequently inviting him to their home for meals and loaning him considerable amounts of money as he struggled to make ends meet. Sometime between 1880 and 1882, Breuer began telling Freud about his hysteria patients, a practice that continued after Freud's return to Vienna from

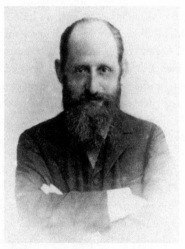

Josef Breuer, c. 1880s.

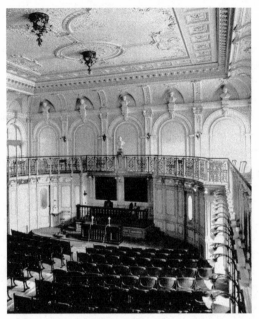

The auditorium of the Vienna Medical Society,
where Sigmund gave his first formal lecture on
hysteria in 1886.

Paris in 1886. Sigmund reciprocated by sharing with Breuer recollections of what he'd seen at the Salpêtrière.

On October 15, 1886, Sigmund delivered his first formal address to the prestigious Vienna Medical Society. He tentatively approached the ornately carved lectern overlooking a white marble, neo-Renaissance auditorium filled with physicians ensconced in narrow seats covered in red velvet. In what many members of the audience interpreted as a pedantic and not terribly data-driven lecture, Freud described a male hysteric he had observed in Charcot's clinic. To Sigmund's dismay, several of the distinguished physicians present, including his beloved psychiatry professor Theodor Meynert, ridiculed the presentation for its faulty scientific reasoning and Freud's failure to locate a precise anatomical lesion explaining the patient's symptoms. How could men become hysterical, one surgeon quarreled, without possessing a uterus? Five weeks later, on November 24, Freud boldly returned to the Vienna

Medical Society to report a case of hysteria in one of his own male patients to an equally dismissive audience.

Freud was disappointed but undeterred. He argued to whoever would listen that hysteria represented the key to solving the great paradigms of the mind-body connection. "Hysterics suffer for the most part from reminiscences," Freud would famously insist. Such individuals transformed their stressful memories and neurotic responses into physical symptoms, many of which were quite debilitating and would mysteriously wax and wane.

One of the most fascinating cases Dr. Breuer shared with Sigmund was that of a young woman named Bertha Pappenheim. She has since become world-famous as "Anna O.," the first patient to undergo what became psychoanalysis. As Breuer told it, thanks to his verbal ministrations Bertha found a temporary reprieve from the many strange symptoms that were dominating her life: a persistent cough, a fear of drinking water, paralysis of the limbs, strange seizures, headaches, an inability to eat, visual and speaking disturbances, and episodes of mania.

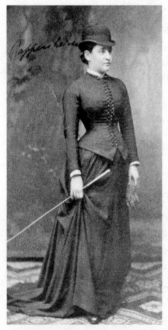

Bertha Pappenheim, a.k.a. Anna O., in 1882, at the age of twenty-two.

Beginning in the summer of 1880, Breuer used hypnosis to explore the connection between Bertha's physical symptoms and the emotional trauma of her beloved father's fatal illness. He spent hours upon hours listening to Bertha in her many altered mental states as she detailed her problems and thoughts. Initially there was some respite. But by the summer of 1882 Bertha's debilitating symptoms were so overwhelming that Breuer resorted to prescribing substantial amounts of the sedatives chloral hydrate and morphine to the point of her becoming an addict.

Eventually, Breuer had little choice but to forcibly commit Bertha to an asylum, where she was weaned off the habit-forming drugs and treated with such modalities as leeches, electrotherapy, and arsenic. The experience so emotionally exhausted Breuer that he began referring similar patients to Sigmund. Nevertheless, Breuer later left the impression in print that he had cured Bertha, despite her frequent stays at asylums long after he stopped seeing her clinically. In subsequent years, Freud and Breuer went as far as to suggest that Bertha's hysterical symptoms resurfaced once she stopped going to daily therapy sessions. Undoubtedly, this was the first time in history that psychoanalysts complained about a patient bailing out on treatment before psychic relief had been achieved.

During the months Bertha did tell all, however, she bragged to her friends and family about her wonderful "talking cure" or "chimney sweeping," setting in motion a profitable and ever-expanding industry of therapeutic confession. Breuer may have stumbled onto a strikingly novel treatment modality, but it was Freud (and his patients) who refined the technique now called free association. It proved to be a perfect combination; Freud's ability to listen and interpret so beautifully meshed with his patients' willingness to speak their minds. He hypothesized that talking at length about one's life, memories, feelings, and virtually everything else that came up generated a catharsis, allowing dormant memories to be recalled, expressed, analyzed, and processed, all to the patient's betterment. Regardless of what critics would say at the time or in retrospect, "the talking cure" turned out to be the great discovery he had been searching for throughout his entire career.

Breuer and Freud went their separate ways not long after they published their book, *Studies in Hysteria,* in 1895. Breuer heatedly disagreed with Freud's insistence that all neuroses were sexual in origin, the result of seduction or sexual abuse during childhood. Some have suggested that Mrs. Breuer grew weary, if not jealous, of hearing her husband confabulate about Anna O. at the dinner table night

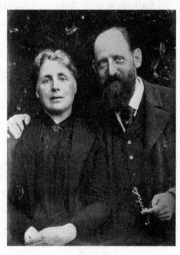

Josef and Mathilde Breuer, c. 1895.

after night. Regardless of the root cause, Dr. Breuer jumped off the psychoanalytical train before it ever left the station, preferring, instead, to pursue a more orthodox medical practice. Predictably, Freud, whose need for acclaim matched his desire to advance scientific inquiry, resented Breuer's failure to support his theories and began to denigrate Breuer's intellectual abilities. In his later years, Freud minimized Breuer's contributions. He told colleagues that the development of psychoanalysis may have cost him his friendship with Breuer but the discovery was so important that the price was justified.

There are many types of warriors. Most prominent are those who risk life and limb on the battlefield. But as anyone who has spent time in a laboratory or a university hospital can attest, the intellectual warfare among doctors can be just as protracted and treacherous, albeit less bloody. Freud's "talk therapy" was, initially, as poorly regarded in staid, scientific Vienna as his ideas about hysteria. Like the reflexive jerk of a knee elicited by the doctor's rubber hammer, the very name Freud incited a ruckus at medical meetings, in coffeehouses, and along the corridors of the Krankenhaus.

This intense disagreement over Freud's theories arose within the context of a remarkably fertile period of medical progress and discovery. The overwhelming majority of Sigmund's investigative colleagues demanded precise, reproducible explanations for every physiological and pathological action, a quantitative, data-driven process that still dominates medical research. Such a rigid intellectual framework, however, posed distinct challenges as he sought to expand his field in such a singularly qualitative manner that broke the bonds of nineteenth-century biology. To be sure, Freud's ideas were presented in a clear, logical prose that made excellent use of language, metaphors, literature, art, and novel psychological models. It was, after all, his luminous texts and cogent explanations that elevated him to the pantheon of intellectual giants. But when first proposed, Sigmund's theories were completely out of synchrony with the very physicians he most wanted to impress. As a result, his work was initially rejected by many of his peers as flighty and without scientific merit.

Like all mavericks, Sigmund paid a high social and personal cost by forging a new path, isolating himself from the academic community to which he'd once aspired. But it is critical to note that during the same period he was thinking about these concepts and coauthoring *Studies in Hysteria,* he was also regularly consuming cocaine. The predictable hangover and generalized grumpiness the drug engenders, once the euphoria disintegrates, could hardly have helped him when he engaged in verbally vicious debates with dismissive doctors and, at times, his closest friends. Such unproductive exchanges frequently led colleagues to avoid and ostracize him. Nevertheless, the alluring siren of cocaine only encouraged him to ignore such warning signs and continue his toxic substance abuse.

IN HIS MASTERWORK, *The Interpretation of Dreams,* Freud admitted:

> My emotional life has always insisted that I should have an intimate friend and a hated enemy. I have always been able to provide myself afresh with both, and it has not infrequently happened that the ideal situation of childhood has been so completely reproduced that friend and enemy have come together in a single individual—though not, of course, at once or with constant oscillations, as may have been the case in my early childhood.

As we have seen, Freud's relationships with Nothnagel, Meynert, and Breuer all had a narrative arc of admiration and adulation followed by irritation and separation. During his long life, Sigmund repeated this pattern of intense closeness and clashes with his friends, colleagues, and acolytes but with no one more spectacularly than a general practitioner from Berlin with an intense interest in the diseases of the nose and throat named Wilhelm Fliess.

Josef Breuer introduced Freud to the twenty-nine-year-old Fliess in the fall of 1887. Fliess hailed from a Sephardic Jewish family and studied medicine at the University of Berlin under the great Helmholz and DuBois-Reymond. Like so many other ambitious doctors, Wilhelm came to Vienna, on a self-rewarded sabbatical, to increase his medical knowledge and connections. Upon meeting Breuer, Fliess inquired after a good course on neurology and was advised to attend a series of lectures Sigmund was presenting at the Krankenhaus.

The meeting coincided with a difficult time in Freud's life. He loved his wife dearly, but his discontent increased with the daily realization that she was far more interested in domestic orderliness than in his pioneering ideas. As he struggled to unlock the secrets of the mind, her chief concern centered on convincing Freud that their expanding family needed a larger flat. Four years later, in 1891, Sigmund finally was able to rent a new and larger abode he'd chosen at Berggasse 19, in the Ninth District of Vienna, a Jewish neighborhood near the Krankenhaus. This now famous second-story apartment served as Freud's clinical, intellectual, and residential headquarters for the next forty-seven years.

On November 24, 1887, a few months after delivering his neurology lectures and after Fliess had returned to Berlin, Freud sent the surgeon a mawkish note of admiration:

> *My letter of today admittedly is occasioned by business, but I must introduce it by confessing that I entertain hopes of continuing the relationship with you and that you have left a deep impression on me which could easily lead me to tell you outright in what category of men I place you.*

Similar in age, religion, demeanor, and desire for success, they were also deeply enamored of creating new ways of understanding the connections among mind, brain, and body. Each had found in the other a soul mate, confidant, friend, and confessor with whom to discuss his desires, ideas, and, literally, dreams. As their novel notions garnered jeers, sneers, and hostility among their colleagues, the two young doctors only drew closer together.

Fliess's speculations about the human body, illness, and sexuality were considered by many physicians of the 1880s and 1890s to be astounding, if not entirely ridiculous. Specifically, Fliess posited that the nose was the major organ of the body, responsible for control of the delicate equilibrium between health and disease, and had a direct connection to the genitals. Moreover, he suggested that both the female body and the male body were governed by biological cycles of twenty-eight and twenty-three days, respectively. Careful nasal examinations at precise points of these cycles, Fliess insisted, would facilitate the diagnostic process as well as eliminate the need for artificial contraception.

As with virtually every surgically inclined doctor since sharp instruments were first placed in their bold hands, it was not enough for Dr. Fliess merely to propose a theory of disease; he was also compelled to develop the means to manipulate or ameliorate the unhealthy circumstances that brought patients to his clinic. Fliess's solution was to treat a compendium of gastrointestinal, neurological, and sexual disorders by applying huge doses of cocaine to the turbinate bones and sinuses of the nose, often followed by intricate, and potentially debilitating, operations on that sensitive region. These, in turn, were followed by more cocaine, for pain relief. Among the many who simultaneously endured and got high off Fliess's misguided therapies was Sigmund Freud.

For most of their relationship, the two men lived apart, Freud in Vienna and Fliess in Berlin, although they frequently met on gentlemen-only Alpine retreats they called congresses. Fortunately for the historical record, they left behind a voluminous correspondence detailing their work, ideas, and lives. Many of their letters were filled with sentiments of mutual admiration and intellectual and emotional support. At others times, they complained about their medical practices and trying colleagues. More intriguing, they explored Fliess's nasal theories, Sigmund's ideas about psychoanalysis and talk therapy, bisexuality, and the role masturbation, coitus interruptus, and condoms played in the development of neuroses.

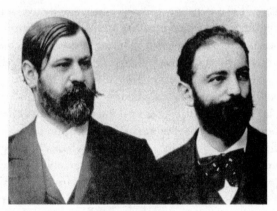

Freud, age thirty-four, and Wilhelm Fliess, age thirty-two, c. 1890.

Freud also dropped clues about a possible physical relationship. In a few letters, he referred to himself as a young woman; in another, when the two were about to meet for a "congress," he remarked that his "temporal lobe [was] lubricated for reception" and that he looked forward to the "introduction of a fertilizing stream." In another still, he eagerly awaited the "thrusts and pushes" of their conversations but worried, "God alone knows the date of the next thrust."

FEW ADDICTS LEAVE BEHIND copious details of their patterns of substance abuse, for reasons ranging from shame, embarrassment, and secrecy to fear of getting caught and its repercussions. Barring an eyewitness or frequent body-fluid screening, it is difficult to document the amount of illicit drugs someone is consuming without complete openness and honesty from the person himself. Moreover, when the individual in question is a world-famous figure, revered by a legion of psychoanalysts, psychiatrists, psychologists, scholars, historians, philosophers, and the general public, there exists a host of reasons to suppress or, at least, gloss over habits or practices that might reflect poorly on the great man's reputation.

Yet in light of the physical symptoms Freud suffered during this period, in my medical opinion, there is ample evidence that he was abusing significant amounts of cocaine during the early 1890s and that he was using it in a dependent, if not outright addictive fashion. In fact, cocaine likely had a negative effect on virtually every aspect of Sigmund's personal relationships, behavior, and health. We can make such a declarative statement because his letters to Wilhelm Fliess tell us precisely so.

In May 1893, Freud suffered a bout of strep throat and tonsillitis resulting in a peritonsillar abscess, a painful and potentially fatal infection in those days before antibiotics. While recuperating, he wrote his "dearest friend" Fliess about the lack of progress he was making and his "incomprehensible disinclination to write (dysgraphia)." A few weeks later, Sigmund explained that he was suffering from a Fliessian syndrome of "crossed reflexes" of the nose, brain, and genitals that had led to severe migraine headaches. The excruciating pain, not surprisingly, could only be interrupted by the multiple doses of cocaine prescribed by Dr. Fliess. Freud reported feeling especially better after cocainizing the side of the nose that corresponded with the side of his head where the migraine originated, followed by generously cocainizing the other nostril as well.

During the next few months, Freud does not mention cocaine explicitly to Fliess, but he does complain about severe nasal congestion. In late November 1893, Sigmund wrote Fliess:

> *The last letter I was able to produce for you immediately thereafter was lost, as we say in Vienna, and then came a period in which I did not feel like writing, my nose was stopped up, and I could not get myself to do it. I again let myself be cauterized, again enjoy working, but otherwise am little satisfied with the success of the local therapy. I am not obeying your order not to smoke; do you really consider it a remarkable boon to live a great many years in misery?*

From a diagnostic standpoint, Sigmund's nasal stuffiness is intriguing. The application of significant amounts of cocaine to the fragile mucous membranes lining the nose causes an intense constriction of the blood vessels feeding that region. Tissue death, copious mucus drainage, and bleeding often ensue. Shortly after, all that sticky detritus dries and hardens inside tortuous sinus passages and produces mucus plugs, which are eventually expelled into one's handkerchief. Although smoking tobacco can set one up for sinus inflammation and infections, few things congest and disturb the nose more than the regular administration of cocaine. Sigmund's need for cauterization—the placement of a hot knife against swollen, blocked nasal tissue to, literally, burn open a passage for air—in concert with his disinclination to write suggests serious cocaine abuse. Incidentally, it was not the last time he would consider resorting to the drastic measures of the cautery to relieve his cocaine-induced nasal congestion.

In April 1894, after three weeks of abstaining from his black cigars, Freud revealed an even more distressing set of symptoms to Fliess:

> *Less obvious, perhaps, is the state of my health in other respects. Soon after the withdrawal* [from nicotine] *there were some tolerable days and I began to write down the state of the neurosis problem for you; then suddenly there came a severe cardiac misery, greater than I ever had while smoking. The most violent arrhythmia, constant*

*tension, pressure, burning in the heart region; shooting pains down
my left arm; some dyspnea* [shortness of breath], *all of it essentially
in attacks extending continuously over two-thirds of the day; the
dyspnea is so moderate that one suspects something organic, and with
it a feeling of depression, which took the form of visions of death and
departure in place of the usual frenzy of activity. The organic
discomforts have lessened during the past two days, the lypemanic
mood* [morbid depression] *persists, having the courtesy to let up
suddenly—as it did last night and at noon today—and leave behind
a human being who looks forward with confidence again to a long
life and unlimited pleasure in resuming the battle.*

Initially, Sigmund diagnosed his problem as due to dilatation
(abnormal enlargement) of the heart or a case of rheumatic myocarditis and prescribed digitalis, a powerful medication for congestive heart
failure. The symptoms failed to abate, prompting Freud—who worried
a great deal about premature death—to cease treating himself and seek
another's medical opinion. The physician he chose to see was his friend
and collaborator the internist Josef Breuer. After a careful history and
physical examination, Breuer explained away Sigmund's symptoms as
the result of nicotine poisoning.

Freud aficionados know that one of the analyst's greatest vices was
cigars. By all accounts, he loved the taste, feel, and aroma of a well-
rolled cheroot and was a heavy smoker. Too often, as Sigmund worked
late into the night in his study on Berggasse 19, accompanied by his
books and antiquities, he desired something to spur him on to complete his nocturnal tasks. Not content to sip multiple cups of coffee or
tea, Sigmund often consumed twenty or more cigars a day.

Nicotine, the active ingredient in tobacco, has long been valued as a
stimulant that produces a mild sense of well-being and alertness.
Highly addictive in its own right, nicotine is cherished for the relax-
ation and concentration it affords. Many a smoker will tell you that
puffing on a cigarette or cigar before embarking on a complex task
affords a useful sense of arousal and attention. Interestingly, in 1897,
Freud characterized tobacco smoking—along with addictions to substances such as cocaine and morphine—as a mere replacement for the
"primary addiction" of masturbation.

Smoking too many cigars or cigarettes can increase the risk of panic attacks, nervousness, tremors, and an annoying awareness of the speed of one's heartbeat. Yet most established smokers, like Freud, develop a tolerance to tobacco that allows them to avoid the unpleasant side effects of what was once termed "nicotine poisoning." An overindulgence in cigars might cause chest discomfort and even anginal pain, especially in an older patient with preexisting atherosclerotic blockage of the coronary arteries. But Freud was a relatively young man, in his late thirties, when he began complaining of his chest pain. Such quibbles aside, nicotine poisoning remained an especially unlikely diagnosis given that he had abandoned cigars for nearly a month before experiencing these problems and was still not smoking in late April and early May, when he wrote Fliess.

If forced to make a retrospective diagnosis, a physician today would be hard-pressed not to consider that Sigmund's cardiac symptoms were related to his cocaine abuse. At first glance, Breuer's failure to make this connection seems puzzling. One assumes that he was well enough acquainted with Sigmund to know something about his colleague's experimentations with cocaine. Moreover, by 1894 the cardiac symptoms associated with cocaine use and the severe depression and headaches after its use—similar to what Sigmund was experiencing—were finally being reported in the medical journals of the day. Yet Dr. Breuer was hardly unique in missing the correct diagnosis. One of the most puzzling scenarios I have observed after a quarter century of medical practice is that physicians, past and present, deny serious signs and symptoms of substance abuse almost as frequently as patients and their family members do.

Despite all the physical problems the drug was causing, Sigmund continued abusing cocaine because it made him feel temporarily better. Throughout this period, he self-medicated away his stomachaches, ennui, depression, fears, migraines, and chest pain with more doses of cocaine followed by the occasional administration of digitalis. Perversely, Freud continued to search for alternative explanations for his chest pain rather than seriously contemplate cocaine's potential role in the matter.

While discussing the issue with Fliess in June 1894, Sigmund again brings up tobacco as a cause but coyly dismisses it:

I would be endlessly obliged to you, though, if you were to give me a definite explanation, since I secretly believe that you know precisely what it is, and that you have been so absolute and strict in your prohibition of smoking—the justification for which is after all relative—only because of its educational and soothing effects.

Six months later, on January 24, 1895, Sigmund wrote Fliess a note singing cocaine's praises:

I must hurriedly write to you about something that greatly astonishes me; otherwise I would be truly ungrateful. In the last few days I have felt quite unbelievably well, as though everything had been erased—a feeling which in spite of better times I have not known for 10 months. Last time I wrote you, after a good period, which immediately succeeded the reaction, that a few viciously bad days had followed during which a cocainization of the left nostril had helped me to an amazing extent. I now continue my report. The next day, I kept the nose under cocaine, which one should not really do; that is, I repeatedly painted it to prevent the renewed occurrence of swelling; during this time I discharged what in my experience is a copious amount of thick pus; and since then I have felt wonderful; as if there had never been anything wrong at all. Arrhythmia is still present, but rarely and not badly.

Later in the year, on June 12, 1895, Sigmund made a disturbing confession of sorts to Fliess about his cocaine consumption:

I need a lot of cocaine. Also I have started smoking again, moderately, in the last two or three weeks, since the nasal conviction [the nasal origin of his cardiac symptoms] *has become evident to me. I have not observed any ensuing disadvantage. If you again prohibit it, I must give it up again. But do consider whether you can do this if it is only intolerance and not etiology. I began it* [smoking cigars] *because I constantly missed it—after 14 months of abstinence—and because I must treat this psychic fellow well or he won't work for me. I demand a great deal of him. The torment, most of the time, is superhuman.*

. . .

FREUD BEGAN COMPOSING a monograph he titled *Project for a Scientific Psychology* in the spring of 1895. In a final effort at appeasing his hidebound medical colleagues, he hoped to construct a theoretical model that would give psychiatry a physiological and quantitative basis. At the same time, he was struggling to clarify and expand his work on neuroses and the tools of psychoanalysis. That fall, Freud feverishly wrote up *Scientific Psychology* and, upon completion, posted it to Fliess for review. Within a few weeks, however, Sigmund reread the manuscript, found it to be grandiose but unrevealing, and buried it in the back of his desk drawer. The literary vehicle to take its place was one that advanced his name and reputation in ways even he could not yet imagine, *The Interpretation of Dreams*.

Although Freud was unable to fully accept the physical and psychic consequences of his cocaine abuse, he was eager to begin a lengthy self-analysis of the subconscious thoughts expressed in his dreams. Freud was a dreamer in the most literal sense in that he dreamed a lot, could remember his dreams upon awakening, wrote them down, and then subjected them to intensive study. He would then rewrite and reanalyze those dreams, over and over again, theorizing that the changes in each version represented his own defenses and psychic conflicts. The more he thought through the meanings of his dreams, the more convinced he became that a careful, systematic interpretation would uncover the archaeology of the unconscious. It was among the ruins of the memory, he posited, where both he and the suffering patients who climbed the iron

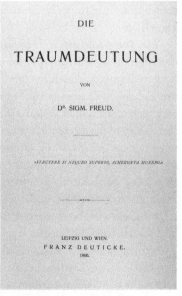

DIE

TRAUMDEUTUNG

VON

D^R. SIGM. FREUD.

»FLECTERE SI NEQUEO SUPEROS, ACHERONTA MOVEBO.«

LEIPZIG UND WIEN.
FRANZ DEUTICKE.
1900.

The title page of The Interpretation of Dreams, *1900.*

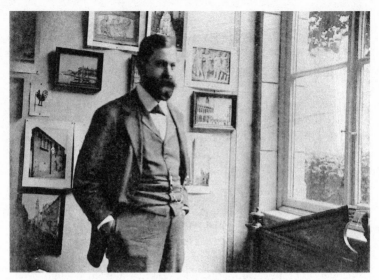

"At the historic corner window": Freud in his study at Berggasse 19, c. 1897.

staircase leading to his consultation room would find a healing self-knowledge.

The Interpretation of Dreams forged the revolutionary path of considering our nocturnal visions as the fulfillment of wishes. It endeavored to describe how the unconscious mind translates these dreams' sources into a fantasy that the awakened dreamer can recall and analyze. And most important, it detailed a novel and comprehensive theory of how the mind works. Sigmund may have begun plotting out his ideas as early as the summer of 1895, but, according to his letters, he did not begin composing the manuscript until late 1897. One reason for the delay, he complained to Fliess, was all the preliminary reading and research he was forced to complete before committing pen to paper. He was also frustrated, depressed, and contemplating leaving both his practice and Vienna.

Freud appears to have curtailed his cocaine consumption beginning in the fall of 1896. During the first half of 1899, however, he briefly took up a more conventional substance of abuse: alcohol. Before and after writing *The Interpretation of Dreams,* he was known to have imbibed sparingly. As he had jovially informed Fliess in 1896, "any trace of alcohol makes me completely stupid." Yet by 1899, he was often finding

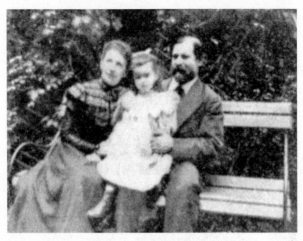

*Martha and Sigmund Freud
with their four-year-old daughter, Anna, 1899.*

temporary solace in a wineglass. In January, he told Fliess of the "restoration" provided by a bottle of Barolo. In mid-June, Sigmund confessed that Martha was counting the bottles of "heavenly Marsala" in their house and "took charge of them lest in loneliness I succumb to the consolation of drink." A few weeks later, he admitted, "I am gradually becoming accustomed to the wine; it seems like an old friend. I plan to drink a lot of it in July." That he did, and in early July Freud informed Fliess that he could not "manage more than two hours a day without calling on Friend Marsala." Eventually, Sigmund realized that his "new vice" was creating more problems than it was solving, and he gave up the libations altogether.

Sigmund soldiered on, and by the late summer of 1899 he'd emerged with a manuscript of more than 250,000 words, the longest book he would ever write. It begins with a bold declarative statement:

> In the pages that follow I shall bring forward proof that there is a psychological technique which makes it possible to interpret dreams and that, if that procedure is employed, every dream reveals itself as a psychical structure which has a meaning and which can be inserted at an assignable point in the mental activities of waking life. I shall further endeavor to elucidate the

processes to which the strangeness and obscurity of dreams are due and to deduce from those processes the nature of the physical forces by whose concurrent or mutually opposing action dreams are generated.

Freud sent Fliess a set of proofs from some of the book's early chapters in August 1899 and explained the volume's organization:

> *The whole thing is laid out like the fantasy of a promenade. At the beginning, the dark forest of authors—who do not see the trees—hopelessly lost on the wrong tracks. Then a concealed pass through which I lead the reader—my specimen [model] dream with its peculiarities, details, indiscretions, bad jokes—and then suddenly the high ground and the view and the question: which way do you wish to go now?*

Cradling a newly published copy of the book in November 1899, Sigmund proudly pronounced it to be his masterpiece. It is a tome leavened with rich metaphors and allusions to great artists ranging from Sophocles, Shakespeare, and Mozart to Goethe, Offenbach, and Heine. Months later, on March 11, 1900, Sigmund painted a slightly different picture of his great achievement for Fliess:

> *After last summer's exhilaration, when in feverish activity I completed the dream [book], fool that I am, I was once again intoxicated with the hope that a step toward freedom and well-being had been taken. The reception of the book and the ensuing silence have again destroyed any budding relationship with my milieu. For the second iron in the fire is after all my work—the prospect of reaching an end somewhere, resolving many doubts, and then knowing what to think of the chances of my therapy. Prospects seemed most favorable in E's case—and that is where I was dealt the heaviest blow. Just when I believed I had the solution in my grasp, it eluded me and I found myself forced to turn everything around and put it together anew, in the process of which I lost everything that until then had appeared plausible. I could not stand the depression that followed.*

Despite Freud's grand hopes, the first edition of *The Interpretation of Dreams* sold only 351 copies in its first six years of life, and a second edition did not appear until 1909. With hindsight, and the century of acclaim that followed, it is easier to see how transformative this book really was. After all, *The Interpretation of Dreams* was the first modern medical treatise to focus on the sleeping individual and, hence, the subconscious or unconscious mind, a striking contrast to virtually all other studies of the mind and brain during Freud's era, which were based on the premise of "the active, rational subject" articulated by the leading thinkers of the Enlightenment. Indeed, the book is widely regarded as the touchstone of Freud's psychoanalytical inquiry of human nature. The Oedipus complex; the notion that neuroses are caused not necessarily by actual events but, rather, by fantasies or inner wishes that are unacceptable to the individual; the importance of free association; and wish fulfillment are all articulated on its pages.

Seven months after the book's publication, in June 1900, the author whimsically asked Fliess about the Belle Vue Castle, a spa hotel on the outskirts of Vienna where he had the "model dream" that figures so prominently in his book: "Do you think that one day there will be a marble tablet on this house saying: Here, on July 24, 1895, the secret of the dream revealed itself to Dr. Sigmund Freud?" Although Freud immediately rejected such a fate in the next line of this letter to Fliess, the "model dream" is today widely known as "Irma's Injection." It was based on a series of all-too-real therapeutic mishaps involving cocaine use on a patient named Emma Eckstein and exacerbated by the fact that before finally getting to bed the night he had this now famous dream, Freud had helped himself to a hefty dose of cocaine.

EMMA ECKSTEIN WAS AN ATTRACTIVE young woman who began consulting Dr. Freud in 1892. Immortalizing her as "Irma" in his book, Sigmund presents a somewhat disingenuous explanation of his late-night reverie concerning cocaine and his patient:

> I was making frequent use of cocaine at that time to reduce some troublesome nasal swellings, and I had heard a few days earlier that one of my women patients who had followed my example

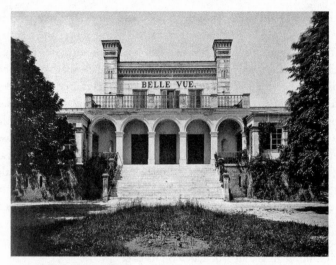

The Belle Vue Castle, outside Vienna, where Freud had his
model dream about Emma Eckstein and cocaine in July 1895.

had developed an extensive necrosis of the nasal mucous membrane. I had been the first to recommend the use of cocaine in 1885, and this recommendation had brought serious repercussions down on me. The misuse of that drug had hastened the death of a dear friend of mine. This had been before 1895 [the date of the dream].

In the dream, a disguised Irma meets Freud at a party hall filled with well-dressed and distinguished guests. She approaches him and complains, in the presence of others, that he had failed to cure her of her ailments and, in fact, had worsened them. Descriptions of scabrous turbinate bones, blood, dirty syringes, injections with a series of agents, including trimethylamine (the organic compound that gives decomposing semen its distinctly fishy smell, a fact recently introduced to Freud by Fliess), infection, and botched surgery abound in this dream.

Upon awakening, Freud was overcome with the unsettling thought that his dream meant he did not take his medical duties seriously enough. After further scrutiny of the fantasy, however, he concluded that this group of thoughts seemed to have put itself at my disposal, so I could produce evidence of how highly conscientious I was, of how deeply I was concerned about the health of my relations, my friends and my patients. There was an unmistakable connection between this more extensive group of thoughts which underlay the dream and the narrower subject of the dream which gave rise to the wish to be innocent of Irma's illness.

When contrasting his interpretation with the actual events that inspired it, one must be prepared to take a deep breath and recall that Sigmund was all too human. Indeed, the dream versus the actual life-events story serves as an ironic proof of one of Sigmund's major tenets: "When the work of interpretation is completed we perceive that a dream is the fulfillment of a wish."

BEFORE SIGMUND EVER DREAMED about "Irma," he was weary from too many days spent listening to Emma's litany of psychosomatic symptoms and too many late nights puzzling out what her thoughts and complaints actually meant. Stumped by the root causes of her psy-

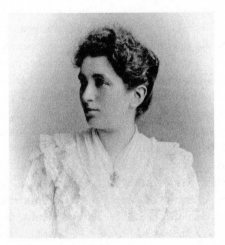

*Emma Eckstein of the "Irma dream" at the
age of thirty, in 1895.*

chological malaise and her relentless digestive complaints, Sigmund worried that he might have overlooked some physical problem in Emma's tortured body. It was also at this time that he was experiencing severe chest pain and worrying about succumbing to a heart attack. Like many a perplexed doctor before and since, he asked a surgeon to search for something that might be removed, amputated, or remodeled in the cause of a cure. The surgeon called into consultation was Freud's good friend and fellow cocaine aficionado Dr. Wilhelm Fliess.

There's an old saying one hears in hospital corridors among those who are disinclined to labor in the operating room: Don't call up a surgeon unless you want an operation. In many cases, specific and sometimes not so specific symptom patterns suggest that an operation is precisely what is called for. Yet there is also the tendency among the less scrupulous, the ill informed, and the simply overeager to perform unnecessary surgical procedures. In these two cases, it turned out to be the last. Considering that Fliess was the surgeon of record, it is not surprising that he diagnosed Sigmund's cardiac pain and Emma's hysteria as being due to a malfunction of the nose requiring surgical manipulation of the nasal turbinates, accompanied by copious applications of cocaine to the surgical wounds.

Dr. Fliess traveled from Berlin to Vienna in late January or early February of 1895 and operated on both Freud's and Emma's noses. Upon leaving Vienna the following day, the surgeon assigned Freud the task of caring for Emma during her postoperative recuperation period. On March 4, 1895, Freud told Fliess that her nasal swelling was persistent, "going up and down like an avalanche." Worse, Emma complained of excruciating pain and suffered massive nosebleeds. At one point, a sneeze yielded a jagged bone chip the size of small coin, no doubt a souvenir from Fliess's recent and ill-conceived surgical expedition. Moreover, Emma's nostrils were loaded with hardened scabs and pools of thick pus that emitted a powerful stench immediately detectable upon entering her bedroom.

On March 8, Sigmund wrote Fliess that Emma was improving somewhat but added that he had to report something that "will probably upset you as much as it did me." Freud was urgently called to Emma's bedside because she was bleeding uncontrollably from her nose. One of Freud's colleagues, a highly regarded surgical man named

Robert Gersuny, had inserted a drainage tube a few days earlier, hoping to clean the infection out of her nose, but was unavailable to take the emergency call until later that evening. Consequently, Freud contacted another ear, nose, and throat man, Ignaz Rosanes, who came to Emma's home at noon to look at her incisions and persistent bleeding from the nose and mouth. At Freud's direction, Rosanes began removing a series of sticky blood clots until his probe came upon a fetid, tangled, threadlike structure that demanded a delicate tug-of-war.

Freud's recollections of these events are absolutely disgusting:

> *Before either of us had time to think, at least half a meter of gauze had been removed from the cavity. The next moment came a flood of blood. The patient turned white, her eyes bulged, and she had no pulse. Immediately thereafter, however, he again packed the cavity with fresh iodoform gauze and the hemorrhage stopped. It lasted about a half a minute, but this was enough to make the poor creature, whom by then we had lying flat, unrecognizable. In the meantime—that is, afterward,—something else happened. At the moment the foreign body came out and everything became clear to me—and I immediately afterward was confronted by the sight of the patient—I felt sick.*

Sigmund and Rosanes restored themselves with a glass of cognac and stayed with the patient until they could have her removed to a sanatorium. In the weeks that followed, Freud grew mortified by the knowledge that his best friend had committed one of the worst surgical errors in the book: Fliess had nicked an artery and left a piece of gauze, a sponge really, inside Emma's surgical incision that had nearly killed her with inflammation, infection, and blood loss. Fortunately, the physically, if not mentally, strapping Emma recuperated, even though the surgical faux pas left her face permanently disfigured. After the bloody event but while still convalescing in bed, Emma admonished a woozy and pale Sigmund with the cutting remark "So this is the strong sex."

The episode was so troubling to Sigmund that he dreamed about it, ruminated over it, and even attempted to cover it up. He had little choice but to adopt such a course. Acknowledging and then revealing the role cocaine had played in his poor medical judgment with Emma would have resulted in professional ruin. To avoid this fate, Sigmund performed a series of mental calisthenics as he obscured responsibility for the fiasco. He reassured Fliess on March 28 that he was hardly to blame, having had to travel to a foreign city to conduct a complex operation, and further noted that the "tearing off of the iodoform gauze remains one of those accidents that happens to the most fortunate and circumspect of surgeons." Sigmund also informed Fliess of Emma's steady improvement, adding that "she is a very nice, decent girl who does not hold the affair against either of us and refers to you with great respect." In retrospect, such agile attempts at burying his malpractice appear to be a superb example of denial—later described to perfection by Freud as a defense mechanism.

On April 20, Freud wrote Fliess about a subsequent hemorrhage during the first week of April, but now Emma finally appeared to be on the mend. It is perhaps more indicative of the emotional toll the mishap was taking that Sigmund also reported that he was suffering from a "horrible attack of sinusitis" demanding copious cocaine applications. A week later, on April 26, he noted that Emma, "my tormentor and yours, now appears to be doing well" but confessed to another round of self-medication with cocaine. He also wondered if Fliess might have to perform another cauterization procedure on him. Apparently not: the following day Freud wrote, "Since the last cocainization three circumstances have continued to coincide: 1) I feel well; 2) I am discharging ample amounts of pus; 3) I am feeling very well." A week later, on May 4, the ever-rationalizing Sigmund speculated that Emma welcomed the bleeding spells as "an unfailing means of rearousing my affection."

At some level, one wonders if the personality that is open to trying mind-altering drugs is more likely to be open to exploring mind-altering ideas. And do such ideas actually emerge when one is under the influence? In terms of the last question, most intellectual historians, not to mention a majority of addiction scientists, psychiatrists, and neurologists, would heatedly answer no. There may well have been a spark of cocaine in Sigmund's misfiring neurons as they disturbed his sleep with the Irma affair. Yet as tempting as it is to singularly ascribe all of Sigmund's revolutionary ideas about dreams and exploring the unconscious to his cocaine use, this tack ultimately constitutes a simplistic and unsatisfying explanation. *The Interpretation of Dreams* covers a skein of thoughts and ideas beyond those set in motion by the Irma episode. Freud's psychological constitution was marked by multiple compulsions, perfectionism, risk taking, resentments, loneliness, alienation, emotional pain, traumatic family experiences, phobias, neuroses, depression, denials and secretiveness about his sexuality, a possible sexual relationship with his sister-in-law, a brief flirtation with excessive drinking, and his self-documented cocaine abuse, to name some of his demons. What makes Sigmund Freud's life and work so remarkable is that instead of sinking under the weight of these psychic challenges, he was able to process them all through his formidable intellect and thereby create a means for exploring the depths of the mind.

On November 2, 1896, several months after Emma's botched surgery and about a year before he began working on his dream book in earnest, Freud wrote a now famous letter to Fliess about the funeral of his beloved father. A father's death, he would observe in the preface

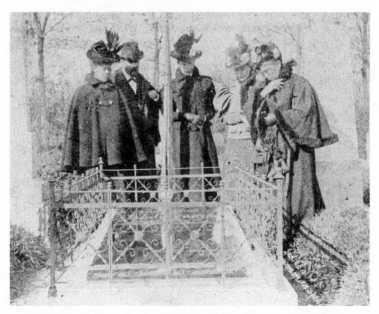

The Freud family at the unveiling of Jacob Freud's grave site, c. 1896–97.

to the second edition of *The Interpretation of Dreams*, is "the most important event, the most poignant loss, of a man's life." On the night following Jacob's funeral, the grieving Freud told Fliess, he had experienced a "nice dream" in which he saw a sign outside his favorite barbershop that declared, "You are requested to close the eyes." Freud interpreted this as a reflection of his filial duty and "the inclination to self-reproach that regularly sets in among the survivors." Distraught by his loss and neuroses, Freud soon after embarked on what he was to call "the most essential thing I have at present": his now famous self-analysis and, of course, the composition of his book.

Less heralded by Freud scholars is a letter he wrote to Fliess only a few days earlier, on October 26, a day after returning from the cemetery. It is the last extant letter in which he documents his cocaine abuse: "Next time I shall write more and in greater detail; incidentally, the cocaine brush has been completely put aside." Many Freudians have concluded that Sigmund was the rara avis of chronic cocaine abusers in that he meant what he said when he pledged a future of abstinence. Alas, the paper trail ends there.

Emma, too, disappears as a topic in the Freud-Fliess correspondence by the spring of 1896. One assumes that Freud's clinical experiences with Emma, if not with Fleischl-Marxow, taught him that cocaine was far too dangerous for any therapeutic application. But in 1896, and probably for the remaining days of his life, Freud had far greater difficulty in fully comprehending the realities of his own substance abuse. He decidedly and repeatedly misinterpreted his famous dream of cocaine. Instead, he chose to elaborate a far more flattering and positive analysis that epitomizes an addiction's power of subterfuge. The man who invented psychoanalysis, a revolutionary pursuit of self-truth, succumbed to the same "big lie" most every practicing addict tells himself.

CHAPTER 10

"The Professor"

THE OPERATING ROOM was pristine and hushed. The tiled floor was spotless and sparkling. The light from the overhead electric lamps gleamed onto the table directly below. Supervising nurses wearing overflowing robes and gauze face masks scurried about making sure every instrument and suture was laid out just so. The patient, still awake and baffled by the strange dance taking place around him, waited nervously while lying perfectly still on the operating table. The muscular resident surgeons held their hands upward, scrubbed and dripping with corrosive antiseptic chemicals, as a harem of student nurses attentively gowned and gloved them.

In strode Professor William Halsted. He rarely spoke to his underlings other than to demand a scalpel or a forceps. If he did venture a comment, it was to criticize a junior surgeon's handiwork or scold an assisting nurse for not anticipating his next move. Decades later, a colleague recalled that Halsted was so "bitingly sarcastic as to completely shrivel those with him at the operating table." He refused to move his body from the operative field to allow interns even one educational peek. This was his theater, his room. In it no one could approach or challenge him. No surgical complication or mishap could distract or distress him. He was in complete control.

Halsted's basement operating room in the Johns Hopkins Hospital's Ward G was relatively small in terms of length and width; nevertheless, it was a place of discovery, miraculous healing, and choreographed action that attracted the most promising surgeons in the country. In 1891, an intern recorded one of the most lyrical accounts of the room's activities:

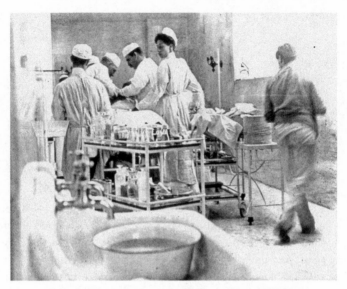

*Halsted in the operating room (Halsted is the middle figure
with his head downward), late 1890s to early 1900s.*

In Halsted's little operating room, with the old wooden table,
the antiseptic technique was so perfect that there was never a
moment of anxiety. I could not believe my eyes. It was like step-
ping into a new world. At the time Halsted's technique was
unique and the sureness and perfection of his results seemed to
me then [to be] the nearest thing to a miracle that had been
given to me to witness.

Unlike in his bold, hurried days while operating at Bellevue, Halsted was now the slowest and most painstaking of surgeons. In the
decades before he first took to the operating table, the years marked by
an absence of anesthesia let alone antiseptic surgery, doctors were
forced to operate as quickly as possible, lest they invite complications
of excruciating pain, shock, and infection. As a young man, Halsted
had learned how to operate from those who valued speed above every
other surgical technique. At Johns Hopkins, however, he elaborated an
extremely gentle but time-consuming means of operating known as the
"School of Safety." His meticulous methods minimized damage to

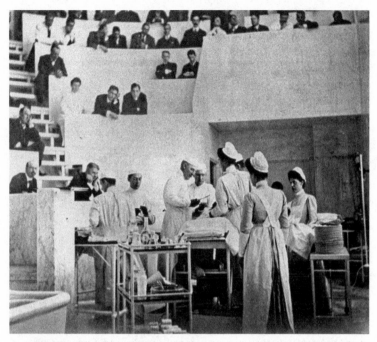

Halsted (center, holding the instrument) in the operating room at the Johns Hopkins Hospital, c. 1905.

blood vessels and nearby tissues and all but eliminated unnecessary traumatic or immunologic injury to the operative field. Halsted also created a series of elegant suturing techniques, always using silk or thin silver wires rather than the traditional catgut, to better conjoin what the surgeon cut apart. Virtually all of his now universally practiced techniques facilitate far better and faster recuperation rates, even after the most aggressive surgical assaults.

Dr. William Mayo, cofounder of the Mayo Clinic, is said to have quipped that the procedures at the Johns Hopkins operating room took so long that the patients typically healed before Dr. Halsted had a chance to close the incision. Perhaps more generously, the surgeon and historian Sherwin Nuland described the critical nature of such gentle techniques in a recent eulogy of another great operator, Dr. Michael DeBakey. Nuland's assessment is equally apt in describing the miracles that transpired in Halsted's operating room: "[His] fingers are engaged in a kind of complicated and tightly coordinated dance with those of [his] colleagues . . . the gentle touch is crucial. Sensitive tissues do not respond well when handled roughly, and may not heal. Living biological structures tolerate very little abuse, and are quick to express their displeasure when treated with less than the consideration that Mother Nature has made them accustomed to. The man or woman who cannot be an artist will never be more than a pedestrian surgeon." Those of us who are not surgeons have little appreciation for this skill; yet all who have successfully sailed through any item on a wide menu of surgical procedures have the artistic Dr. Halsted to thank.

Some have suggested that the marked shift in Halsted's surgical technique was due either to his active cocaine use or to his recovery from it; the most convincing arguments tend to side with the latter explanation. Dating back to the days when Sigmund Freud wrote his monograph *Über Coca,* physicians often believed that cocaine enhanced one's powers of intellectual concentration and physical strength. Like many other stimulants, it might do so in small doses but only for short periods of time. Long-term cocaine use and surgical craftsmanship, on the other hand, are contradictory activities. Given Halsted's history of cocaine consumption, it is impossible to imagine him operating so delicately and perfectly while actively under the influence. Cocaine would make his hands (and his brain) jitter and tremor too much to so expertly apply his scalpel.

IN FEBRUARY 1889, Halsted was offered a one-year appointment as chief of the surgical dispensary and acting surgeon of the hospital. Yet even with this promotion, William's future was far more tenuous than Welch had led him to believe. The trustees had other ideas about whom to appoint as the permanent surgeon-in-chief. In this quest, they approached Sir William Macewen, the accomplished professor of surgery at the University of Glasgow. The arrangement fell apart over control of the surgical nurses, a prerogative the hospital was not prepared to relinquish. The vacuum created by Macewen's rejection led to an eloquent plea by Welch, who vouched for his protégé's sobriety. After a series of lengthy conferences, the trustees finally acceded. In October 1889, Halsted was named associate professor of surgery and, in

March 1890, surgeon-in-chief at the Johns Hopkins Hospital and chief of the surgical dispensary. Two years later, on April 4, 1892, the mollified trustees rewarded Halsted's exemplary work with the lifetime appointment of professor of surgery at the medical school. In a little more than two decades, he had gone from Yale undergraduate and College of Physicians and Surgeons medical student to becoming, seriatim, the surgical wunderkind of New York City, a raging cocaine addict, an asylum inmate, a brittle recovering and relapsing addict, a distinguished surgical scientist, and, finally, holder of the most prestigious professorship of its kind in North America and, soon, the world.

Beginning in 1889 and continuing through the 1890s, Dr. Halsted worked to create a remarkably aggressive means of battling breast cancer. His bold operation called for removing the breast and lymph nodes in the affected region as well as the major and minor pectoral muscles lying underneath. This drastic, disfiguring procedure became one of Halsted's most famous contributions to surgery, even though it is, thankfully, no longer performed. In an era before early detection, radiation, and chemotherapy, a diagnosis of breast cancer was essentially a death sentence, and those stricken had few options available. At the opening of the twentieth century, Halsted performed his radical mastectomy at the Hopkins with the full expectation that his procedure worked to tame the cancer, if not cure it; that it should be offered to all women with breast cancer; and that it needed to be performed in a timely, precise, and uniform manner.

But this was hardly Halsted's only surgical interest. During these years, he perfected new treatments for thyroid gland goiters, huge, unsightly growths on the neck once common in the United States before the development of iodized salt. He also created several virtuoso techniques for correcting inguinal hernias and aneurysms of large arteries, and the safe removal of gallstones. All of these problems counted among the most common (and once most vexing) of surgical maladies known to humankind.

After the last suture was stitched on each of these thousands of procedures, Halsted immediately dictated their precise details to a secretary, who just as quickly typed them up for the professor's review, analysis, and eventual conversion into widely read and authoritative journal articles. His surgical word was law; every practitioner of the

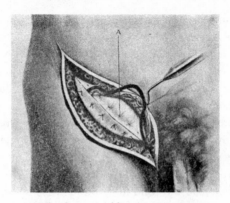

Halsted's inguinal hernia repair, 1893.

craft followed what Halsted of Baltimore decreed. As a result of his renown, he maintained a voluminous correspondence with a legion of surgeons and patients around the the globe seeking his help.

LONG A DEVOTEE OF PERFORMING SURGERY under the most germ-free, or aseptic, conditions possible, Halsted, as one might expect, was among the first surgeons in the world to insist that he, his assistants, and all his nurses completely remove their street clothes before entering the operating room. The uniform Halsted chose for himself consisted of a freshly steam-laundered and sterilized short-sleeved white duck suit with white tennis shoes and a white skullcap. Over this garb he wore a sterile white gown tied from behind by his chief nurse. Such a uniform would hardly raise an eyebrow in today's operating rooms, with the exception of its bright white color, which was later discarded for scrubs dyed greenish-blue, to cut down on the glare generated by the operating room's intense lights. But in the late 1890s, when many could still recall surgeons who operated in frock coats spattered with the blood and sinew of operations past, Halsted's sartorial choices represented a true advance. If scrupulously adhered to, it did and does reduce unnecessary infections introduced into the open bodies of unsuspecting patients.

Halsted insisted on a ritual of painting the incision site with alcohol, iodine, and other disinfectants, followed by an elaborate draping with sterile cloth, leaving only the operating field in view. Soon after

these preparations were completed,
the master surgeon nodded to the
residents to securely strap the patient to the operating table. He then
asked the anesthetist, typically one
of his junior residents, to begin the
onerous task of placing an "ether
cone," a funnel covered with oiled
silk and a towel, over the patient's
nose and mouth. Because a nearly
strangling dose of ether was employed, a period of intense struggle
often followed this action, forcing
the residents, nurses, and orderlies
to throw their bodies across the
patient in order to keep him still.
Eventually, the ether did its work,
and within minutes the patient was
"under," insensate, and the operation began.

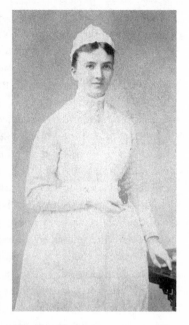

Caroline Hampton as a nurse, 1889.

For procedures requiring local anesthesia, weak solutions of cocaine
were "not infrequently used" by residents in the Hopkins operating
room, even if William rarely prescribed it. One morning during the
late 1890s, while examining an agitated patient who'd undergone hernia repair with cocaine anesthesia, Halsted told a resident surgeon to
administer some morphine as an antidote. "If you knew how terrible
the suffering is with that restlessness after cocaine," Halsted remarked,
"you would not stint his morphia." Yet even with the power to medically counteract cocaine, keeping his addictive archenemy so close at
hand was akin to lighting a cigarette in a gas station. Such daily proximity to cocaine may well have constituted one of the greatest risk factors in Halsted's episodic relapses in the years to come.

Medical historians have fiercely debated whether it was true love or
William's fetish for cleanliness that led him to create the iconic symbol
of modern surgery: the rubber glove. Like all Listerians, William
insisted that everyone entering his operating room vigorously scrub
their hands in abrasive toxic chemicals that killed microbes. At Johns
Hopkins, Halsted's assistants immersed their hands in a basin filled

with permanganate, followed by a dip in a basin of oxalic acid, and then a five-minute soak in a corrosive bichloride of mercury solution. They used stiff brushes, along with plenty of soap and water, to scrape and clean every millimeter of their hands, from the nail beds and crevices between their fingers all the way up to the elbows. The fastidious Dr. Halsted preferred to wash his hands with a sterilized cloth in a special basin filled with rubbing alcohol.

In 1889, one of the Hopkins surgical nurses caught William's eye. Her name was Caroline Hampton. A tall woman with piercing eyes, she hailed from a distinguished family of planters that included her uncle Wade Hampton III, a decorated Confederate general. A photographic portrait of Caroline in her nurse's uniform exhibits a bright air of confidence and a prematurely pear-shaped figure. Robust and horsey, Caroline was especially good at maintaining the various mechanical gadgets then in use at the hospital. By some accounts, she was difficult, spirited, prone to haughtiness, and high-strung. But Dr. Halsted saw her worth and appointed her to be the head nurse in his operating room.

The abrasive chemicals Caroline doused her hands in every day rendered her skin rough, cracked, and marred by red, angry rashes. None of these traits appealed to either the southern belle or the surgeon who pursued her. As the dermatitis traveled up her fingers and hands and extended to her forearms, a besotted William grew determined to do something therapeutically definitive and sweetly chivalrous. In the winter of 1889–90 (in later years he could never recall precisely when), the surgeon took a train up to New York and met with an executive at the Goodyear Rubber Company. Armed with drawings of prototypes, he asked the rubber man if he would kindly manufacture "two pairs of thin rubber gloves with gauntlets." Soon after, all the surgeons and nurses in his operating room donned them. William's invention may have begun as a means to win Caroline's heart, but it ultimately changed the way doctors operate, much to the benefit and safety of their patients.

In March 1890, William proposed marriage to Caroline. Whether this reveals his caustic sense of humor or signs of a conflicted inner life, a few weeks later he wrote to his Johns Hopkins colleague, the acerbic anatomist Franklin P. Mall: "I know that you will be astounded to hear that I am engaged to be married. A good joke for you I know. I wish that I could see you chuckle. Miss Hampton reminds Booker and me very much of you. I suppose that is the reason that I proposed to her."

The couple wed in Columbia, South Carolina, at the Hampton family–endowed Trinity Episcopal Church on June 4, 1890, with William Henry Welch standing up as the best man. Before the nuptials, Caroline resigned from her post at the hospital.

In later years, colleagues would comment on Dr. and Mrs. Halsted's distant marriage. Theirs was a type of relationship that was rather common in the late nineteenth and early twentieth centuries: spouses lived together and shared emotional connections but pursued activities that did not include the other. Some criticized her mannish dressing style and his general avoidance of any close contact with her. It was well known in Baltimore that the Halsteds occupied separate floors of their enormous town house at 1201 Eutaw Place. He lived on the second floor, with his books, papers, and a secretary desk stocked with boxes of freshly filled fountain pens, Pall Mall cigarettes, cigarette holders, and eyeglasses. She resided on the third floor, with their beloved black dachshunds, Sisly, Fritz, Nip, and Tuck. The union produced no chil-

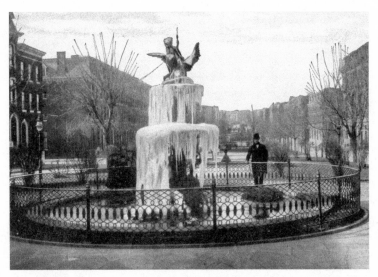

Eutaw Place, Baltimore, c. 1900; the street where the Halsteds lived.

dren. They supped as a couple, followed by a brief conversation of the day's events and withdrawal to their separate quarters. According to those familiar with the couple's domestic routine, they never had breakfast together.

As exacting about his home environment as he was about his operating room, William made the sort of incessant demands that proved particularly grating for Caroline. The surgeon's Turkish coffee had to be ground and brewed just so; the table linens were always to be freshly laundered and flatironed. He typically interfered with the management of dinner parties by insisting on ordering groceries from nearby Lexington Market, planning the menu, arranging the flowers and china, and, even though he rarely drank, selecting the wines. William's ceaseless search for perfection often exhausted the migraine-prone Mrs. Halsted.

In 1898, Harvey Cushing, then a surgical resident of Halsted's and soon to be a founder of modern neurosurgery, wrote his mother that William's "stone-cold" lair reminded him of Charles Dickens's Bleak House. The house overflowed with antiques, Oriental rugs, blooming dahlias, leatherbound books, telescopes, knickknacks, and an intricate telephone system linking each room in the house and connected to an

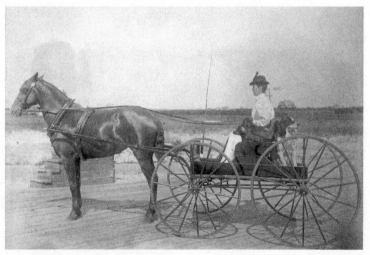

Mrs. Halsted, out for a carriage ride, c. 1910s.

outside line, the latter strictly guarded by servants ordered to tell any callers that the Halsteds were unavailable. It was an unwritten law among his residents at the hospital that the chief was not to be disturbed at home, no matter how dire the situation. Once his castle's heavy door was slammed shut for the evening, William intended it to stay that way.

Even at his healthiest, Dr. Halsted did not operate often: three mornings a week at the most and rarely more than one patient in a single morning. In the latter years of his career, he operated far less frequently. The cases he chose were selected from among the many patients seeking care at the Hopkins's surgical clinic, but Halsted limited his practice to the conditions he was studying at the time.

Those days he did operate, he left the surgical theater promptly at the stroke of noon. From there he beat a hasty retreat to his rooms on the second floor of the hospital for a light and solitary luncheon. This suite was where he'd lived in 1889 and 1890, until he'd married Caroline. William was so finicky about the decor of his pied-à-terre that he ordered the painting of its walls to be done over and over again until the color suited his aesthetic sensibilities. Equally central to the setting was a marble-manteled fireplace that was kept well stoked by an orderly assigned to fulfilling his every wish. The small suite of rooms, with its overstuffed Victorian furniture and a large photograph of Michaelangelo's *Madonna of Bruges,* was his refuge from the tumult and stress of his surgical world.

Halsted organized his hospital service into a hierarchy of men and offered them an unparalleled training experience. Composing the base were several interns and junior residents. As the pyramid rose to its apex, the surgical wheat was separated from the chaff. Those still standing assumed increasing responsibilities in and out of the operating room. At the end of a term of eight or more years, the most able trainee was handpicked to become Halsted's chief resident. This lofty position, one that held the keys to the fabled Hopkins operating room, invariably led to a professorship and chief of surgery post at a premier hospital. Rigorous, entirely exhausting, and challenging to even the hardiest of men, this system was quickly adopted by virtually every surgical residency program in the United States and, for decades, produced many thousands of qualified surgeons.

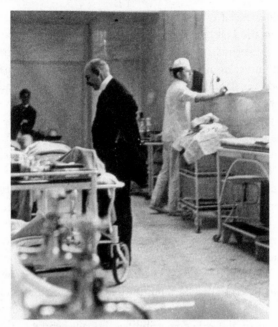

Halsted (center, in black) on ward rounds
at Johns Hopkins Hospital, c. 1914.

Once patients left the operating room, Halsted relegated their care to his residents. These young doctors stayed up night and day, paying scrupulous attention to the operative wounds with frequent dressings and bandage changes. They were also on the lookout for signs of the surgeon's greatest nemesis: postoperative fevers, the sometimes subtle, sometimes raging indication of infection brewing below the surface of the skin.

Halsted's visits to the hospital wards were erratic and rarely comprehensive in terms of walking from bed to bed. On some days, he inquired after only a few cases. On other occasions, he discussed unusual conditions and diseases. One morning a week during the school year, Dr. Halsted was required to conduct rounds on one or several wards for the sake of his attention-hungry students. His visits might last fifteen to thirty minutes or as long as an hour or two. Some weeks, he skipped them entirely.

With the "public" patients, drawn from the neighborhoods sur-

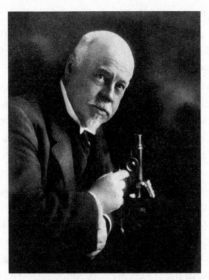

*William H. Welch at the pinnacle
of his career, c. 1905.*

rounding the hospital, Halsted was unfailingly polite but aloof and distant. He rarely discussed precise diagnoses or treatments with these patients. In accordance with the manner of the patrician white American male of the time, he may have assumed that the immigrants, African Americans, and working stiffs he saw on the public wards were intellectually incapable of understanding such complex matters. When attending private patients, armed with both social standing and the resources to meet his outsized fee schedule, he was a bit more solicitous. But even among the very rich, William was quick to assert that he was in command and it was a privilege to be placed on his operating table. Years later, in 1940, Harvey Cushing eulogized William's bedside manner with the observation that "he spent his medical life avoiding patients."

AT THE DAWN OF THE GAY NINETIES, Baltimore boasted many amenities, including a burgeoning port, thriving theatrical companies, booming businesses, and a determined zest for consuming meals captured from the "immense protein factory" better known as Chesapeake

Bay. In terms of propelling the ancient craft of medicine into modernity, however, it was considered by many toiling in the hospitals of Vienna, Paris, London, and even New York to be little more than a provincial outpost.

Such derisive assessments began to ebb after the Johns Hopkins Hospital officially opened its doors in 1889 and, even more definitively, in 1893, when the medical school was inaugurated. Before the century turned, crowds of young men with stars in their eyes and ambition in their loins flocked to 601 North Broadway to participate in what historians universally regard as one of the most important developments in American medical education. In fact, Halsted was just one of many distinguished doctors practicing there.

As the story is told to each intern the night before he takes his first call on the wards of the Johns Hopkins Hospital, in the beginning there were four physicians—each of them under the age of forty—who set out to transform the stodgy and deleterious American medical profession. By every imaginable metric, they succeeded wildly. Almost immediately, the Hopkins assumed its place at the vanguard of a fin de siècle revolution where doctors abandoned a blind allegiance to centuries-old, not infrequently toxic medications and deadly surgical measures in favor of the scientific and evidence-based enterprise that characterizes modern medical practice.

First among equals, of course, was the majordomo and initial hire of the hospital, the rotund William Henry Welch, whose Vandyke beard grew pointier and whiter with each passing year. At the laboratory bench, Dr. Welch failed to make a lasting mark, although one species of bacteria he described, *Clostridium welchii,* carried his name for decades. He was an indifferent administrator who often forgot to return phone calls or telegrams and was notorious for misplacing memoranda and manuscripts for weeks on end. Where Welch shined, however, was as the nation's preeminent medical statesman, with the ability to identify and nurture scientific talent in others long before they knew they had it in themselves. He enjoyed impeccable connections. An executive officer or board member of virtually every major American medical society and research institute, Welch knew everyone who was worth knowing; and virtually every doctor alive wanted to know him.

In the years before and long after the medical school's opening, Welch attended countless scientific meetings, trolled the best hospitals

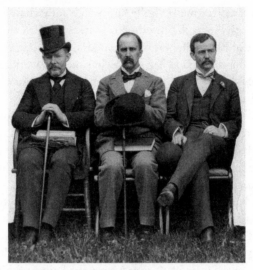

Drs. Halsted, Osler, and Kelly, c. 1889.

and medical schools in the nation, and enticed the brightest doctors to abandon the workaday world of medical practice for exciting careers in the laboratory. It has often been said that William Henry Welch had enough charm to sell a furnace in the middle of a Baltimore summer. It served him well when recruiting the ambitious men who populated Johns Hopkins. In dulcet tones, he described the rich purse his institution was dedicating to medical research. Long before he finished his pitch, Welch convinced most of these listeners to pack their bags and board the next train for Baltimore. Every year until his retirement at the onset of the Great Depression, Welch's laboratory and pathology residency program attracted a stellar cadre of eager young trainees, the vast majority of whom came to dominate the next generation of academic medical leaders in the United States and around the world.

Then there was Howard Atwood Kelly, the ebullient and talented gynecologist from the University of Pennsylvania. In surgical circles, Dr. Kelly is best recalled for inventing several operating tools, including a clamp that still bears his name and is requested every day in operating rooms all over the world. His superb descriptions of diseases ranging from appendicitis to cervical cancer continue to inform physicians who take the time to go to the library stacks and pull down his richly illustrated textbooks. Kelly also wrote authoritative tomes on medical history, biography, mushrooms, snakes, reptiles, and canoeing.

The love of Kelly's life was his savior, Jesus Christ. So tightly intertwined was the connection between Kelly's medical work and his religious beliefs that he often knelt down in prayer before examining a patient or beginning an operation—until, that is, many of his uncomfortable colleagues and patients asked him to stop. A crusader for a number of civic reform movements, Kelly had an odd nocturnal habit of visiting Baltimore's most notorious street corners. Once there, he approached many a prostitute, not in search of a business transaction but, instead, to facilitate a direct path to the Lord.

In 1926, Kelly wrote a widely selling book "proving" the compatibility of Christian faith with the tenets of science and evolution, a thesis the famed Baltimore journalist H. L. Mencken publicly dismissed as "completely insane." Perhaps an even sharper slice at Kelly's mental status came in the form of a private query the Pulitzer Prize–winning novelist Sinclair Lewis posed to the Harvard neurosurgeon Harvey Cushing. In discussing Kelly's dual devotion to scientific inquiry and religious faith, Lewis asked, "My dear Harvey, what does an obstetrician know about the Virgin Birth?"

Dr. Kelly was a neighbor of the Halsteds' and maintained a profitable practice at his home on Eutaw Place, where he employed radium as a treatment for cervical cancer. In 1898 one of his resident physicians described him as "effulgent as an X-ray tube, he is distinctly phosphorescent." Such a description may have turned out to be more than metaphor. As Baltimore legend has it, long after Kelly died, when the time came to raze his abandoned house, the amount of radioactive waste left behind in the ground was so great that a team of hazardous materials experts had to come in and abate it.

The undisputed star of the faculty, however, was William Osler, a Canadian by birth who was formerly professor of the Institutes of Medicine at McGill University, in Montreal (1874–84) and of clinical medicine at the University of Pennsylvania, in Philadelphia (1884–89). The author of the best-selling medical textbook *The Principles and Practice of Medicine,* Osler was widely known as one of the greatest diagnosticians ever to wield a stethoscope. So remarkable was his personality and presence that it has been said Osler changed the atmosphere of every room he entered. Learned, compassionate, accomplished, and fun, William Osler inspired a cult of hero worship that has never ended.

At nine o'clock each morning, the great physician heaved open the great wood-and-glass doors of the Johns Hopkins Hospital's main entrance. He was always impeccably dressed in a silk hat and black frock coat, accessorized by a splendidly striped cravat, a freshly cut flower in his lapel, and an imperious gold chain hanging from his expansive waistcoat. Handing his gloves, hat, and umbrella to a waiting nurse, Osler warmly greeted the weary resident physician on duty, who reported on the patients he had admitted the night before.

Having gathered this critical intelligence, Osler raced around an imposing marble statue, *Christus Consolator* (the Divine Healer), and up a quarter-sawn oak staircase centered in a domed octagonal atrium that, quite possibly, constitutes the grandest hospital lobby in the history of medicine. Upon entering the house officers' quarters, he joyfully spent several minutes offering salutations to an admiring group of junior doctors. Eventually, he descended the stairs and made his way to the wards to visit his patients and enlighten the students assigned to their care. By insisting that his pupils observe, perform, and then teach clinical lessons to others more junior down the line, Osler trained them to think and act like doctors before John Dewey became famous for the educational method he called "learning by doing."

One Saturday evening a month, Dr. Osler invited the most promising students to his home for beer and sandwiches. After greeting them warmly in the vestibule of his expansive town house on West Franklin Street, he ushered his acolytes into a richly paneled library that contained a five-thousand-volume collection of the greatest medical and scientific works ever published. "To study the phenomena of disease without books is to sail an uncharted sea," Osler told them between bites of Virginia ham, sips of pilsner, and the regaling of great medical tales. But he always concluded this point with the warning that "to study books without patients is not to go to sea at all." Their destiny, the physician insisted was "a calling not a profession."

HALSTED'S PUPILS' educational experience was poles apart from Osler's. All week long, the students labored on the surgical wards, dressing wounds, examining patients, conducting laboratory tests, and

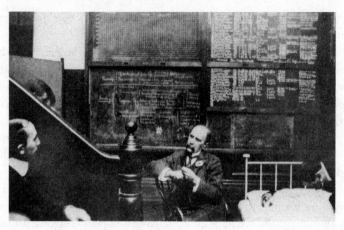

Dr. Osler teaching students at Johns Hopkins, c. 1900.
The blackboard behind him lists all the typhoid fever patients
admitted to the Johns Hopkins Hospital that year.

reading up on their cases in the hope of impressing their elusive teacher. The copious notes they took on each patient's progress became "part of the permanent hospital record and the need for careful work was stressed and the work itself checked by the interns and residents." The stakes were high, and no student wanted to be caught committing an error or omission. This practical experience was supplemented by attending ward rounds, an operative clinic conducted by one of Halsted's associates, work in the surgical dispensary (or outpatient clinic), an operative surgery course performed on animals (typically stray dogs caught near the hospital), and, most important, a "dry clinic" conducted each Friday at noon by the eminent professor of surgery.

At these formal affairs, Halsted eschewed the traditional discourse on pathology, clinical symptoms, diagnosis, and treatment, assuming that the interested student could easily read about these topics. Instead, he presented an array of surgical problems and experimental questions he was examining in his laboratory. To some, "it was an impressive demonstration of wide reaching, profound knowledge and fertility of suggestion—a keen scientific mind at work." But for most of his students, it was a boring and intimidating ordeal. There may have been a few inspiring axioms, but there were no moments of kindness in Halsted's classroom. Crusty and mordant, he was referred to by his students behind his back as "the Professor" because of his scolding and intimidating ways. William detested the nickname, which recalled the title appropriated by many a late-nineteenth-century dancing instructor and vaudeville orchestra conductor. Other medical students took to calling his ward rounds "Shifting Dullness," a play on the term used to describe a maneuver whereby the physician examines a supine patient for evidence of ascites, or excess fluid, in the abdomen.

Halsted often came to class late and unprepared. As medical students are all but genetically programmed to do, they complained about this habit to their dean, William Welch. From time to time, Welch angrily pledged to "come down on Halsted who ought to see that they have systematic instruction in surgical pathology as was advertised." Rarely, if ever, did Welch act upon those threats.

During many of the Friday afternoon dry clinics, Halsted spoke for the entire hour with his back to the audience, so immersed was he in the undecipherable drawings he chalked up on the blackboard. Cruelly, he took pleasure in speaking in a rapid-fire, prolix manner as he watched his students scribble furiously in their notebooks about surgical procedures they had never performed and did not yet quite understand. Unlike the generous instructor he'd once been in New York, Professor Halsted was frequently condescending and insulting at the Hopkins. Those few brave or completely uninformed students who dared ask him a question soon discovered whether or not their queries were up to Halsted's intellectual standards. If they received a lengthy and not entirely clear answer, they knew they were on the right track; if they were shot down with a stern rebuke or a sarcastic quip, they knew otherwise. Down the hallway, Osler's lecture room was filled with the sounds of laughter, learning, and discovery; in Dr. Halsted's amphitheater, the only voice that mattered was his own, and the only mirth that emerged was the nervous, inappropriate laughter of students forced to watch the humiliation of one of their peers.

OUTSIDE THE OPERATING ROOM and lecture hall, Halsted's behavior was even more strange. When walking through the corridors of the hospital, he cast his head and gaze downward. Upon spying someone approaching in the distance, he would duck into a stairwell or an empty patient room to avoid any form of contact. If pressed to explain his misanthropy, Halsted gruffly stated that he avoided those he did not care for or who he felt wanted something; those who would delay or bore him; and the multitudes he judged as simply not up to his intellectual rigor.

The medical staff, students, and resident physicians at Johns Hopkins tolerated William's rude and quirky behavior because of his surgical wizardry. His endless capacity for generating new, life-saving operative procedures was truly amazing. Indeed, many seasoned Johns Hopkins doctors advised the offended to thicken their epidermis with the tacit understanding that they were encountering the best surgeon in the world.

Beyond the sharp remarks, reclusive behavior, and rambling lectures, however, were far more troubling behaviors suggesting that Halsted was never quite as clean a recovering addict as the trustees had hoped when they'd appointed him surgeon-in-chief in 1892. To begin, there was Halsted's erratic attendance at work, due to a slew of vague illnesses and his extended vacations in North Carolina and Europe. Such absences without leave wreaked havoc on the daily routines of the hospital and prompted numerous meetings of and reports to the hospital board. In fact, Halsted's absenteeism would surely have resulted in immediate dismissal were he a lesser surgeon.

One odd morning, for example, an entire team of scrubbed nurses and surgeons, along with a nervous and not yet anesthetized patient, waited ninety minutes for his arrival. The flimsy excuse Halsted offered was that he and his wife had been otherwise preoccupied killing rats in their cellar.

On other mornings in the operating room, "with the scalpel in his hand ready to begin the operation, [Dr. Halsted] paused, stood perfectly still, his face gray with anxiety and suffering. Without referring to his condition, he handed the knife to his assistant with an apology and with the request that he continue the operation." Sometimes, Halsted simply sat on a nearby stool for a few minutes, watching the procedure he'd been slated to perform; other times, he exited the operating room, scurried to his office, changed into his street clothes, and left the hospital entirely.

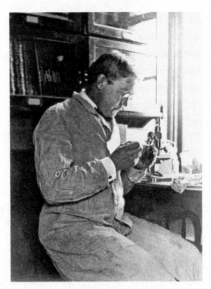

*Joseph Colt Bloodgood, M.D.,
late 1910s to 1920s.*

The aptly named Dr. Joseph C. Bloodgood, one of William's former chief surgical residents, recalled that Halsted often complained of severe tachycardia, an excessively rapid heartbeat, or, as Bloodgood described it, a "thumping of his heart" that Halsted ascribed to smoking too many cigarettes. His staff universally accepted such excuses. Gossiping in early 1931 to H. L. Mencken, Bloodgood described William's many departures of duty in a positive vein:

> This gave me an extraordinary amount of experience, and did me a lot of good. So long as Halsted smoked, whoever was surgical resident at the Johns Hopkins had his hands full. When he stopped smoking he began to do all of his own work. The residents then got less experience, and hence amounted to less when they left.

Halsted was an incurable chain-smoker, and, as noted in the case of Freud's legendary cigar habit, consuming large amounts of nicotine can yield a rapid beating of the heart and even chest pain. Still, it is not surprising that he preferred to blame the cigarettes that stained his snowy-white mustache a sickly yellow for his debilitating symptoms.

With clinical retrospection, however, it seems likely that Halsted's absences and abrupt exits from the operating room had a great deal to do with the other substances he was actively abusing. Taking cocaine, for example, can easily yield trembling hands and annoying heart palpitations, which would prevent a surgeon from operating well. Explaining the effects of morphine is a bit more complicated. If William took too small a dose for his daily morphine requirement or if he tried to abstain completely, he may have experienced withdrawal symptoms, including shaky hands, sweating, and rapid heartbeat, resulting in his professed inability to operate. On the other hand, if he still felt inebriated from the dose of morphine he'd injected the evening before, Halsted might be slow to rise from bed or not show up at the hospital at all.

Professional or pedagogic rationales aside, one compelling reason William may have been so motivated to organize his famously competitive residency training program was an unending taste for morphine and cocaine. Sitting atop a pyramid of eager young doctors willing to stay up to all hours tending to his patients was the perfect vehicle for a surgeon with severe addiction problems. Halsted needed the nightly comfort of his narcotics or the occasional cocaine binge without having to worry that those he operated upon while sober in the morning might suffer from his indisposition that evening. In essence, his drug-induced absences were covered and enabled by the residents. Given the effects of morphine and cocaine on the size and appearance of one's pupils, the days he made the least eye contact with his colleagues, or avoided them outright, may have correlated with his recent drug use and fear of discovery. Those periods in which William "began to do all of his own work," and was all the grumpier for it, likely corresponded with the days, weeks, or months when he was able to abstain from cocaine and could tightly control, if not completely eliminate, his daily dose of morphine.

For decades, almost all the skilled physicians of the Johns Hopkins Hospital failed to put his actions together, diagnose his continued use of morphine and cocaine, or find a means of keeping him away from patients. Even William Osler, who did suspect that something was amiss early in their professional relationship, was hesitant to speak his

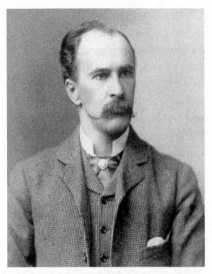

William Osler, c. 1888.

mind freely about Halsted's problem. Public knowledge of his addiction would destroy Halsted and seriously injure the reputation of the Hopkins. Instead, Osler honored Halsted's need for privacy and, in proper historical fashion, left behind an intriguing volume of notes, which was sealed for fifty years. In fact, it contains one of Dr. Osler's most startling clinical discoveries: Halsted's continuing and active addiction to morphine.

OSLER'S MEMOIR HAS LONG reposed in the library bearing his name at McGill University, in Montreal. Bound in black leather, tied with a red ribbon, originally sealed with wax and a now broken silver lock, the text makes the hearts of medical historians instantly beat faster. The "secret" manuscript was willed by Osler to his wife, Lady Grace Revere Osler, in 1919 and, upon her death, in 1928, to her sister and executrix, Susan Revere Chapin. Mrs. Chapin, in 1931, donated the manuscript to the care of W. W. Francis, the dean of Osler's alma mater the McGill Medical School and Sir William's bibliographical protégé. It has been cherished by the McGill faculty ever since.

Titled "The Inner History of the Johns Hopkins Hospital," the memoir is jam-packed with sensitive revelations about the early days of the Hopkins. As a result, Dr. Osler instructed his survivors to neither discuss nor open the manuscript "until preparations are being made to celebrate the hospital's centenary in 1989." Dr. Osler cleverly concealed his furtive essay in a "dummy" copy of a fictional journal he titled *Archives of Medical Sciences* and produced as a practical joke in 1893. The volume was elaborately bound, embossed, and included a fake table of contents listing "articles" by William Welch, Howard Kelly, William Halsted, and himself, under the nom de plume "Egerton Y. Davis."

Some have speculated that Mrs. Chapin and Dean Francis broke the original seal of the manuscript for a prolonged peek sometime in 1928. Whether they read the manuscript or not, we do know that the manuscript was resealed around this time by Mrs. Chapin and that Francis kept his oath of confidentiality. As soon as he died, in 1959, however, scholars began agitating to study and publish the memoirs. The historical record trumped privacy in 1969, and "The Inner History" appeared in the *Johns Hopkins Medical Bulletin,* a full twenty years ahead of the hospital's centennial.

Osler may have composed his stunning observations as early as the 1890s or as late as 1902 to 1905, but the physician did not leave behind enough evidence for a more precise dating. For example, Osler offers an amendment to his remarks about Halsted that is dated January 10, 1898, suggesting that the manuscript may have been written before that date. Seven years later, in 1905, when delivering his valedictory, and inadvertently scandalous, address "The Fixed Period" before leaving Hopkins for a prestigious post at Oxford University, Osler cursorily mentioned that he had recently written about the early days of the hospital. The speech was widely reported in newspapers across the nation, but not because of his announcement of a secret history of the Johns Hopkins Hospital; instead, it was Osler's humorous comment on how men do their best work before the age of forty and how society might be better served if all men over sixty were "chloroformed" that created a media maelstrom.

Dr. Osler probably wrote his "Inner History" late at night in his library on West Franklin Street, at the sturdy, polished library table he'd had imported from England. When he got around to discussing Halsted, Osler began by noting the surgeon's "sharp tongue and a very cynical manner." The epitome of every pupil's most adored professor, Osler could not have appreciated Halsted's refusal to play to the gallery or welcome the medical students into his home. Osler complained that Halsted could be quite "standoffish" until one got to know him personally and detailed his tortured relationships with the local medical community of Baltimore, amicable interactions being an essential aspect of attracting goodwill and patient referrals for the fledgling hospital.

Osler loved a crisp dollar and what it could buy. Not surprisingly, he waxes a tad envious when describing the fees Halsted charged his wealthy patients. After referring one dowager to the surgeon for removal of bile duct stones, Osler complained that Halsted had had the gall to submit a bill for $10,500, or almost $260,000 in 2010 dollars. He did add, however, that the woman recovered from both her financial and her surgical extractions quite nicely.

During the winter of 1893, however, only six months after William's surgical coronation as a Johns Hopkins professor, Osler witnessed telltale signs that his colleague's addiction was active and thriving. Somewhere in the hospital, perhaps in the stairwell, in the library, or along the corridor to his rooms, Osler noticed Halsted shivering as if stricken by a "severe chill." Suffering from neither a cold nor a physical response to the last thrills of a mildly snowy season, Halsted was withdrawing from morphine. He either had run out of the drug he'd first been introduced to at Butler Hospital in Rhode Island or had miscalculated his last dose and was in desperate need of another. This was Osler's "first intimation" that his colleague was "still taking morphia," a habit he'd previously been certain Halsted had abandoned because "he had worked so well and so energetically that it did not seem possible that he could take the drug and do so much."

The benevolent physician took it upon himself to win Halsted's "full confidence" and gain a better understanding of his affliction. After many candid conversations, Osler confirmed his worst suspicions. "He had never," Osler wrote in his secret diary, "been able to reduce the amount to less than three grains daily; on this he could work comfortably and maintain his excellent physical vigor (for he was a very muscular fellow). I do not think that any one suspected him not even

Welch." Three grains, incidentally, is equal to 195 milligrams of morphine, a robust amount that speaks volumes about the level of drug tolerance Halsted had developed because of his chronic and frequent use. On a surgical ward, the typical dose ranges from 5 to 20 milligrams every four hours, depending on the severity of the pain experienced by the patient. For moderate to severe pain (after a major operation, for example), the optimal intramuscular dose is 10 to 20 milligrams per 70 kilograms (154 pounds) of body weight every four hours.

One final but puzzling clue demands to be recounted: on an otherwise blank page of the manuscript, dated January 10, 1898, Osler noted, "Subsequently he got the amount down to 1.5 grains, and of late years (1912) has possibly gotten on without it." On the basis of Osler's recollections, it seems likely that, at a minimum, Halsted was injecting himself with morphine at relatively high doses between the autumn of 1893 and 1898, and probably for much longer than that.

After his intense struggle for resurrection, why did Halsted continue to abuse drugs? Everything he had hoped and worked for was now at his fingertips to enjoy, savor, and perpetuate. Why couldn't he simply stop? For addicts' loved ones this is a familiar quandary. Those fortunate not to have any firsthand knowledge of addiction may never understand it. As for millions of drug addicts, it was never a question of morals, character, intellect, or physical stamina for Halsted; by all accounts he was among the most honorable, vigorous, and hardworking of men. Still, as Dr. Osler attested, at least once a day the surgeon was compelled to satiate his constant hunger for morphine.

Surgeons are consummate risk takers. They never really know, after ordering a patient to be anesthetized, whether or not that person will awaken, let alone recover from the operation about to be performed. The surgeon needs to deny all those risks. He must banish them from his mind in order to muster the courage to invade a patient's body and fix the problem at hand.

Addicts are accomplished at denial and risk taking, too. For William the addict, intoxicating injections of morphine (and, less frequently, cocaine) loomed far more important to his sense of well-being than all of his surgical accomplishments, medical titles, accolades, scientific papers, students, patients, and considerations of personal health and professional reputation combined. Just as they deadened physical

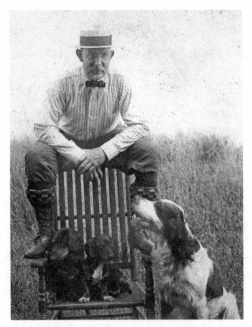

*Halsted, impeccably dressed while relaxing in
North Carolina with his dogs, c. 1904.*

pain, his drugs of choice placed his troubled mind at ease. Halsted routinely gambled his life and career on whether a morphine or cocaine dose might yield a high or permanent oblivion. Perhaps better than any physician alive, he could explain the long-term ravages of addiction on the body and its predictable path to ruin and death. As a consummate medical scientist, he prided himself on being scrupulously honest about a particular technique or medical statement. But William the addict remained unconvinced that the dose he was about to take might bring about his demise. At such moments of intense drug craving, he simply did not care. The unenlightened might demean Halsted's behavior as dishonest; those more acquainted with addiction know that the denials and outright lies—to himself and others—were sentinel symptoms of his illness.

CHAPTER 11

Dr. Freud's Coca Coda

IT WAS INEVITABLE that Freud's relationship with Wilhelm Fliess would end badly. Although their once-amiable accord began to fray before the publication of *The Interpretation of Dreams,* a thunderstorm of animosity erupted in August 1900 when the two met for a "congress" at the Achensee, a lake near Innsbruck. During the trip, they fought constantly. As happens with many good friends who descend into hatred, the taunts and criticisms each hurled at the other were perfectly pitched. Fliess scored his most brutal points by questioning the scientific validity of Freud's psychoanalytical theories. The thin-skinned Sigmund fumed at such impudence, refusing to see Fliess again in person and sharply curtailing their legendary correspondence. A year later, Freud admitted his intellectual debts to Fliess but cruelly reopened their rift: "There is no concealing the fact that the two of us have drawn apart to some extent. . . . [You] have come to the limit of your perspicacity."

The final winds blew on July 20, 1904, after Fliess picked up a copy of a recently published book titled *Sex and Character.* Its author, Otto Weininger, was a twenty-three-year-old convert from Judaism to Protestantism with a Ph.D. from the University of Vienna. Depressed over the tepid reviews his book initially inspired, on October 3, 1903, Weininger retired to his room in the same house where Beethoven had died decades earlier and shot himself in the heart. Taken immediately to the Krankenhaus, he succumbed the following day. Otto's melodramatic end appears to have improved his royalty statements; soon after his funeral, the book became the talk of Vienna's literary and intellectual salons.

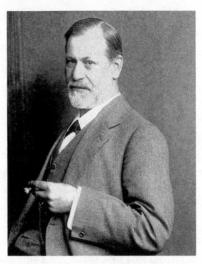

The famous Dr. Freud, 1910.

Sex and Character is a sprawling, racist treatise in which Weininger espoused that women and Jews were bereft of a rational and moral self and, therefore, were unequal to Aryan men and undeserving of simple liberty. Far more troubling to the egocentric Fliess, however, was that Weininger's tome speculated about bisexuality in a manner strikingly similar to what he had discussed with Freud but not yet published. Consequently, in the summer of 1904, Fliess confronted Sigmund about the book.

Freud denied Fliess's charges and described Weininger as "a burglar with a key he had picked up." While he did admit to telling a troubled young man named Hermann Swoboda about Fliess's theories on bisexuality, Freud denied all responsibility and suggested, instead, that Swoboda had conveyed these ideas to Weininger, who'd then incorporated them into his book. Astoundingly, Freud went as far as to imply that Weininger's suicide was "out of fear of his criminal nature."

Fliess subsequently heard from a mutual friend that Weininger had shown Freud an early version of his manuscript and that Sigmund had declared it to be "nonsense" and advised against publishing. Refusing to be placated by even this explanation, Fliess complained that his intellectual property had been stolen and accused Sigmund of being the fence. "I believe," he wrote angrily on July 26, 1904, "in this case you should have called his attention and mine to this 'burglary.' "

A somewhat disingenuous Freud admitted the next day that while he had "forgotten" about meeting with Weininger and regretted handing "over your idea" (via Hermann Swaboda),

> *I do not believe . . . that I should have shouted "Stop, thief" at that time. Above all, it would have been no use because the thief can just as well claim it was his own idea; nor can ideas be patented. One can withhold them—and does so advisedly if one sets great store by one's right of ownership. Once they have been let loose, they go their own way.*

Their now famous correspondence ends at this point. Some historians have generously suggested that Freud felt guilty about this episode as well as a subsequent instance when he appropriated some of Fliess's thoughts on bisexuality for his popular 1901 book, *The Psychopathology of Everyday Life.* Still, one wonders how Freud would have responded if the tables were turned and Fliess had helped himself to some of Sigmund's ideas without proper credit. Certainly, Sigmund's long-held grudge over Carl Koller's primacy in discovering cocaine anesthesia suggests that he would not have reacted terribly well. In later years, Freud rarely, if ever, mentioned Fliess's name; nor was he willing to fully acknowledge the role his once-cherished companion played at the dawn of psychoanalysis. In her dotage, Anna Freud, Sigmund's daughter and the zealous defender of his intellectual legacy, revealed that her father "never talked to her about Fliess."

ANOTHER SOURCE FOR DISSECTING the Fliess-Freud split is Princess Marie Bonaparte. One of Sigmund's favorite analysands and followers, Princess Marie was a disinherited relative of Napoleon Bonaparte's who, thanks to her mother's family fortune, had the funds to pay the ransom for Freud's escape from Nazi-occupied Vienna to England in 1938. She initially consulted Dr. Freud in 1925, her chief complaint being an inability to achieve orgasm while in the missionary position. Historians better recall Princess Marie as the woman who bought and preserved for posterity the Freud-Fliess letters, despite Sigmund's strenuous objections and desire for their destruction. In an unpublished notebook she composed near the end of her long life, Marie wrote:

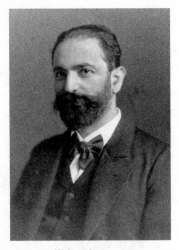

> The friendship with Fliess began to decline as early as 1900 . . . when Freud published the book on dreams. Freud had not realized this! I taught it to him. His friendship with Fliess made him reluctant to impute envy to Fliess. Fliess could not bear the superiority of his friend. Nor could he tolerate, this time according to Freud, Freud's scientific criticisms. . . . Ida Fliess, moreover . . . out of jealousy, did everything possible to sow discord between the two friends, whereas Martha Freud understood very well that Fliess, according to Freud, had as passionate a friendship for Freud as Freud had for Fliess.

Wilhelm Fliess, c. 1904.

Princess Marie offers an insightful analysis of the ultimately corrosive relationship. Doctors are a competitive breed. Few things irritate and disturb a physician's internal balance more than being left behind by the professional successes of a close colleague. These were the years when psychoanalysis was just beginning to be accepted by a small but enthusiastic body of practitioners and patients. Only a decade later, Freud's name would be internationally recognized, albeit often during conversations shrill with controversy and contention. Dr. Fliess simply could not compete with his intellectual juggernaut of a friend. Envious of such medical greatness, Fliess must have grasped that Sigmund's lofty accomplishments would never be his, which likely rankled him. At the same time, Freud seemed incapable of fully acknowledging the important role Fliess played in helping him to articulate so many of his ideas.

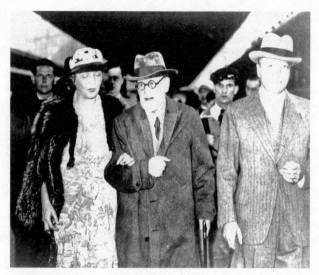

*Freud, with Marie Bonaparte and U.S. ambassador to France
William Bullitt, fleeing Nazi-dominated Vienna via Paris
to London, 1938.*

Others have speculated about the precise boundaries of Fliess and
Freud's relationship, one that may have extended into a physical realm
that could not even be discussed, let alone reconciled, in early-
twentieth-century Vienna. On October 6, 1910, years after the Freud-
Fliess dissolution, Freud wrote a confession of sorts to his colleague and
acolyte Sándor Ferenczi:

> *You have not only noticed, but also understood, that I no longer
> have any need to uncover my personality completely and you correctly
> traced this back to the traumatic reason for it. Since Fliess's case,
> with the overcoming of which you saw me occupied, the need has
> been extinguished. A part of homosexual cathexis has been
> withdrawn and made use of to enlarge my own ego. I have succeeded
> where the paranoiac fails.*

A little more than a week later, Freud wrote Ferenczi, "You probably
imagine that I have secrets quite other than those I have reserved for

myself, or you believe that my secrets are connected with a special sor-
row, whereas I feel capable of handling everything and am pleased with
the greater independence that results from having overcome my homo-
sexuality." The following year, Freud wrote Ferenczi, and made his final
mention of Fliess in his copious correspondence: "I have now overcome Fliess, about whom you were so curious."

TO BE SURE, the effects of professional jealousy or a love affair gone
sour eat away at the most stable of human relationships. Yet still
another explanation is worth considering. Freud may have felt a need
to pull away from Fliess in the years after forsaking cocaine. Many substance abusers predictably share drugs or alcohol with others. Addiction experts today characterize such acquaintances as "using buddies"
and insist that terminating these relationships is the sine qua non of
successful recovery. This is especially true for a tantalizing drug like
cocaine. As recovering addicts have learned the hard way, spending significant time with one's using buddies all but invites relapse. Any doctor in Vienna at the turn of the last century could have procured as
much cocaine as his pocketbook allowed. But there is no question that
Freud's cocaine abuse was often facilitated by Wilhelm Fliess. The two
doctors may have even abused the drug together during their many
"congresses." One only wonders if Freud, at some level, appreciated
this risk to his sobriety as he converted Fliess from an "intimate friend"
into his "hated enemy."

Sigmund represented many fields of inquiry during his long and
productive life, but for much of it he enjoyed his standing as a member
of the medical profession. In 1925, Freud glibly recalled that as a young
man he did not feel "any particular predilection for the career of a doctor. I was moved rather by a sort of curiosity, which was, however,
directed more towards human concerns, than towards natural objects."
Retrospective recollections aside, there can be no question about his
profound commitment to being a healer. He was immersed and social-
ized into the profession during the most formative years of his adult
life, a period that coincided with one of the most progressive periods in
the history of medicine. Even after years of enduring hostility and verbal abuse from his colleagues, he devoted his life to caring for patients

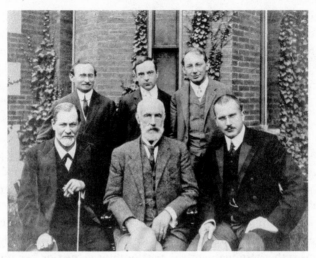

*Freud with G. S. Hall and Carl Jung, front row. Second row, left
to right, are some of Freud's best pupils: A. A. Brill, Ernest Jones,
and Sándor Ferenczi. The occasion was the Clark University
Vigentennial Celebration, which featured Freud's lectures on the
origins and development of psychoanalysis as well as
a symposium on psychology and pedagogy, 1909.*

and developing new ways to make them feel better. In 1908, for example, an associate declared his desire to elevate Sigmund's status to that
of a revolutionary moral philosopher. Freud replied, "We are doctors,
and doctors it is our intention to remain."

By understanding the depth of Sigmund's identity as a doctor, one
begins to appreciate why Emma Eckstein so thoroughly haunted his
dreams. The cunning Freud, always with his eyes aimed toward posterity, was often less than candid about the actual details of the episode.
Nevertheless, it seems almost inevitable that a soul as sensitive as Sigmund's would frequently revisit it in a distressed state of mind or during his late-night hours of self-analysis. Even as late as 1910, Sigmund
confessed to Ferenczi that he continued to be troubled by his relationship with Fliess and, perhaps by extension, the Emma Eckstein fiasco:
"That you surmised I had great secrets, and were very curious about
them, was plain to see and also easy to recognize as infantile. . . . My

dreams at that time were concerned, as I hinted to you, entirely with the Fliess affair, which in the nature of things would be hard to arouse your sympathy."

When contemplating or dreaming about the botched nose operation, Sigmund must have realized at some level that had Emma Eckstein died, much of the blame and consequences would have rested upon his painfully rounded shoulders. Such an act of malpractice could only have added to the guilt he felt over the death of his friend Fleischl-Marxow, whom Sigmund had accidentally transformed into a cocaine addict a few years earlier.

At some point in every addict's life comes the moment when what started as a recreational escape devolves into an endless reserve of negative physical, emotional, and social consequences. Those seeking recovery today call this drug-induced nadir a "bottom." Caught in a maelstrom of catastrophe, many substance abusers can be inspired or forced into taking the necessary steps to quit or, at least, temporarily abstain. The bottom that Sigmund experienced featured far more than the physical and mental ravages of consuming too much cocaine; it involved Wilhelm Fliess, Emma Eckstein, and the misguided surgical procedure that nearly took Emma's life and destroyed Freud's hard-won career. If he was ever to rid himself of these destructive forces, he needed to abandon cocaine, sever his friendship with Fliess, and alter his experiences with Emma from a clinical debacle into the dazzling thesis that helped shape *The Interpretation of Dreams.*

BETWEEN 1896 AND HIS DEATH IN 1939, Freud rarely discusses cocaine in his letters or published work. Indeed, he did his best to distance himself from the subject. On occasion, he comments on Koller and the events of 1884–86, spinning tales about missing an important discovery that was literally in front of his nose. At a few other points in time, he mentions recent publications about cocaine that caught his eye. But there are a few instances where he offers far more alluring references to the drug.

In June 1908, Jung was treating a patient named Otto Gross, a physician, psychoanalyst, and colleague of Freud's, for acute paranoia. Gross also had a long history of active addiction to both cocaine and morphine. Writing to Jung, Freud observed, "I attributed it [Gross's behavior] to the medication, especially cocaine, which, as I well know, produces a toxic paranoia." The phrase "as I well know" is alluring, to say the least, but with the distance of time it is difficult to discern whether Freud was referring to his own experiences with cocaine or was basing this comment on his clinical observations of either Gross or Fleischl-Marxow.

Nearly a decade later, in June 1916, Freud explained to Sándor Ferenczi that cocaine, "if taken to excess," could produce symptoms of paranoia and that those who stopped using the drug experienced severe withdrawal symptoms, often leading to a relapse. He further observed that drug addicts were not very suitable for analytic treatment because every backsliding or difficulty in the analysis led to further recourse to the drug. Only a few months earlier, in February 1916, Sigmund had obliquely written to Ferenczi that his love of cigars kept him from working out specific psychological problems. One wonders whether his compulsive cocaine abuse from 1884 to 1896 was one of those unexplored problems.

Most recovering addicts insist that two touchstones of a successful recovery are daily routines and rigorous accountability. Fortunately for Freud, Martha managed the household at Berggasse 19 with precision. She may have complained of relentless domestic tasks, but her close attention to the schedules, meals, and virtually every other activity in their spacious flat allowed Sigmund to focus exclusively on his work and patients. Because he conducted most of his career in a set of three rooms directly attached to the family quarters, Martha orchestrated reliable but controlled contact with his children, whom he numbered among the great joys of his life.

From Monday through Saturday, during his working life as a psychoanalyst in Vienna, Freud rose from his bed promptly before seven a.m., bathed, partook of a light breakfast and coffee, and sat for a daily trim of his beard and hair by a barber who made house calls. At eight a.m., Freud greeted his first patient and began a fifty-five-minute analytic session. Once his practice started to flourish, Sigmund saw twelve or more patients a day. He typically took a break from one to three p.m.,

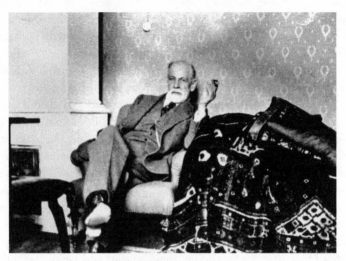

Freud and the famous couch, c. 1932.

enjoying a family lunch and a walk to clear his head before returning to his consulting room with the famous couch and more patients to analyze. There were also brief visits with colleagues and his children, trips around the corner to the tobacconist for his daily fix of cigars, perhaps another cup of coffee for energy, lectures to his medical students at the University of Vienna, and an evening meal with the entire family. Virtually every week, he attended meetings of the Vienna Medical Society and the Vienna B'nai B'rith men's lodge, as well as gatherings of his like-minded colleagues and acolytes eager to discuss psychoanalysis.

This overflowing agenda does not even begin to account for the time he spent each night, and well into the early morning, reflecting on his psyche and those of others. These were the critical hours when he composed and ruminated over the many books and papers containing his claim to intellectual immortality. From fall to late spring, he limited his recreation to Saturday nights, attending lectures and plays or playing cards and chess, although later in life he claimed to find the latter too stressful a leisure activity. Sundays were supposed to be a sacrosanct day of rest in the company of his beloved children, mother, wife, and friends. More often than not, he managed to steal a few hours away from his self-imposed, secular Sabbath to write a few pages of his latest

manuscript. Every summer, Sigmund and his family took a long vacation filled with restorative hikes in the mountains, playful activities
with his children, and reading for pleasure.

With Freud's intense work schedule and the daily demands he made
on his mind and body, one could easily argue that there was little room
for cocaine abuse. Cocaine may have briefly picked him up and given
him energy during the early years of his career, but, especially as he
aged, his body began to rebel against the intensely draining peaks and
valleys of mood the drug instigated. Cocaine highs resulted in a disjointed prose that was best relegated to the wastebasket. The lows of
cocaine abruptly halted the productive commitment of pen to paper
and thwarted his ability to complete useful thoughts about the complex topics he tackled. The ever-driven Sigmund, one of the most prolific and persuasive intellectual authors of the twentieth century, simply
did not have the time for cocaine's hour-stealing and rapidly debilitating effects.

All of these exercises—the never-ending demand for new manuscripts, students and patients to see, friends and colleagues to talk with,
thinking about his mental health as well as the mental health of others,
packaged in predictable routines and demanding constant accountability to so many—served as the ideal therapeutic program he required for
his recovery from substance abuse. Admittedly, the precise means
Freud used to keep his mind off cocaine were markedly different, if not
unique, when compared to the methods of the overwhelming majority
of recovering addicts.

One only wishes that he'd had similar fortitude to put down his
addictive and cancer-producing cigars, which, beginning in 1923, at age
sixty-seven, robbed him of an intact, functioning mouth and forced
him to undergo multiple painful surgeries and wear ill-fitting prosthe-
ses. On September 21, 1939, a year after he fled Nazi-dominated Austria
for London, a cancer-riddled Freud asked his physician Max Schur for
a fatal dose of morphine to end his life. Freud was reported to have
said, "Schur, you remember our 'contract' not to leave me in the lurch
when the time had come. Now it is nothing but torture and makes no
sense." Dr. Schur administered a large dose of morphine that day, after
which Freud sank into a deep sleep but did not die; a second (and perhaps a third) dose was given the following day, and Freud went into a

coma from which he did not awake. He died at three a.m. on September 23, 1939.

THE DIVIDENDS OF SIGMUND'S "recovery program" from 1896 to 1939 are easily quantifiable. These were the years when he became one of the greatest intellectuals of his generation and provided a modern language for understanding the unconscious mind; when his fertile mind brimmed over with new ideas about neuroses, psychoses, sexuality, the development and refinement of the psychoanalytic relationship, and the interpretation of just about everything; and when he delivered countless lectures and led seminars for aspiring therapists, students, and acolytes. All of these accomplishments grew out of his Herculean ability to summon the intense concentration and mental acuity to write book after book—works that continue to shape our beliefs about human behavior and incite heated debate among great minds.

Just as there have been multiple arguments over the veracity of Freud's ideas, there have been contentious discussions about his cocaine abuse and its influence on his work. One of the most controversial studies was published in 1983 by a British librarian named E. M. Thornton. In a book entitled *Freud and Cocaine: The Freudian Fallacy,* she presents a disjointed ad hominem brief claiming that all of Freud's "bizarre set of hypotheses" resulted exclusively from cocaine intoxication and should, therefore, be considered invalid. In recent years, other scholars have offered more nuanced contemplations on the connection of Sigmund's cocaine abuse to his signature ideas about accessing unconscious thoughts with talk therapy; the division of how our mind processes pleasure and reality; the interpretation of dreams; the nature of our thoughts and sexual development; the Oedipus complex; and the elaboration of the id, ego, and superego. Most intriguing is a theory articulated by the historian Peter Swales that "Freud's [concept of the] libido is merely a mask and a symbol for cocaine; the drug, or rather its invisible ghost, haunts the whole of Freud's writing to the very end."

It is enticing to suggest a causal relationship between Sigmund's cocaine abuse and the thinking that produced the origins of psychoanalysis. Such a singular answer appeals to the way we humans think but rarely, if ever, explains the human predicament. Although his dependence on the drug and the behavioral highs and lows produced by its abuse were certainly factors in his complex intellectual and psychological life between 1884 and 1896, I remain hesitant to consign Freud's entire body of work during that period to an endless line of cocaine. For all the reasons enumerated, it appears unlikely that Sigmund used cocaine after 1896, during the years when he mapped out and composed his best-known and most influential works, significantly enriched and revised the techniques of psychoanalysis, and, in keeping with his identification with Sophocles' Oedipus Rex, attempted to "explain some of the great riddles of human existence."

That said, we also know that the last four years of the nineteenth century marked a significant period of depression for Freud. Many addicts who give up their drug of choice seek other intoxicants or pleasures, and Sigmund was no exception. There remains the suggestive evidence of a rather risky sexual relationship with Minna Bernays, especially during the summer of 1898 in the Swiss Alps. A year later, Sigmund engaged in a brief attempt to self-medicate away his melancholia by consuming dozens of bottles of wine. It is all but certain that his depression, cocaine urges, occasional binge drinking, sexual affairs, caustic behaviors, and emotional absence negatively affected his wife, children, colleagues, and friends. Recovering alcoholics and addicts today might recognize the Freud of these years as a "dry drunk," a person who has quit drinking or abusing his drug of choice but is unhappy about it and often makes everyone else around him miserable. In the decades that followed, Sigmund's constant endeavor at self-analysis may have helped tamp down his desire to abuse cocaine or engage in counterproductive behaviors. But during the early years after quitting cocaine, he must have been difficult to live with.

The clinical odds of beating cocaine dependency are daunting; recent studies of addicts have found that, statistically speaking, fewer than one in four remain sober after five years. One doubts that the chances were that much better in 1896 when Freud testified to putting aside his cocaine brush. Yet many cocaine abusers, past and present, do enter recovery successfully. And with Sigmund Freud, we are describing a self-controlled individual highly motivated to protect grand professional ambitions and treasured personal relationships that were imminently threatened by cocaine.

It is also clear that Freud kept his own counsel as his id battled his ego and superego and he attempted to divine the secrets of others. The precise details of his cocaine use both before and after 1896 may well be among those secrets. Such elusive puzzles recall the historian's basic dilemma: the absence of evidence does not always signify evidence of absence. In the end, we will likely never know.

CHAPTER 12

Dr. Halsted in Limbo

IN 1905 MARY ELIZABETH GARRETT, heiress to the fortune generated by the Baltimore and Ohio Railroad and a major benefactress to the Johns Hopkins Medical School, commissioned John Singer Sargent to paint a portrait of William Welch, William Osler, Howard Kelly, and William Halsted. That June, Welch, Kelly, and Halsted sailed for Southampton and traveled to London. There they reunited with Osler, who had left Johns Hopkins a year earlier to become the Regius Professor of Medicine at Oxford, and all four made their way to Sargent's famous studio at 33 Tite Street, near the Chelsea Embankment.

For days, the physicians sat under a sunlit skylight in a stifling hot, poorly ventilated room redolent with the noxious fumes of oil paint, turpentine, and sweat. Some afternoons all four were in the studio; others, they each came alone. All four doctors agreed to pose in their heavy woolen academic robes and hoods, resplendently lined in satin with the class colors of their alma maters: McGill, Yale, the University of Pennsylvania, and Columbia.

Initially, Sargent could not make up his mind about the painting's composition. He paced up and down the room, chain-smoking cigarettes, while the doctors, none of them known for their patience, allowed themselves to be positioned and repositioned according to the artist's latest whim. Sargent was said to have pulled at his hair, exclaiming, "It won't do. It isn't a picture. I cannot see just what to do."

By the time his subjects left the studio and returned to their demanding work, Sargent was on his way to creating a divine gem of portraiture; the painting captures the men's characters and insatiable

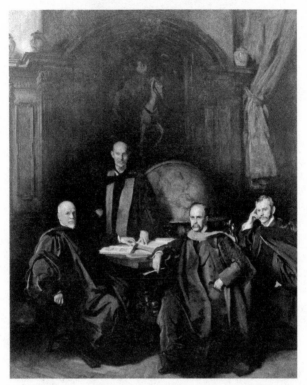

The Four Doctors *by John Singer Sargent (1906).*
From left to right: Welch, Halsted, Osler, and Kelly.

lust for inquiry. On a canvas measuring roughly eleven by nine feet, the four doctors are arranged around a book-strewn reading table and an antique Venetian globe so large that Sargent had to chop open the doorway and surrounding wall of his studio to allow for its entry. In the painting's background hangs a facsimile of El Greco's *Saint Martin and the Beggar.* Osler appears as if about to leap to his feet to aid a patient; Welch, the kingmaker, sits satisfied, his fingers resting on the leaves of an open tome; Kelly is beatific, as if he has just "saved" another soul for Jesus. Even truer to life, standing in Welch's shadow, with a dark, brooding pall cast over his face, is William Stewart Halsted.

Legend has it that Halsted was difficult and argumentative during the sittings, and that the artist threatened to use shoddy paints so that

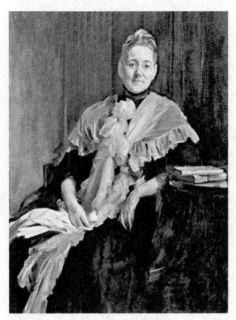

*Mary Elizabeth Garrett; 1904 portrait
by John Singer Sargent.*

in the years to come the surgeon's face would gradually fade from the picture. Fortunately, Sargent never made good on his threat. More than a century later, Dr. Halsted's visage is still powerfully visible. And while gazing intently at his stunning portrait, a viewer can easily imagine that he is peering into the soul of a troubled man.

As gifted an artist as Sargent was, however, he was not qualified to diagnose Halsted's addiction during his visual inspections of the surgeon's face and body. Instead, that onerous task—one that required more than the eyes alone—fell to William's former chief resident, a talented surgeon named George J. Heuer.

AFTER GRADUATING FROM the Johns Hopkins Medical School in 1907, Dr. Heuer spent the next seven years toiling away on Halsted's elite surgical service. In 1915, he sailed for Germany, but his studies there were abbreviated because of the events we now call World War I.

A captain in the American Expeditionary Force, Heuer distinguished himself as a combat surgeon specializing in penetrating chest wounds and thoracic surgery. After the war, Heuer returned to the Hopkins as an associate professor and thence to appointments as surgeon-in-chief and professor, first at the Cincinnati General Hospital and University of Cincinnati (1922–32) and then at the New York Hospital and Cornell Medical College (1932–47).

Devoted to his mentor until his dying day, Heuer knew deep in his doctor's gut that something was not right about Halsted. And true to his professional calling, Heuer was determined to uncover just what was at the root of Dr. Halsted's countless bad days. He wanted to explain what was behind the anguish and pain Sargent had portrayed. Why the stinging gibes in which the surgeon directed his inner hatred, a sharp knife indeed, out toward others? What about all the episodes of too shaky hands or too rapid a heartbeat that prevented him from operating? Why was William so often absent at critical times in the lives of his patients and students? What did he do when he disappeared every summer? And most peculiarly, why was William routinely incommunicado from approximately four-thirty each afternoon until nine or ten the next morning, while his vaunted residents ran the Johns Hopkins Hospital's world-famous surgery service?

By the time Heuer walked the wards at the Hopkins, Halsted's earlier battles with cocaine were the stuff of heroic legend. Interns and medical students had long murmured and bruited about Halsted's "New York episode." Many assumed that this part of William's life had ended precisely when Welch finagled his appointment to the faculty at Johns Hopkins. As the story went, William abandoned his old habits and, while a bit more the cantankerous for it, proceeded on to greater things. Osler's "Inner History," of course, had not yet seen the light of day. Consequently, when looking objectively at William's remarkable record of accomplishment, his development of so many surgical procedures, his creation of the surgical residency program, and his publication of so many lucidly written and pathbreaking papers, many subscribed to this version of abstinence. Or as lawyers like to quip, *res ipsa loquitur*—the thing speaks for itself.

This was precisely the tale told in the authorized biography *William Stewart Halsted, Surgeon* by the eminent Johns Hopkins pathologist

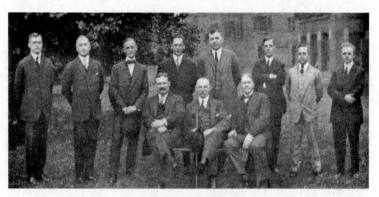

*Dr. Halsted with his early associate and resident surgeons at the twenty-fifth
anniversary of the opening of the Johns Hopkins Hospital, October 7, 1914.
Standing, left to right: Roy D. McClure, Hugh H. Young, Harvey Cushing,
James F. Mitchell, Richard H. Follis, Robert T. Miller Jr., John W. Churchman,
George J. Heuer; seated, left to right: John M. T. Finney, William S. Halsted,
Joseph C. Bloodgood.*

W. G. MacCallum. Published in 1930 and widely distributed to medical libraries across the nation, the book was read by countless aspiring
surgeons for the next several decades. The biography's introduction,
written by William Henry Welch, acknowledges Halsted's cocaine
episode of the late 1880s but does so in a somewhat heroic style:

> In the pages of this narrative will be found the story of the
> break-down in Halsted's health and of the circumstances which
> brought him to me in Baltimore. I had guarded unviolated for so
> many years the confidence which Halsted had placed in me that
> I confess I was surprised to learn that the secret was more widely
> known than I had suspected, and its publication after his death
> shocked me. I now realize that not only should the facts be made
> known, but that instead of reflecting injuriously upon Halsted's
> character, they bring out a triumphant issue of hard struggle
> rarely exemplified in similar circumstances.

Yet despite Welch's provocative introduction, the book devotes only
a few pages to exploring Halsted's addiction. Even when MacCallum

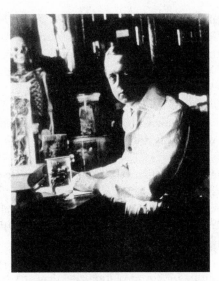

*William G. MacCallum, professor of
pathology at Johns Hopkins and Halsted's
first biographer, c. 1903–04.*

describes Halsted's cocaine bottom, he effectively closes the discussion
with a theme of permanent triumph:

> Dr. Halsted did not escape. Those who knew of it kept it for
> many years a secret, and perhaps some of them may still feel that
> it would be better forgotten, but it is with no thought of uncov-
> ering a disgrace or belittling him that we speak of it freely. For,
> first of all, those early victims were quite innocent of any knowl-
> edge of its habit-forming character, and secondly, he almost
> alone of the many who fell under its influence, conquered it
> through superhuman strength and determination and came back
> to a splendid life of achievement. . . . After this interval he came
> back to a far more thoughtful, leisurely life, with time for reflec-
> tion and contemplation of his surgical problems, a life in the end
> far more fruitful than could ever have been the strenuous rush of
> his existence in New York if he had kept on at that pace. After all,
> in his case it was probably no misfortune but rather the reverse.

This "official history" as articulated by MacCallum, however, failed to tally with George Heuer's firsthand observations. As such, Heuer decided to research and write his own biography, a book that garnered interest from a New York publisher during the 1940s but only appeared in print after Heuer's death as a special supplement of the *Johns Hopkins Hospital Bulletin* in 1952. For more than two decades, Dr. Heuer dissected his boss's disease with the same care and attention William devoted to the women suffering from breast cancer in his famous operating room.

The surgeon began his literary postmortem by reviewing Dr. Halsted's enormous collection of papers and manuscripts carefully cataloged and filed in the archives of the Johns Hopkins Medical Institutions. Piquing his curiosity were a series of letters to Halsted's friend Rudolph Matas, a distinguished professor of surgery at Tulane University. In early 1920, Dr. Matas petitioned the National Dental Association to recognize "the Professor" for revolutionizing dentistry by introducing nerve blockade, or local anesthesia. For months, Matas pestered Halsted to write down his thoughts and recollections of the cocaine episode of 1884–85 in order to gather the evidence needed for the judging committee, which ultimately ruled in Halsted's favor.

William freely described the surgical details to Matas but remained less than forthcoming about his personal experiences with cocaine. For example, in May 1921 he vaguely, if not dishonestly, jotted to Matas:

> You are indeed a sturdy friend. I wrote very little on the subject of my cocaine experiments, which for a year were carried on vigorously. Then my health gave way, due primarily to an infected finger and the horrible pains from the neuritis that resulted. For more than a year, I was incapacitated, and thereafter for two years worked in the Pathological Laboratory of Dr. Welch at the Johns Hopkins. Thus my misfortune has its bright as well as its gloomy side.

Less than a year later, after a grand dinner celebrating his contributions held at the Maryland State Dental Association on April 1, 1922, Halsted wistfully wrote his friend Matas:

> How can I ever express my gratitude to you for this act of unparalleled kindness—an act which has covered two years. . . .

Not a wink of sleep did I get during the night of Saturday, I was too exhilarated for repose. Once before in my life was I kept awake by great happiness; this was the night that I passed successfully the examination for Bellevue Hospital in 1876. Then, it was in contemplation of the future, now in reflection upon the good fortune that led to our friendship. The reaction from this great joy seems to be setting in tonight and my happiness is tinged with regret for the lost opportunities—for the time wasted from loss of health.

Unsatisfied by these scant archival remnants, Dr. Heuer dashed off dozens of letters to the doctors, nurses, secretaries, librarians, medical students, and former residents who'd spent significant time with Halsted. The scandalous nature of addiction during this era combined with a desire to protect Halsted's reputation generated a resounding silence—most of the recipients simply refused to answer. Nonetheless, a few responses did make their way back to Heuer.

One reply was from W. G. MacCallum, Halsted's authorized defender and biographer. Only days earlier, Heuer had written asking MacCallum about the evidence he had with respect to William's abstinence from cocaine and respectfully inquired if the aging pathologist might have glossed over evidence to the contrary. In a frosty reply handwritten on December 18, 1940, Dr. MacCallum insisted that he had thoroughly investigated the matter and discussed it with several of Halsted's former residents:

> _All_ [MacCallum's underline] *said there was no direct evidence of his having still taken any cocaine and all agreed that he could not have maintained such activity and keenness of intellect if he had continued all those years as an addict. There was not in the least disagreement about it and I feel and did feel at that time, that they were correct about it and never believed that he continued to take any cocaine. I did not hesitate in writing as I did about his recovery. I would like to know on what basis of reliable evidence all these surgeons are still discussing it.*

Similarly, two of Mrs. Halsted's nieces and several secretaries who worked in his home all swore on a proverbial stack of Bibles that "never

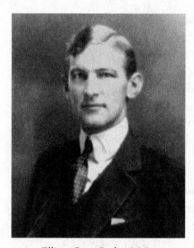

*Elliott Carr Cutler, M.D.,
age thirty-six, in 1924.*

in their association with him was there the slightest evidence of drug addiction."

The most damning testimony came in the form of some handwritten notes of a conversation with the world-renowned neurosurgeon Harvey Cushing on March 1, 1931, several months after the publication of MacCallum's biography. The notes actually represent a roundabout piece of historical documentation in that they were recorded by Dr. Elliott Carr Cutler, a cardiovascular surgeon and one of Cushing's favorite colleagues at Harvard's Peter Bent Brigham Hospital, where Cushing was long surgeon-in-chief.

Dr. Cutler scribbled down Cushing's confidential musings and secreted them away in his files for almost nine years. On November 10, 1939, just over a month after Cushing died of a heart attack, Cutler allowed Heuer to copy the notes. So powerful and controversial were the claims that when Heuer's biography finally appeared in print they were slightly amended as being the remarks of a "well-known surgeon" rather than directly attributed to Harvey Cushing. While this is not a perfect line of evidence, none of these individuals was prone to exaggeration or lying, nor was there any secondary gain to be had, some seventeen years after Halsted's death, by vilifying or embarrassing their teacher, a man they had deeply respected if not always understood.

Cushing was particularly qualified to bear witness because of the many years he'd spent as Halsted's resident, surgical disciple, and key associate at the Johns Hopkins Hospital, from 1896 to 1912. During that time, Cushing often stood directly next to Halsted at his famous wooden operating table. Moreover, Cushing labored at the Hopkins for several years after Osler wrote his hidden memoir of Halsted's

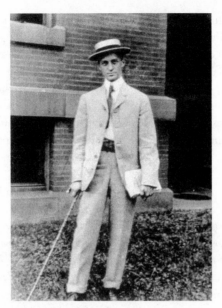

*Harvey Cushing as a young surgical resident
at Johns Hopkins Hospital, c. 1900.*

morphine use. Finally, the multitalented neurosurgeon was also an obsessively detail-oriented historian. In addition to many hundreds of surgical papers, books, research reports, and medical monographs, Cushing wrote the critically acclaimed biography *Life of Sir William Osler,* which won the Pulitzer Prize in 1926. In all his pursuits, Cushing was regarded as a skilled physician and an astute observer determined to get it right—whether deftly removing a rapidly expanding brain tumor, correctly ascertaining a particularly elusive diagnosis, or accurately recounting the history of medicine and surgery.

Long after leaving Baltimore for Boston, Dr. Cushing kept in close contact with Halsted and frequently wrote his chief solicitous letters. Earlier in his career, however, Cushing had often been frustrated by Dr. Halsted's mysterious airs, his inability to quickly make up his mind, his frequent absenteeism accompanied by odd excuses, and his too easy relegation of surgical cases to his assistants. As a junior surgical resident at the Hopkins, Cushing went as far as to misjudge Halsted as lazy. In

March 1898, the young surgeon complained to his then sweetheart and soon-to-be-wife, Kate Crowell: "Here I am, a youth, doing surgical work that not one of my school confreres will hope to do for years. It frightens me sometimes. The Chief rarely operates. Today I did all of his cases."

In the years that followed, however, Cushing revised his diagnosis of Dr. Halsted from slothful to something far more serious. In fact, Cushing's comments to Elliott Cutler comprise some of the most intriguing clues to be found on William's heavily shrouded addiction and, while a bit hyperbolic, merit quoting in their entirety:

> In a discussion of MacCallum's book, the Chief [Cushing] pointed out the very abrupt change in Halsted's nature when he moved from New York to Baltimore; that he had been a rigorous, rather showy, didactic, bustling individual. He became a very refined and most punctilious and fastidious individual. In the interim between New York and Baltimore, he acquired the cocaine habit. The real truth of the matter is that he never conquered it. There are several proofs of this and perhaps MacCallum should have faced this, for he must have known it and should have published it in his book, for it would have been a wonderful story of a person who, like De Quincey, acquired a precarious habit to death and old age unbeknownst to the rest of the world.
>
> There are many instances in support of this. Shortly after accepting the Hopkins post he took a big trip to South America and took with him not quite enough cocaine to make the trip, hoping that he could cut his daily dose down. But he could not do this and found himself about the Equator sailing home with no cocaine. He rifled the captain's store and stole what was there—a fact which has not got out.
>
> Moreover, his change in philosophy is entirely in keeping with the cocaine habit. The story of his going home at 4:30 every day and locking himself in his room an hour and a half before dinner, the stories of his many trips to Europe each summer when he never saw anyone but locked himself in a hotel room and took his drug, and the fact that Reid Hunt [a professor of pharmacology at Harvard and formerly a Johns Hopkins faculty member] knew all along that he was taking cocaine, leaving to those who know this the

feeling that MacCallum failed to write one of the greatest romances of modern life.

There is another very interesting side to this Jekyll and Hyde character. That is that it might even seem that the whole Halsted school of surgery which I have called a School for Safety in surgery may have been due to this drug addiction. Note that Halsted before this addiction with cocaine was a brilliant, rapid, spectacular operator, that just as he changed his character and his dress to that of a fastidious person, paying great attention to details—a matter which characterizes cocaine addicts—so his outlook on surgery itself was changed and he in turn devoted himself to the infinite precision of little details of surgery. There was no longer the picture of the brilliant operator but the cautious individual with tremendous and profound devotion to the little things. His fastidiousness in disposition was carried to fastidiousness in technical surgery and this change in character, which has given rise to the greatest school in surgery this country has ever seen, may have been due to cocaine addiction. What a romance! And what a wonderful example of how destinies of men are influenced by extremely little things!

ONE OF THE GREAT IRONIES to be found in the lives of many physicians is that their final illnesses often mirror the pathological conditions they pursued during their careers. Dr. Halsted is no exception. Three years before his death, on September 7, 1919, he underwent a protracted operation to remove his gallbladder and clean out his common bile duct, which was filled with "an abundance of putty-like material." His convalescence was tumultuous, and within a few months, his body rebelled with bouts of severe abdominal pain. By early August 1922, while he was relaxing at High Hampton, North Carolina, the episodes had progressed to daily ordeals. The riot of excruciating gallstones lodged in his liver, causing nausea, chills, fever, vomiting, and jaundice, was unrelenting. On August 21, he had little choice but to make a perilous and jostling journey by horse-drawn carriage, automobile, and train from his remote country home in North Carolina to Baltimore.

Dr. Karl Schlaepfer, the surgeon who admitted William to the Johns Hopkins Hospital on August 23, 1922, described him as "in a condition which terrified every doctor who saw him: deeply jaundiced, dehydrated, under the effect of the constant use of morphia for weeks due to the fact that no day passed without a severe attack." Initially, Halsted feared the risks of submitting to an operation he had perfected, if not invented. The worsening jaundice accompanied by spiking fevers—all signs of obstruction, infection, and impending death—eventually persuaded him to proceed.

His former chief residents Mont Reid and George Heuer, now prominent surgeons in their own right, entrained from Cincinnati to perform the procedure. Once he was out of the operating room on August 25, William's course only became stormier. In early September, he developed pancreatitis, pneumonia, and a series of gastrointestinal hemorrhages. Despite multiple blood transfusions and valiant efforts by his physicians, he died on September 7, 1922.

At this point in the narrative, the evidentiary trail diverges somewhat. In Heuer's biography, Dr. Mont Reid, one of the two physicians of record for Halsted's last illness, insisted that he "was certain that [Halsted] was not addicted" to cocaine or morphine. Similarly, the nurses who took care of "the Professor" during his last illness are collectively quoted as stating that "he failed to show any deprivation symptoms." The other doctor attending Halsted during his last illness, George Heuer, leaves no direct comment on William's requirements for morphine or cocaine, perhaps feeling bound to his Hippocratic oath of never divulging the treatment of a patient to others.

Sometime in the early 1950s, the Johns Hopkins ear, nose, and throat surgeon Samuel J. Crowe peeked at Halsted's final hospital chart while writing a book about his life and surgical legacy. Like Heuer's book, it, too, was published posthumously. In this account, however, Crowe asserted that for the last three months of his life Halsted was self-administering a quarter grain (about 16 milligrams) a day of morphine, divided into four or more doses, for the painful biliary colic he was experiencing. Halsted, Crowe claims, brought an extremely dilute solution of morphine with him to Baltimore, and it appears that it was from this supply that his injections were derived during his hospitalization. Such a small dosage suggests that William was able to cut down his daily morphine requirement considerably over the years, especially when compared to the hefty three grains (195 milligrams) he was consuming daily in the 1890s when Osler wrote about him in his "Inner History." Interestingly, as a practicing surgeon, Halsted worried about drug toxicity and addiction, always insisting that if morphine was to relieve postoperative pain, "a very small dose will do it just as effectively as a large dose and with less side effects." Consequently, his patients at Johns Hopkins were rarely given more than one-tenth of a grain, or 6.4 milligrams, without his express permission. Conversely, there exists the possibility that as Halsted confessed his own doses to his Johns Hopkins physicians he minimized and obscured the exact amounts he was injecting.

In 1971, Emile Holman, a prominent professor of surgery at Stanford University, published yet another fascinating account of Halsted's addiction. In it, Holman quotes the more than thirty-year-old memories of a urologist named David Sprong. In 1934, Dr. Sprong was a house officer (or training physician) at the Johns Hopkins Hospital taking care of William Henry Welch. Sometime before Welch's death on April 30, 1934, Sprong reported, Welch had told him:

> Although it has been widely reported that Halsted conquered his addiction, this is not entirely true. As long as he lived he would occasionally have a relapse and go back to the drug. He would always go out of town for this and when he returned he would come to me, very contrite and apologetic, to confess. He had an idea that I could tell what he had done. I couldn't but I let him go on thinking so because I felt it was good for him to have somebody to talk it over with.

This, of course, is an astounding statement. Yet even if the words ring as true as a well-cast bell, it does raise a question: Why would Welch, who zealously protected Halsted's secret for more than a half a century, make such a convicting admission to a junior physician?

Whether one believes that Dr. Welch made this last statement or not, after weighing all the evidence, Dr. Cushing's posthumous diagnosis remains the most compelling: "The real truth of the matter is that he never conquered it." Indeed, the biographical, archival, and clinical

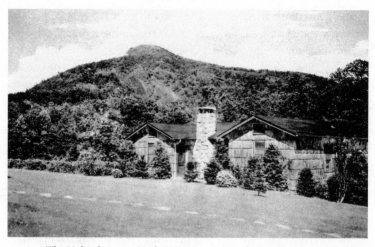

The Halsted cottage High Hampton, in North Carolina, c. 1920.

data strongly suggest that William remained an active morphine and cocaine addict until the final days of his life. Few would doubt that nearly thirty-eight years of morphine and cocaine exacted a harsh toll on his physical health. Less measurable at this late date are the psychic wounds he incurred by living a double life for such a long time. Every day, he was forced to spin a web of falsehoods obscuring the fact that the world's greatest surgeon was a ravenous drug addict.

Halsted, of course, had a vested interest in submerging his thoughts, urges, and actions about cocaine and morphine to avoid the slightest risk of dimming his lustrous reputation. Yet one can imagine that on many mornings he awoke hoping that this day would be different. That he would not succumb to his body's desperate need for self-medication. That he would not have to lie to everyone he encountered about his clandestine drug abuse. That, instead, he would simply suit up in his white surgical scrubs and focus intensely, if not obsessively, on advancing the craft that would—and continues to—save millions of lives every year.

But every afternoon, when the clock struck four-thirty, William

Halsted hurried home to his study. There, more times than not, he took out his own morocco case containing a syringe and a soothing dose of morphine. Ever the measured surgeon, he worked hard to calibrate his dosage to calm his jitters and angst but not cloud his senses or interfere with his medical judgment; on not a few occasions, however, he miscalculated and sailed off to narcotized oblivion, abandoning his responsibilities.

On many mornings after, he awoke to gnawing guilt, remorse, and a stomach full of acid. His hungover sensorium fueled his penchant for verbalizing the most curmudgeonly of thoughts and acting on his anger-filled impulses. And with each biting barb, he inexorably harmed personal relationships with those who cared for him. Later each afternoon, he returned to his home to repeat the same slow-motion cycle of self-destruction. There may have been days when Halsted could tell his demons to cease and desist or, at least, accept a smaller dose of morphine; but there were many, many more when he invited the demons into his locked study.

Most likely, William was able to abstain from cocaine for long periods of time, but he presumably pursued many prolonged binges in the years after he left Butler Hospital. These relapses probably coincided with his isolated summer vacations in Europe and North Carolina and his many frequent absences from the Johns Hopkins Hospital. Such episodes also may have included balancing the stimulant effects of cocaine with injections of morphine.

The long-term course for most active cocaine and morphine addicts is uniformly bad. Eventually, the limbic system telling such addicted brains to "go-go-go" for the immediate gratification of mind-altering drugs completely conquers the inhibiting frontal cortex, which would normally stop them from engaging in foolish or dangerous acts. The result is a constant search for and consumption of the addictive drug of choice and a steady downhill course toward death.

Halsted, on the other hand, was a remarkably high-performing addict for almost four decades. Armed with a controlling personality of epic proportions, more times than not the surgeon restricted satisfying his drug hunger to a precise schedule of furtive morphine injections. He also managed to contain his cocaine cravings to those safe periods when he was far away from the hospital and could afford to binge.

What remains extraordinary about Halsted's substance abuse was that he was able to escape on his morphine and cocaine holidays so well, so often, and for so long, while so few knew of his habit. Sadly, the ashamed, guarded, and lonely Halsted concealed this part of his life to the very end.

Epilogue

ADDICTIVE AGENTS, when taken chronically and copiously, can transform anatomy. Like an overloaded power switch, an insurgency of bad judgment and risky behavior hijacks the brain's delicate circuitry, inducing temporary states of well-being and release from all inhibitions. Long after the high has disappeared, a neurologically mediated form of bondage forces the addict to pursue his own destruction. His body progressively demands greater amounts in exchange for briefer moments of escape amid a growing cascade of physical and mental health breakdowns. In the end, for the witness it is death at its most repellent and for the addict at its most seductive.

For many people, the use of mind-altering drugs is nothing more than a guilty little pleasure that provides a brief, occasional reprieve from life's emotional battles. But predictably, 5 to 10 percent of humans develop serious abuse problems after discovering their substance of choice. Imagine this susceptibility as a wheel of misfortune that includes wedges depicting risks related to genetics, environment, mode of administration, and emotional or physical trauma. The addict's luck runs short when the wheel stops at the most harmful wedges.

When Freud and Halsted first became acquainted with their chemical bête noire, they fully expected cocaine to be the wonder drug of modern medicine. Neither had any idea of its potential to dominate and endanger their lives. Addiction as a bona fide medical diagnosis was not yet in the doctor's lexicon, let alone his textbooks. Quite simply, these talented medical investigators studied the effects of cocaine by experimenting on themselves, consumed great quantities of it, and eventually encountered serious problems because they had done so.

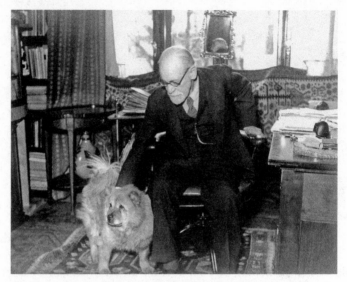

*Sigmund Freud with one of his beloved chow dogs
in his London study, c. 1939.*

Each man actively participated in the birth of the modern addict, and their clinical histories prefigure the ever-challenging spectrum of substance abuse, addiction, and recovery. Freud somehow escaped from his cocaine dependency even as he was plagued by periods of sexual turmoil, increased alcohol consumption, and depression. Decades after Halsted restricted his cocaine abuse to occasional binges, he still availed himself of daily morphine injections to quell his addictive urges, often with negative results.

In years past, some scholars have been eager to discount Freud's and Halsted's so-called cocaine episodes, citing their vast work output as evidence that cocaine posed only inconsequential problems, ignoring the reality that even fervent substance abusers can achieve greatness. Others have highlighted the accidental aspect of their maladies—as if anyone becomes an addict on purpose. Even at this late date, it is tempting for some to wonder why these two men's brilliance, social position, specialized knowledge, or determination failed to immunize them against cocaine's indiscriminate ravages. But in reality, their vulnerability to the disease of addiction demonstrates that the two intellectual giants were all too human.

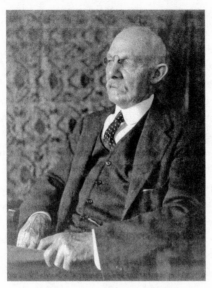

Halsted's formal portrait, 1922.

Cocaine failed to make either man more productive, happier, or smarter. They often recklessly practiced medicine while under the influence, and their most fallow professional years coincided with their most prodigious substance abuse. Each in his own fashion confessed regret over the physical and emotional tolls cocaine exerted, the valuable time it consumed, and the harm its abuse inflicted on others.

Yet cocaine no more explains the sum total of their lives and occupational achievements than a diagnosis of diabetes or hypertension would define others. Chronology alone does not imply a direct equation of causation between mind-altering drugs and creativity. Pharmacologically enhanced flashes of uninhibited thought alone do not result in intellectual progress over long periods of time; nor do they allow for the fine motor control one needs to conduct intricate surgical operations. Genius is not found in a bottle, pill, or potion. It arises from within and in most cases must be discovered and nurtured by others. The titanic legacies of Sigmund Freud and William Halsted were ground out page by page, stitch by stitch, patient by patient, insight by insight, day after day, year after year.

Today, neither man can claim the ultimate authority they held in their respective fields while alive. Long after Freud composed his last sentence, mental health professionals advanced, disputed, and replaced his theories and methods. In the decades since Halsted quit the operating room, surgeons have superseded his work in ways he could only have dreamed about. Still, none of us can approach an understanding of modern psychology or surgery without at least taking their work into serious consideration. Without fear of exaggeration, it can be said that each man changed the world.

History repeatedly reminds us that great accomplishments are often accompanied by great risks, just as personal tragedy often gives birth to inspirational growth. In their quest to change the course of medicine, Freud and Halsted imperiled their lives with cocaine, initially as a potential means to revolutionize science and ultimately from its abuse. In defiance of the malady that nearly destroyed them—or perhaps because of their struggle to overcome it—neither man ever lost his zeal for delivering his healing gifts to the world.

Notes

Prologue

4 The orderlies rushed: Allan E. Dumont, "Halsted at Bellevue, 1883–1887," *Annals of Surgery* 172, no. 6 (1970): 929–35. The laborer's case is logged into a volume of surgical records entitled "Bellevue Hospital Record Book, 1883–1897," which is the basis of Dumont's 1970 report. For similar contemporary accounts, see also William H. Rideing, "Hospital Life in New York," *Harper's New Monthly Magazine,* July 1878, pp. 171–89; and "The Bellevue of Today: Sights in the Wards of the Great Charity Hospital," *New York Times,* November 23, 1884, p. 6.

4 Before X-ray technology: X-rays were discovered by the German physicist Wilhelm Roentgen in 1895. This remarkable technology has aided physicians and surgeons in diagnosing organic diseases ever since. Stanley J. Reiser, "Enigmatic Pictures: How Patients and Doctors Encountered the X-Ray," *Technological Medicine: The Changing World of Doctors and Patients* (New York: Cambridge University Press, 2009), pp. 14–30; Stanley J. Reiser, *Medicine and the Reign of Technology* (New York: Cambridge University Press, 1981); Bettyann Kevles, *Naked to the Bone: Medical Imaging in the Twentieth Century* (New Brunswick, N.J.: Rutgers University Press, 1997).

4 Discounting the attendant risks: Allen O. Whipple, *The Evolution of Surgery in the United States* (Springfield, Ill.: Charles C. Thomas, Publisher, 1963), pp. 86–88; quote is from p. 87; J. C. O. Will, "On Fracture of the Tubercle of the Tibia," *British Medical Journal* 1, no. 1360 (1887): 152–53; "Orthopaedic Surgery," in *The History of Surgery in the United States, 1775–1900,* ed. Ira M. Rutkow, vol. 1, *Textbooks, Monographs, and Treatises* (San Francisco: Norman Publishing, 1988), pp. 243–86; Alfred R. Shands, *The Early Orthopaedic Surgeons of America* (St. Louis: C. V. Mosby Co., 1970); Mark M. Ravitch, ed., *A Century of Surgery: The History of the American Surgical Association,* vol. 1 (Philadelphia: J. B. Lippincott, 1981), pp. 34, 36, 118, 122, 124, 127, 129, 133, 137, 183, 203–04, 206; and G. H. Brieger, "A Portrait of Surgery: Surgery in America, 1875–1889," *Surgical Clinics in North America* 67 (1987): 1181–216.

4 It read, in six-inch-high black letters: "The Bellevue of Today: Sights in the Wards of the Great Charity Hospital," *New York Times,* November 23, 1884, p. 6.

4 Otherwise, the broken leg: William S. Halsted, "Adduction and Abduction in Fractures of the Neck of the Femur," *New York Medical Journal* 39 (1884): 317–19.

This paper was also reprinted in the *Medical Record of New York* (25 [1884]: 248) and in the *Medical News of Philadelphia* (44 [1884]: 288). It can be found more easily in William S. Halsted, *Surgical Papers in Two Volumes,* ed. Walter C. Burket (Baltimore: The Johns Hopkins Press, 1924), vol. 1, pp. 19–26.

6 an up-and-coming neurologist: Sigmund Freud to Martha Bernays, May 17, 1885, Ernst L. Freud, ed., *Letters of Sigmund Freud* (New York: Basic Books, 1960), pp. 145–46 (Letter 65). For a superb synopsis of Freud's training and work as a neurologist and neuroanatomist between 1876 and 1896, see Oliver Sacks, "The Other Road: Freud as Neurologist," in *Freud: Conflict and Culture: Essays on His Life, Work, and Legacy,* ed. Michael S. Roth (New York: Alfred A. Knopf, in association with the Library of Congress, 1998), pp. 221–34.

6 On May 17, 1885: Freud to Martha, May 17, 1885, Freud, *Letters,* pp. 145–46 (Letter 65). The paper Sigmund is referring to in this letter is *"Zur Kenntnis der Olivenzwischenschicht"* (Concerning the Knowledge of the Intermediary Layer of the Olive), *Neurologisches Zentralblatt* 4, no. 12 (1885): 268. The term "olive" refers not to the fruit but to a brain structure that has the shape of an olive, or, more specifically, the "inferior olivary eminence, a smooth oval prominence of the ventrolateral surface of the *medulla oblongata* (brainstem) corresponding to the *nucleus olivaris,"* as defined by *Stedman's Medical Dictionary,* 23rd ed. (Baltimore: Williams and Wilkins, 1976), p. 977. Freud's paper discussed his histological tracing of the acoustic nerve and the connection of the interolivary tract with the crossed trapezoid body.

7 Such individuals were mandated: The *Oxford English Dictionary's* first entry under "addiction" defines it as a term from Roman law meaning "a formal giving over or delivery by sentence of court. Hence, a surrender or dedication of anyone to a master." *The Compact Edition of the Oxford English Dictionary,* vol. 1 (Oxford: Oxford University Press, 1981), p. 26; John A. Crook, *Law and Life of Rome* (Ithaca, N.Y.: Cornell University Press, 1984), pp. 61, 172–76; Barry Nicholas, *An Introduction to Roman Law* (Oxford: Clarendon Press, 1962), pp. 2–15. I am indebted to my colleague Michael Schoenfeldt, professor and chairman of English literature and language at the University of Michigan, for introducing me to the word's fascinating history.

7 Alcohol abusers, too: Such is the stark contrast to our current era, when the application of the word "addiction" has opened up significantly to include not only a large number of habit-forming drugs but also a number of behaviors ranging from excessive gambling to promiscuous sexual activity. See, for example, William Osler, *Principles and Practice of Medicine* (New York: D. Appleton, 1892), pp. 1001–07; David T. Courtright, *Dark Paradise: A History of Opiate Addiction in America* (Cambridge, Mass.: Harvard University Press, 2001), pp. 79–101; Sarah Tracy, *Alcoholism in America: From Reconstruction to Prohibition* (Baltimore: Johns Hopkins University Press, 2007). For engaging essays on the origins of terms for alcoholics, see, for example, H. G. Levine, "The Discovery of Addiction: Changing Conceptions of Habitual Drunkenness in America," *Journal of Studies on Alcohol* 39 (1978): 143–74; William L. White, "The Lessons of Language: Historical Perspectives on the Rhetoric of Addiction," in *Altering American Consciousness: The History of Alcohol and Drug Use in the United States, 1800–2000,* ed. Sarah W. Tracy and Caroline J. Acker (Amherst: University of

Massachusetts Press, 2004), pp. 33–60; Timothy Hickman, "The Double Meaning of Addiction: Habitual Narcotic Use and the Logic of Professionalizing Medical Authority in the United States, 1900–1920," in Tracy and Acker, *Altering*, pp. 182–202.

8 For example, epidemiological studies: David T. Courtright, *Dark Paradise: A History of Opiate Addiction in America* (Cambridge, Mass.: Harvard University Press, 2001), p. 36; O. Marshall, "The Opium Habit in Michigan," *Michigan State Board of Health Annual Report* 6 (1878): 63–73; Charles Warrington Earle, "The Opium Habit: A Statistical and Clinical Lecture," *Chicago Medical Review* 2 (1880): 442–46; Charles Warrington Earle, "Opium-Smoking in Chicago," *Chicago Medical Journal and Examiner* 52 (1886): 104–12; J. M. Hull, "The Opium Habit," *Iowa State Board of Health Biennial Report* 3 (1885): 535–45.

8 A survey of Boston's drugstores: Courtright, *Dark Paradise*, p. 38; and Virgil G. Eaton, "How the Opium Habit Is Acquired," *Popular Science Monthly* 33 (1888): 663–67.

8 During this period: Alas, criminalizing these agents in the decades since has not had nearly the success that reformers once hoped for, and substance abuse continues to present global health problems of gargantuan proportions. See David F. Musto, *The American Disease: Origins of Narcotic Control*, 3rd ed. (New York: Oxford University Press, 1999); Howard Markel, "When Teenagers Abuse Prescription Drugs, the Fault May Be the Doctor's," *New York Times,* December 27, 2005, p. D7; and David F. Musto, *Drugs: A Documentary History* (New York: New York University Press, 2002).

Chapter 1. Young Freud

10 On a June morning in 1884: Karl Baedekker, *Baedekker's Southern Germany and Austria,* 7th ed. (Leipzig: Karl Baedeker, 1891), pp. 188–89; *Illustriertes Landtmann Extrablatt,* no. 5, 2007 (Vienna: Cafetiers Familie, Querfeld, 2007); and Café Landtmann website, www.cafe-wien.at/ldt-start_ENG_HTML.html (accessed May 4, 2010).

10 Freud had been studying: Sigmund's given name was Sigismund Schlomo Freud, but he soon dropped the middle name, after his paternal grandfather, and formally adopted Sigmund by the time he matriculated into the University of Vienna, in 1872. Peter Gay, *Freud: A Life for Our Time* (New York: W. W. Norton, 1998), pp. 4–5.

11 One of the most famous: Erna Lesky, *The Vienna Medical School of the 19th Century* (Baltimore: Johns Hopkins University Press, 1976); Hortense Koller Becker, "Carl Koller and Cocaine," *Psychoanalytic Quarterly* 32 (1963): 309–73; Sherwin B. Nuland, *The Doctors' Plague: Germs, Childbed Fever and the Strange Story of Ignac Semmelweis* (New York: W. W. Norton, 2004); and Irvine Loudon, *The Tragedy of Childbed Fever* (Oxford: Oxford University Press, 2000).

12 It was a line: Ernest Jones, *The Life and Work of Sigmund Freud,* vol. 2, *1901–1919* (New York: Basic Books, 1955), pp. 13–14; in the same courtyard, there now is a bust of Freud bearing the Sophocles inscription. The bust's placement was arranged by Ernest Jones and unveiled in 1955.

13 Popular and pretty: Louis Breger, *Freud: Darkness in the Midst of Vision* (New York: John Wiley and Sons, 2000), pp. 55–56.

14 In his later life: Gay, *Freud*, pp. 6–9; quote is from p. 6.

14 Yet even as a child: Eli Zaretsky, *Secrets of the Soul: A Social and Cultural History of Psychoanalysis* (New York: Alfred A. Knopf, 2004), pp. 26–27; and M. Huttler, "Jewish Origins of Freud's Interpretation of Dreams," *Journal of Psychology and Judaism* 23 (1999): 5–48. The inscribed Pentateuch is on display at the Sigmund Freud Museum in Vienna.

15 A widow deeply concerned: For example, Sigmund warns Martha not to listen too closely to her "mama's complaints against him and their relationship," Sigmund Freud to Martha Bernays, February 21, 1883, Ernst L. Freud, ed., *Letters of Sigmund Freud* (New York: Basic Books, 1960), pp. 37–40 (Letter 13).

16 "Now and again I see a girl": Freud to Martha, March 31, 1885, Freud, *Letters,* pp. 138–39 (Letter 60); quote is from p. 139.

17 "Defending my case valiantly": Freud to Martha, August 23, 1883, Freud, *Letters,* pp. 44–47 (Letter 16); quote is from p. 44.

17 "the things that go": Freud to Martha, June 6, 1885, Freud, *Letters,* pp. 148–49 (Letter 67); quote is from p. 148.

17 "I am preparing myself": Freud to William Knöpfmacher, August 6, 1878, Freud, *Letters,* pp. 6–7 (Letter 2).

18 Once there, he would enjoy: Lesky, *Vienna;* Ernest Jones, *The Life and Work of Sigmund Freud,* vol. 1, *1856–1900* (New York: Basic Books, 1953), pp. 36–77.

19 But the cause, Dr. Osler explained: "The Master Word in Medicine," in William Osler, *Aequanimitas and Other Addresses* (Philadelphia: P. Blakiston's Sons and Co., 1904), pp. 363–88.

20 Failures of this magnitude: William F. Bynum, *Science and the Practice of Medicine in the Nineteenth Century* (Cambridge: Cambridge University Press, 1994); Lesky, *Vienna,* pp. 228–42; and Henry Sigerist, *The Great Doctors: A Biographical History of Medicine* (New York: W. W. Norton, 1933), pp. 303–11.

20 Some have suggested: Peter Gay, for example, intuits a sense of discontent over both the research and with Claus. See Gay, *Freud,* pp. 30–31. The main project Sigmund worked on under Claus appeared as S. Freud, *Beobachtungen über Gestaltung und feineren Bau der als Hoden beschriebenen Lappenorgane des Aals* (Observations on the Formation and More Delicate Structure of Lobe-Shaped Organs of the Eel Described as Testicles) (Vienna, 1877).

20 When Brücke, the son of a painter: Brücke maintained an interest in art and later in life wrote treatises on the theory of pictorial art, the physiology of colors in applied art, and how motion is represented in art.

21 Müller is credited: Bynum, *Science;* Lesky, *Vienna,* pp. 228–42; Sigerist, *Doctors,* pp. 303–11.

21 One afternoon in the late 1870s: Jones, *Life,* vol. 1, p. 39.

22 Freud also often referred: Ibid., p. 43; see also Gay, *Freud,* p. 32.

22 The historian Peter Gay: Gay, *Freud,* p. 30.

22 Anti-Semitism remained: Ibid., p. 27.

22 At the end of each week: A kymograph is a revolving drum with carbon-coated paper wrapped around it. Late-nineteenth- and early-twentieth-century physi-

ologists used kymographs to record data in the laboratory, such as blood pressures, cardiac pulses, muscle contractions, and respirations. A needle connected to a subject's pulse point, chest, or other area would transmit activity and etch a series of squiggles, spikes, and valleys on the carbon-coated paper. The device was invented by the famed physiologist Carl Ludwig of the University of Leipzig and, formerly, the University of Vienna. See Horace W. Davenport, "Physiology, 1850–1923: The View from Michigan," *Physiologist* 25, Supp. 1 (1982): 1–100.

22 A few of his studies: See, for example, Sigmund Freud, *Über den Ursprung der Hinteren Nervenwurzeln im Ruckenmark von Amnocoetes (Petromyzon Planeri)* (On the Origin of the Posterior Nerve Roots in the Spinal Cord of Amnocoetes [*Petromyzon Planeri*]), 1877; and Sigmund Freud, *Über Spinalganglien und Ruckenmark des Petromyzon* (On the Spinal Ganglia and Spinal Cord of the Petromyzon), 1878. For a superb synopsis of Freud's training and work as a neurologist and neuroanatomist between 1876 and 1896, see Oliver Sacks, "The Other Road: Freud as Neurologist," in *Freud: Conflict and Culture: Essays on His Life, Work, and Legacy*, ed. Michael S. Roth (New York: Alfred A. Knopf, in association with the Library of Congress, 1998), pp. 221–34.

23 One had to then carefully "fix": Freud to Martha, August 23, 1883, Freud, *Letters,* pp. 44–47 (Letter 16); and Freud to Martha, October 15, 1883, Freud, *Letters,* pp. 69–70 (Letter 25).

23 Specifically, neurons are independent: Stanley Finger, *Origins of Neuroscience: A History of Explorations into Brain Function* (New York: Oxford University Press, 1994), pp. 43–50.

24 He then craftily submitted: Ibid., pp. 203–05. See also "Early Psycho-Analytic Publications," in *The Standard Edition of the Complete Psychological Works of Sigmund Freud,* vol. 3, *1893–1899,* ed. J. Strachey (London: The Hogarth Press and the Institute of Psychoanalysis, 1962), pp. 223–57.

24 To quote Sigmund's career self-assessment: Jones, *Life,* vol. 1, p. 43; Gay, *Freud,* pp. 36–37. Sigmund took a year of compulsory military service in the Austrian army from late 1879 until the end of 1880.

25 On July 31: Jones, *Life,* vol. 1, p. 63.

25 Worse, his pedagogic bigotry: Ibid.; N. McLaren and R. V. Thorbeck, "Little-Known Aspect of Theodor Billroth's Work: His Contribution to Musical Theory," *World Journal of Surgery* 21 (1997): 569–71; and Theodor Billroth and Johannes Brahms, *Letters from a Musical Friendship,* ed. Hans Barkan (Norman: University of Oklahoma Press, 1957). Billroth's anti-Semitic tirades appear most infamously in Theodor Billroth, *The Medical Sciences in the German Universities: A Study in the History of Civilization* (New York: Macmillan, 1924); and Sherwin B. Nuland, "An Austrian Jew" (Letter to the editor), *New York Review of Books,* November 17, 1994, available at www.nybooks.com/articles/archives/1994/nov/17/an-austrian-jew/ (accessed May 4, 2010).

25 As an example of this behavior: Freud to Martha, January 6, 1885, Freud, *Letters,* pp. 131–32 (Letter 55); quote is from p. 131.

26 "Whoever needs more": Lesky, *Vienna,* p. 280; see pp. 279–90 for a description of Nothnagel's career.

26 Freud served under Nothnagel: Gay, *Freud,* p. 42; Jones, *Life,* vol. 1, p. 64.

26 Freud called him: Jones, *Life,* vol. 1, p. 65.

28 Dermatologists of the late nineteenth century: Claude Quétel, *The History of Syphilis,* trans. Judith Braddock and Brian Pike (Baltimore: Johns Hopkins University Press, 1992), p. 136.

28 He embarked on this clinical course: Jones, *Life,* vol. 1, pp. 66–67.

28 In the end, Freud did not find dermatology: Freud to Martha, October 5, 1882, Freud, *Letters,* pp. 30–34 (Letter 12); quote is from p. 33.

29 In late January 1884, Sigmund wrote to his "Fräulein Martha": Freud to Martha, January 29, 1884, Freud, *Letters,* pp. 94–96 (Letter 36); quote is from p. 95.

29 "You will certainly be surprised": Freud to Martha, April 21, 1884, Freud, *Letters,* pp. 107–09 (Letter 43); quote is from p. 107. See also Freud, *Letters,* p. 66, footnote 1.

Chapter 2. Young Halsted

32 Late in life: William G. MacCallum, *William Stewart Halsted, Surgeon* (Baltimore: Johns Hopkins University Press, 1930), pp. 9–10. MacCallum is quoting a series of "long letters" that Halsted wrote in the summer of 1922 about his upbringing and life to William H. Welch as the latter was preparing to write a foreword for an edition of Halsted's collected papers. See also Gerald Imber, *Genius on the Edge: The Bizarre Double Life of Dr. William Stewart Halsted* (New York: Kaplan Publishing, 2010).

33 Both Mary Louisa and William Jr.: The four Halsted children in birth order were William (born on September 23, 1852), Bertha, Mary Louisa, and Richard. A successful Wall Street stockbroker, Richard was an alcoholic who died in 1915 of a gastrointestinal hemorrhage secondary to esophageal varices and cirrhosis of the liver. J. Scott Rankin, "William Stewart Halsted: A Lecture by Dr. Peter D. Olch," *Annals of Surgery* 243 (2006): 418–25.

33 Perhaps the singular exception: MacCallum, *Halsted,* pp. 4–8; Rankin, "Halsted," pp. 418–25.

34 Upon acceptance: Quote is from *Catalogue of the Officers and Students of Yale College, 1870–1871* (Collections of the Yale University Manuscripts and Archives Collection, New Haven), p. 39; see pp. 38–39 for descriptions of the entrance examinations and curriculum. General information is also from George J. Heuer, "Dr. Halsted," *Johns Hopkins Hospital Bulletin,* Supp. 90 (1952): 1–104; Sherwin B. Nuland, "Medical Science Comes to America: William Stewart Halsted of Johns Hopkins," *Doctors: The Biography of Medicine* (New York: Vintage Books, 1988), pp. 386–421; MacCallum, *Halsted,* pp. 1–28; *The Yale Banner, 1870* (Yale University Class Book), vol. 27, no. 1 (New Haven: Tuttle, Morehouse and Taylor, 1870), pp. 20–23, 40–43; "Commencement Week," *New York Times,* July 20, 1870, p. 4; "Commencements," *New York Times,* July 22, 1870, p. 5. To convert 1870 dollars into 2010 values, I used a formula based on the consumer price index from the economic history–focused website Measuring Worth, www .measuringworth.com/index.html (accessed February 25, 2010).

34 In 1873, he served: One of the best sources of information on Halsted's student days, as well as his internship and postgraduate training, is a letter Halsted wrote

for Welch as the latter prepared an introduction for a collected volume of Halsted's surgical papers: Halsted to Welch, July 14, 1922, Series II, Notes, Box 31, W. H. Welch Papers, Alan Mason Chesney Archives, Johns Hopkins Medical Institutions, Baltimore. See also Edwards A. Park, "Notes of an Interview with Reverend Samuel Bushnell on February 23, 1927," William Halsted Papers, Alan Mason Chesney Archives, Johns Hopkins Medical Institutions, Baltimore.

34 At Yale, William was a member: Even late in life, Halsted drank sparingly, if at all. Nuland, "Medical Science," pp. 386–88; Samuel J. Crowe, *Halsted of Johns Hopkins: The Man and His Men* (Springfield, Ill.: C. C. Thomas, 1957); Peter D. Olch, "William Stewart Halsted: Legendary Figure of American Surgery," *Review of Surgery* 20 (1963): 83–90; and MacCallum, *Halsted,* pp. 11–14. With respect to his clothes, Halsted was an avid consumer of expensive and well-tailored suits, shirts, ties, and shoes for the remainder of his life.

35 "He was generally popular": Halsted was noted to enjoy popular fiction and may have taken a few books out of the local Brothers Library of New Haven during this time; Park, "Notes," William Halsted Papers, Alan Mason Chesney Archives, Johns Hopkins Medical Institutions, Baltimore. This interview with Bushnell, who at one point was Halsted's roommate, is extensively quoted in Edwards A. Park, "A Pediatrician's Chance Recollections of Dr. Halsted," *Surgery* 32 (1952): 472–78; Heuer, "Dr. Halsted," pp. 6–7; Peter D. Olch, "William S. Halsted's New York Period, 1874–1886," *Bulletin of the History of Medicine* 60 (1966): 495–510; Nuland, "Medical Science Comes to America," pp. 386–88; Crowe, *Halsted of Johns Hopkins;* Olch, "Halsted: Legendary Figure," pp. 83–90; and MacCallum, *Halsted,* pp. 11–14.

35 "Devoted myself solely": Halsted to Welch, July 14, 1922, Series II, Notes, Box 31, W. H. Welch Papers, Alan Mason Chesney Archives, Johns Hopkins Medical Institutions, Baltimore; and Nuland, "Medical Science," pp. 386–88.

36 The first volume William mentions: Henry Gray, *Anatomy, Descriptive and Surgical* (Philadelphia: H. C. Lea, 1870).

36 The other book: John Call Dalton, *A Treatise on Human Physiology: Designed for the Use of Students and Practitioners of Medicine* (Philadelphia: Blanchard and Lea, 1859); and W. Bruce Fye, *The Development of American Physiology: Scientific Medicine in the 19th Century* (Baltimore: Johns Hopkins University Press, 1987), pp. 15–53.

36 "Dr. Dalton is one of the few": The review is credited to Holmes by medical historian W. Bruce Fye in his book *Development,* p. 30. For the original review, see "Bibliographical Notices: A Treatise on Human Physiology by John Call Dalton," *Boston Medical and Surgical Journal* 60 (1859): 80.

36 So persuasive were Dalton's powers: S. Weir Mitchell, "Memoir of John Call Dalton, 1825–1889," *Biographical Memoirs* (Washington, D.C.: National Academy of Sciences, 1890), pp. 177–85.

36 But there also existed: Kenneth M. Ludmerer, *Learning to Heal: The Development of American Medical Education* (New York: Basic Books, 1985).

38 Given the state of medical education: John Call Dalton, *History of the College of Physicians and Surgeons in the City of New York: Medical Department of Columbia College* (New York: Columbia College, 1888); John Shrady, ed., *The College of*

Physicians and Surgeons of New York and Its Founders, Officers, Instructors, Benefactors, and Alumni, 2 vols. (New York: Lewis Publishing Co., 1904); William H. Rideing, "Medical Education in New York," *Harper's New Monthly Magazine,* October 1882, pp. 668–80; and Charles F. Gardiner, "Getting a Medical Education in New York City in the Eighteen-Seventies," *Academy Bookman* 8, no. 2 (1955): 3–11.

38 The medical students: Gardiner, "Getting a Medical Education," pp. 3–11; Rideing, "Medical Education," pp. 668–80; and Olch, "New York Period," pp. 497–98.

38 Halsted delivered a sterling performance: To convert 1876 dollars into 2010 values, I used a formula based on the consumer price index from the economic history–focused website Measuring Worth, www.measuringworth.com/index .html (accessed February 25, 2010).

39 In such an institutional atmosphere: Charles E. Rosenberg, *The Care of Strangers: The Rise of America's Hospital System* (New York: Basic Books, 1987), p. 36; and Howard Markel, "When Hospitals Kept Children from Parents," *New York Times,* January 1, 2008, p. F6.

40 "[The area was] plentifully dotted": William H. Rideing, "Hospital Life in New York," *Harper's New Monthly Magazine,* July 1878, pp. 171–89; quote is from p. 180. See also J. West Roosevelt, "In the Hospital," *Scribner's Magazine,* October 1894, pp. 472–86; A. B. Ward, "Hospital Life," *Scribner's Magazine,* June 1888, pp. 697–716; A. B. Ward, "The Invalid's World," *Scribner's Magazine,* January 1889, pp. 58–73; H. M. Silver, "Surgery in Bellevue Hospital Fifty Years Ago," *Medical Journal and Record* 120 (1924): pp. 551–57; Helen Campbell, "Hospital Life in New York," in *Darkness and Daylight; or, Lights and Shadows of New York Life: A Pictorial Record* (Hartford, Conn.: Hartford Publishing Co., 1898), pp. 279–304; and Gardiner, "Getting a Medical Education," pp. 3–11.

41 Adjacent to the hospital: Rideing, "Hospital Life," pp. 171–89; see also MacCallum, *Halsted,* pp. 15–16.

41 "The picture has many changes": Rideing, "Hospital Life," p. 180.

42 The most desperately ill: Robert J. Carlisle, ed., *An Account of Bellevue Hospital with a Catalogue of the Medical and Surgical Staff from 1736 to 1894* (New York: Society of the Alumni of Bellevue Hospital, 1893); Page Cooper, *The Bellevue Story* (New York: Thomas Y. Crowell Co., 1948); Salvatore R. Cutolo, with Arthur Gelb and Barbara Gelb, *This Hospital Is My Home: The Story of Bellevue* (London: Victor Gollancz, 1956); John Starr, *Hospital City: The Story of the Men and Women of Bellevue* (New York: Crown Publishers, 1957); and Rideing, "Hospital Life," pp. 171–89.

42 The seven-day-a-week job: Silver, "Surgery in Bellevue," pp. 551–57.

43 In later life Halsted noted: For evidence of his activities, it is worthwhile reviewing Halsted's surgical cases, which were recorded in a bound ledger entitled "Bellevue Hospital History Book for the Winter of 1877–1878" and can be found at the Ehrman Medical Library, New York University. There we find intricate descriptions written in what A. E. Dumont described as "a stylized Spencerian script by short-term prisoners who served as clerks and transcribed, verbatim, information contained on the hospital chart." Many of these pages

describe how Halsted and his colleagues treated patients with traumatic fractures, burns, abscesses, congenital malformations, and strangulated hernias. Among these meticulously kept case ledgers are copious descriptions of the use of chloroform and ether as surgical anesthetics. We also find evidence that many Bellevue surgeons still doubted the existence of disease-causing microbes and the role they played in thwarting surgical procedures. Indeed, the teachings of Joseph Lister, the Scottish surgeon who insisted on conducting surgical explorations only after dousing his hands and the wound with powerful antiseptic chemicals, were only sporadically practiced in the vast operating theaters of Bellevue. See Allan E. Dumont, "Halsted at Bellevue, 1883–1887," *Annals of Surgery* 172, no. 6 (1970): 929–35. (Dumont describes the record book for 1883–87, but the volume for 1877–78, as well as several others during that era, were similarly dictated to and transcribed by recuperating prisoners facile with an ink pen.) See also Olch, "New York Period," pp. 495–510; Carlisle, *An Account of Bellevue;* MacCallum, *Halsted,* pp. 39–57; S. Smith, "Reminiscences of Two Epochs—Anesthesia and Asepsis," *Bulletin of the Johns Hopkins Hospital* 30 (1919): 273–78; and Gert H. Brieger, "American Surgery and the Germ Theory of Disease," *Bulletin of the History of Medicine* 40 (1966): 135–45.

43 There he briefly flirted: James J. Walsh, *History of Medicine in New York,* vol. 1 (New York: National Americana Society, 1919), pp. 224–25; and MacCallum, *Halsted,* pp. 19–20. Halsted and his roommate Thomas McBride even invited Seguin to live with them after the suicide of the neurologist's wife.

43 Between 1870 and 1914: Thomas N. Bonner, *American Doctors and German Universities: A Chapter in International Intellectual Relations, 1870–1914* (Lincoln: University of Nebraska Press, 1963), pp. 23–68.

44 Every evening, he washed down: Bonner, *American Doctors;* see also Thomas N. Bonner, *Becoming a Physician: Medical Education in Great Britain, France, Germany, and the United States, 1750–1945* (New York: Oxford University Press, 1995); and Charles D. O'Malley, ed., *The History of Medical Education* (Los Angeles: University of California at Los Angeles, 1970).

44 Each morning, Professor Meynert: Halsted to Welch, July 14, 1922, W. H. Welch Papers, Series II, Notes, Box 31, Alan Mason Chesney Archives of the Johns Hopkins Medical Institutions, Baltimore; and MacCallum, *Halsted,* p. 22.

45 As his Johns Hopkins colleague William Osler: Bonner, *American Doctors,* pp. 99–101; and William Osler, "The Inner History of the Johns Hopkins Hospital," ed. D. G. Bates and E. H. Bensley, *Johns Hopkins Medical Journal* 125 (1969): 184–94.

Chapter 3. Über Coca

46 Along the way,: Margaret Haney, "Neurobiology of Stimulants," in *The American Psychiatry Publishing Textbook of Substance Abuse Treatment,* ed. Marc Galanter and Herbert D. Kleber, 4th ed. (Washington, D.C.: American Psychiatry Press, 2008), pp. 143–55; and D. A. Gorelick, "The Pharmacology of Cocaine, Amphetamines and Other Stimulants," in *Principles of Addiction Med-*

icine, ed. R. A. Ries, D. A. Fiellen, S. C. Miller, and R. Saitz, 4th ed. (Philadelphia: Wolters Kluwer / Lippincott Williams and Wilkins, 2009), pp. 133–57.

46 So cherished a staple: Sigmund Freud, *Cocaine Papers,* ed. Robert Byck (New York: Stonehill, 1974); William Golden Mortimer, *Peru: History of Coca; "The Divine Plant" of the Incas* (New York: J. H. Vail and Co., 1901); and George Andrews and David Solomon, eds., *The Coca Leaf and Cocaine Papers* (New York: Harcourt Brace and Jovanovich, 1975). The story of cocaine—and its use by Peruvian Indians and its so-called discovery by Europeans—is, of course, far more complex and nonhegemonic; for an analysis of this global history, see Paul Gootenberg, *Andean Cocaine: The Making of a Global Drug* (Chapel Hill: University of North Carolina Press, 2009); *Cocaine: Global Histories,* Paul Gootenberg, ed. (London: Routledge, 1999); Dominic Streatfeild, *Cocaine: An Unauthorized Biography* (New York: Picador, 2001); and Curtis Marez, "The *Coquero* in Freud: Psychoanalysis, Race, and the International Economics of Distinction," *Cultural Critique* 26 (Winter 1993–94): 65–93.

47 Manco Cápac's other gift: Quote is from Sigmund Freud, *Über Coca,* in Freud, *Cocaine Papers,* p. 50; see also Mortimer, *History of Coca,* pp. 28–54.

47 They brought with them: Guenter B. Risse, "Medicine in New Spain," in *Medicine in the New World: New Spain, New France, and New England,* ed. Ronald L. Numbers (Knoxville: University of Tennessee Press, 1987), pp. 12–63; and William H. McNeill, *Plagues and Peoples* (New York: Anchor Books, 1977).

48 The Spanish conquerors of Peru: Mortimer, *History of Coca,* pp. 265–89.

48 "I shall collect": Alexander von Humboldt, *Personal Narrative of a Journey to the Equinoctial Regions of the New Continent,* abridged ed. (New York: Penguin Classics, 1996), p. ix.

48 The two men forged ahead: Kirkpatrick Sale, *Christopher Columbus and the Conquest of Paradise* (New York: Longitude Books, 1990).

49 He was impressed: Alexander von Humboldt, *Personal Narrative of a Journey to the Equinoctial Regions of the New Continent During the Years 1799–1804,* 2nd ed., trans. Helen Mona Williams (London: Longman, Rees, Orme, Brown, and Green, 1827), p. 648.

50 Parenthetically, Humboldt erroneously hypothesized: The traditional chewing of the coca leaf with *llipta,* most commonly the ash of a quinoa plant, tones down its rather bitter taste and activates the alkaloids in the leaf, which contain coca's active ingredient. Eleanor Carroll, "Coca: The Plant and Its Use," in *Cocaine: 1977,* ed. Robert C. Petersen and Richard C. Stillman, NIDA Research Monographs 13 (Rockville, Md.: U.S. Department of Health, Education, and Welfare, 1977), pp. 35–44.

50 Before long Humboldt's fascination: Mortimer, *History of Coca,* pp. 168–71.

50 "[The Indians] masticate": Quoted in Mortimer, *History of Coca,* p. 169. See also *Gentleman's Magazine,* 1814, vol. 84, p. 217; and Streatfeild, *Cocaine,* pp. 50–51.

51 A few years later, he developed: "William Hickling Prescott," in *Dictionary of American Biography,* vol. 15, ed. Dumas Malone (New York: Charles Scribner's Sons, 1935), pp. 196–200; and Donald Darnell, "William Hickling Prescott," in *American National Biography,* vol. 17, ed. John A. Garraty and Mark C. Carnes (New York: Oxford University Press, 1999), pp. 835–36.

51 He became a best-selling author: William H. Prescott, *History of the Reign of Ferdinand and Isabella, the Catholic, of Spain* (Boston: Richard Bentley, 1858).

51 From there, he turned to writing: "Prescott," *American Biography,* vol. 15, pp. 196–200; "Prescott," *National Biography,* vol. 17, pp. 835–36; and William H. Prescott, *History of the Conquest of Mexico and History of the Conquest of Peru* (New York: Modern Library, 1936).

51 "Even food the most invigorating": Prescott, *History of the Conquest,* p. 803.

52 "Yet, with the soothing charms": Ibid.

53 During much of the 1850s: Mortimer, *History of Coca,* pp. 295, 299.

53 By the close of the nineteenth century: Ibid., pp. 294–98. Other sources of information that Niemann used in his studies were the work of a University of Pennsylvania chemist named John Maisch and that of the German chemist Friedrich Gaedcke.

54 "I sneered at all the poor mortals": A translation of excerpts of this monograph appears as Paolo Mantegazza, "Coca Experiences," in *The Coca Leaf and Cocaine Papers,* pp. 38–42; quote is from p. 41. This was a paper Freud read and incorporated into his monograph *Über Coca.*

55 "Each race has its fashions": Angelo Mariani, *Coca and Its Therapeutic Applications,* 2nd ed. (New York: J. N. Jaros, 1892), p. 5; see also Angelo Mariani, *Coca erythroxylon: Its Uses in the Treatment of Disease with Notes and Comments by Prominent Physicians,* 4th ed. (Paris: Mariani and Co., 1886). Two intriguing yet marginal notes emerge from this essay. The first is Mariani's claim that South Americans chewed coca leaves in their sleep, which runs counterintuitive to its regard as a stimulant. Second is Mariani's reference to a "certain therapeutist," who was, as it turned out, Sigmund Freud's former professor Hermann Nothnagel. Dr. Nothnagel publicly declared cocaine to be worthless in Hermann Nothnagel and M. J. Rossbach, *A Treatise on Materia Medica, Including Therapeutics and Toxicology,* trans. H. N. Heinemann (New York: Bermingham's Medical Library, 1883–84); originally published as *Handbuch der Arzneimittellehre* (Berlin: A. Hirschwald, 1878).

55 In the decades that followed: Cocaethylene has the same affinity for dopamine receptors as cocaine, but the time it holds on to these receptors greatly exceeds that of cocaine. This means that a combination of cocaine and alcohol can keep one inebriated longer than taking cocaine alone. Steven B. Karch, *Karch's Pathology of Drug Abuse* (Boca Raton, Fla.: CRC Press, 2001), pp. 3–5.

56 Around the same time: Mortimer, *History of Coca,* p. 180; and A. LaLauze, ed., *Portraits from Album Mariani* (New York: Mariani and Company, 1893).

58 In the years to come: See, for example, *Portraits from Album Mariani;* and Streatfeild, *Cocaine,* pp. 59–61.

58 Such positive buzz: Mariani, *Therapeutic Applications;* see also Mariani, *Coca erythroxylon.*

59 That first year: To convert 1886 dollars into 2010 values, I used a formula based on the consumer price index from the economic history–focused website Measuring Worth, www.measuringworth.com/index.html (accessed February 25, 2010).

59 In 1887, he abruptly sold: The convoluted history of the ownership of Coca-Cola is nicely described in Mark Pendergrast, *For God, Country and Coca-Cola:*

The Definitive History of the Great American Soft Drink and the Company That Makes It (New York: Basic Books, 2000); and Streatfeild, *Cocaine,* pp. 80–82. Late-nineteenth-century dollars were converted into 2010 values using a formula based on the consumer price index from the economic history–focused website Measuring Worth, www.measuringworth.com/index.html (accessed February 25, 2010).

59 In 1892, Candler prevailed: The merchandising and use of all these coca products reached epidemic proportions until 1906, beginning with the U.S. Congress's passage of the Pure Food and Drug Act and, more definitively, with a series of municipal, state, and, ultimately, federal laws, such as the Harrison Narcotic Act of 1914, which introduced national drug prohibition. Specifically, the Harrison Act decreed that all dangerous drugs, including cocaine and morphine, be prescribed by physicians, dispensed by registered pharmacists, and taken by specific patients along with strict, accurate record keeping. After the passage of this law, any other type of cocaine or opiate sales became a federal crime. See Joseph E. Spillane, *Cocaine: From Medical Marvel to Modern Menace in the United States, 1884–1920* (Baltimore: Johns Hopkins University Press, 2000), pp. 67–104; and Streatfeild, *Cocaine,* pp. 79–82, 155–56.

60 Such chemical developments: Fran Hawthorne, *The Merck Druggernaut: The Inside Story of a Pharmaceutical Giant* (New York: John Wiley, 2003); and Tom Mahoney, *The Merchants of Life: An Account of the American Pharmaceutical Industry* (New York: Harper and Brothers, 1959).

61 But while they all became adept: David T. Courtwright, *Forces of Habit: Drugs and the Making of the Modern World* (Cambridge, Mass.: Harvard University Press, 2001), pp. 46–52.

62 In the decades before Henry Ford: Duffield left the firm in 1866, and the name Parke, Davis and Company was adopted in 1871. Weirdly, Hervey Parke's middle name was Coke. The other major industries in Detroit during this era included timber and the manufacture of ships, cast-iron stoves, metal products, and railway cars. See Mahoney, *Merchants of Life,* pp. 69–73; Olivier Zunz, *The Changing Face of Inequality: Urbanization, Industrial Development and Immigrants in Detroit, 1880–1920* (Chicago: University of Illinois Press, 1982); Arthur Pound, *Detroit: Dynamic City* (New York: D. Appleton–Century Co., 1940); Stephen Meyer, *The Five Dollar Day: Labor Management and Social Control in the Ford Motor Company, 1908–1921* (Albany: State University of New York Press, 1981); and Steven Watts, *The People's Tycoon: Henry Ford and the American Century* (New York: Alfred A. Knopf, 2005).

62 Instrumental to Parke, Davis and Company's attempt: Courtwright, *Forces of Habit,* p. 48.

62 Nearly half a century later: Henry Hurd Rusby, *Jungle Memories* (New York: McGraw-Hill, 1933), p. 3.

63 It was, as Rusby later described: Ibid.; *Fifty Years of Manufacturing Pharmacy and Biology: Jubilee Souvenir, 1866–1916* (Detroit: Parke-Davis, n.d.), Collections of the Bentley Historical Library, University of Michigan; *Parke-Davis, 1806–1966: A Backward Glance* (Detroit: Parke-Davis, 1966), Collections of the Bentley Historical Library, University of Michigan; and Mahoney, *Merchants of Life.* For

an extensive reprinting of most of the cocaine papers published in the *Therapeu-tic Gazette* during this period, see Freud, *Cocaine Papers;* a complete set of the *Therapeutic Gazette* (or, as it has often been referred to, the *Detroit Therapeutic Gazette*) has been preserved and stored in the University of Michigan Libraries, Ann Arbor. A subsequent blockbuster drug developed by Parke, Davis was adrenaline, or epinephrine, which was discovered by the great Johns Hopkins pharmacologist John Jacob Abel.

64 With such ready access: Jill Jonnes, *Hep-Cats, Narcs, and Pipe Dreams: A History of America's Romance with Illegal Drugs* (Baltimore: Johns Hopkins University Press, 1996), pp. 11–58; and Courtwright, *Forces of Habit,* pp. 31–52.

64 During the early 1880s: Marez, "The *Coquero* in Freud," pp. 65–93. Marez notes that during the first six months of 1885, the elite *British Medical Journal* featured more than sixty-seven separate articles about cocaine. See, for example, Robert Christison, "The Effects of *Cuca* or Coca, the Leaves of *Erythroxylon coca*," *British Medical Journal* 1 (1876): 527–31; see also Atherton P. Mason, "*Erythroxy-lon coca*: Its Physiological Effect, and Especially Its Effect on the Excretion of Urea by the Kidney," *Boston Medical and Surgical Journal* 107 (1882): 221–23.

64 Indeed, this now forgotten and crumbling periodical: A bibliography of these *Therapeutic Gazette* articles, as well as reprints of many of them, can be found in Freud, *Cocaine Papers.*

64 For a brief period: Mahoney, *Merchants of Life,* pp. 69–73. The other, and per-haps more important, index of the medical literature of this era was the *Index-Catalogue of the U.S. Surgeon General's Office,* a publication of the United States Government. Freud himself noted that the *Index-Catalogue* was the first major index source he consulted when he began his study of cocaine.

Chapter 4. An Addict's Death

67 They were inscribed: Ernest Jones, *The Life and Work of Sigmund Freud,* vol. 1, *1856–1900* (New York: Basic Books, 1953), pp. 66–68; the aphorisms are quoted on p. 66, and a diagram of the chamber appears on p. 67. The actual letter is in the collection of the Library of Congress, Washington, D.C. Three years later when Freud was setting up his clinical practice, he asked Martha to embroider a third panel quoting Jean Martin Charcot: "Il faut avoir la foi" ("One must have faith").

68 Sigmund, who hardly needed any incentive: Freud worked on Scholz's nervous disease service for fourteen months, but the two never really got along and the senior physician wanted Freud transferred to another service some six months before his term was up. Freud then went on to complete a three-month stint in the ophthalmology department and applied for another three-month rotation in dermatology. He was spared this last task when he received permission to spend those last three months as a locum tenens physician for 100 gulden a month, plus room and board, in Heinrich Obersteiner's private neurology clinic just outside Vienna; Jones, *Life,* vol. 1, pp. 73–74.

68 Instead, his main inspiration: Ibid., pp. 78–97; E. M. Thornton, *Freud and*

Cocaine: The Freudian Fallacy (London: Blond and Briggs, 1983), pp. 36–47; and Peter Gay, *Freud: A Life for Our Time* (New York: W. W. Norton, 1998), p. 44. See also Robert C. Fuller, "Biographical Origins of Psychological Ideas: Freud's Cocaine Studies," *Journal of Humanistic Psychology* 32 (1992): 67–86; Richard Karmel, "Freud's Cocaine Papers (1884–1887): A Commentary," *Canadian Journal of Psychoanalysis* 11 (2003): 161–69; Siegfried Bernfeld, "Freud's Studies on Cocaine, 1884–1887," *Journal of the American Psychoanalytic Association* 1 (1953): 581–613; George Andrews and David Solomon, eds., *The Coca Leaf and Cocaine Papers* (New York: Harcourt Brace Jovanovich, 1975); and Sigmund Freud, *Cocaine Papers*, ed. Robert Byck (New York: Stonehill, 1974).

69   Despite a series of operations: Jones, *Life*, vol. 1, pp. 89–92.

70   "an unending torture": Ibid., p. 44.

70   "I could not rest": Ibid., p. 89.

70   "Cunning, baffling, and powerful": *Alcoholics Anonymous: The Story of How Many Thousands of Men and Women Have Recovered from Alcoholism*, 4th ed. (New York: Alcoholics Anonymous World Services, 2001), pp. 58–59.

71   His was an addiction: Some might argue that while Fleischl-Marxow was physically dependent on morphine, he might not be diagnosed today with *DSM*-IV criteria for true addiction; instead, he might be considered to suffer from the poorly named "pseudoaddiction," which suggests that the treatment of severe pain can yield many aberrant drug-taking behaviors that look like addiction but often disappear if the source of pain is adequately treated with other agents. I am grateful to my colleague Professor Kirk Brower, medical director of the University of Michigan Addiction Treatment Service, for pointing out this distinction to me.

71   Most of these medical doctors: The well-known mild pain reliever aspirin merits mention. Willow bark, rich in salicin, the active ingredient of aspirin, had been prescribed since the days of Hippocrates, but aspirin was not mass-produced and marketed until 1899, by the Bayer Company of Germany. As superb a medication as it is for mild pain and headaches, however, aspirin is not effective against more severe forms of pain, such as that experienced by Fleischl-Marxow. See Diarmuid Jeffreys, *Aspirin: The Remarkable Story of a Wonder Drug* (New York: Bloomsbury, 2004).

71   During the mid-1800s: Barbara Hodgson, *In the Arms of Morpheus: The Tragic History of Laudanum, Morphine, and Patent Medicines* (Buffalo, N.Y.: Firefly Books, 2001), pp. 14–15, 79–101; Martin Booth, *Opium: A History* (New York: Thomas Dunne Books / St. Martin's Press, 1996), pp. 1–34; W. Travis Hanes and Frank Sanello, *The Opium Wars: The Addiction of One Empire and the Corruption of Another* (Naperville, Ill.: Sourcebooks, 2002); and Jack Beeching, *The Chinese Opium Wars* (San Diego: Harcourt Brace Jovanovich, 1975).

71   "If the whole *materia medica*": Oliver W. Holmes Sr., "Currents and Counter-Currents in Medical Science," in *Medical Essays* (Boston: Houghton, Mifflin, 1883), pp. 202–03. *Materia medica,* a term that dates back to the era of the Roman Empire and was still in use at the opening of the twentieth century, referred to the body of knowledge on various therapeutics used for healing purposes. It has since been replaced by the modern scientific field of pharmacology.

72   A German pharmacist: Hodgson, *Arms of Morpheus,* p. 79.

72 Morphine's popularity and profitability: Eric C. Schneider, *Smack: Heroin and the American City* (Philadelphia: University of Pennsylvania Press, 2008). Heroin was first extracted in 1874 by a London pharmacist in search of a nonaddictive alternative to morphine. By boiling morphine with acetic anhydride he produced a powerful narcotic, twice as potent as a dose of morphine, which the Bayer Company began to market as heroin in 1898.

72 Especially in the decades after the development: G. Lawrence, "The Hypodermic Syringe," *Lancet* 359, no. 9311 (March 23, 2002): 1074; George L. Servoss, *The Hypodermic Syringe* (Newark, N.J.: Physicians Drug News, Publishers, 1914); and Roberts Bartholow, *Manual of Hypodermic Medication: The Treatment of Diseases by the Hypodermic Method,* 4th ed. (Philadelphia: J. B. Lippincott, 1882).

72 In O'Neill's play: Eugene O'Neill, *Long Day's Journey into Night* (New Haven: Yale University Press, 1955). See also Barbara Gelb and Arthur Gelb, *O'Neill: Life with Monte Cristo* (New York: Applause Books, 2000); and Hamilton Basso, "Profiles: The Tragic Sense," *New Yorker,* February 28, 1948, pp. 34–45; parts 2 and 3 of this article appear in the March 6, 1948, issue, pp. 34–49, and the March 13, 1948, issue, pp. 37–47. See also David T. Courtright, *Dark Paradise: A History of Opiate Addiction in America* (Cambridge, Mass.: Harvard University Press, 2001); Richard Davenport-Hines, *The Pursuit of Oblivion: A Global History of Narcotics* (New York: W. W. Norton, 2001); Jill Jonnes, *Hep-Cats, Narcs, and Pipe Dreams: A History of America's Romance with Illegal Drugs* (Baltimore: Johns Hopkins University Press, 1996); Caroline J. Acker, *Creating the American Junkie: Addiction Research in the Classic Era of Narcotic Control* (Baltimore: Johns Hopkins University Press, 2002); and Booth, *Opium: A History.*

72 Interestingly, morphine addicts: Courtright, *Dark Paradise,* pp. 35–60; and Hodgson, *Arms of Morpheus,* pp. 14–15, 79–101.

73 As the late comedian: *Lenny Bruce: Swear to Tell the Truth,* film documentary, 1998 (produced, written, and directed by Robert B. Weide; edited by Geof Bartz and Robert B. Weide; released by Whyaduck Productions in association with HBO Documentary Films, 1998); P. Krassner, "The Busting of Lenny," *Index on Censorship* 6 (2000): 78–85; and Albert Goldman, *Ladies and Gentlemen, Lenny Bruce!!* (New York: Random House, 1974).

74 Ramped-up versions: Mary Jeanne Kreek, "Neurobiology of Opiates and Opioids," in *The American Psychiatry Publishing Textbook of Substance Abuse Treatment,* 4th ed., ed. Marc Galanter and Herbert D. Kleber (Washington, D.C.: American Psychiatry Press, 2008), pp. 247–64; Soteri Polydorou and Herbert D. Kleber, "Detoxification of Opiates and Opioids," in *Textbook of Substance Abuse Treatment,* pp. 265–87; L. Borg, I. Kravets, and M. J. Kreek, "The Pharmacology of Long-Acting as Opposed to Short-Acting Opioids," in *Principles of Addiction Medicine,* 4th ed., ed. R. A. Ries, D. A. Fiellen, S. C. Miller, and R. Saitz (Philadelphia: Wolters Kluwer/Lippincott Williams and Wilkins, 2009), pp. 117–31; Robert M. Julien, *A Primer of Drug Action: A Concise, Nontechnical Guide to the Actions, Uses, and Side Effects of Psychoactive Drugs* (New York: Holt/Owl Books, 2001), pp. 173–81; and S. M. Stine and T. R. Kosten, "Opioids," in *Addictions: A Comprehensive Guidebook,* ed. Barbara S. McCrady and Elizabeth E. Epstein (New York: Oxford University Press, 1999), pp. 141–61.

74 "I am also toying": Sigmund Freud to Martha Bernays, April 21, 1884, Ernst L. Freud, ed., *Letters of Sigmund Freud* (New York: Basic Books, 1960), pp. 107–09 (Letter 43); quote is from p. 107.

75 Elsewhere in this letter: Freud notes in his monograph *Über Coca* that his first source of material was the section on *Erythroxylon coca* in the *Index Catalogue of the Library of the U.S. Surgeon General's Office*, vol. 4, 1883, which he considered to be the most complete index of the literature up to that time.

75 For example, he refers: Freud, *Über Coca*, in Freud, *Cocaine Papers*, p. 73; see also a paper Freud read and referenced by the Italian physician Paolo Mantegazza, "Sulle virtù igieniche e medicinali della coca," *Memoria Annali Universali di Medicina*, 1859, cited by Byck in *Cocaine Papers*. An English translation of parts of this paper appears in Andrews and Solomon, *The Coca Leaf*, pp. 38–42.

75 He also describes: T. Aschenbrandt, "Die Physiologische Wirkung und Bedeutung des Cocain insbesondere auf den menschlichen Organismus," *Deutche medizinische Wochenschrift*, no. 50 (December 12, 1883): 730–32.

76 Two years later: W. H. Bentley, "*Erythoxylon coca* in the Opium and Alcohol Habits," *Therapeutic Gazette* 1 (1880): 253, reprinted in Freud, *Cocaine Papers*, pp. 14–19.

76 Substituting one addictive drug: Andrews and Solomon, *The Coca Leaf*; Freud, *Cocaine Papers*; and Thornton, *Freud and Cocaine*. Today, addiction physicians routinely prescribe the less severely but nonetheless addictive drug methadone for opiate addicts, with great success; the difference is that with this modern substitution the medical repercussions are significantly less than when trading cocaine for morphine. A newer agent, buprenorphine, blocks opiate receptors and, thus, the high one might get upon taking a subsequent dose of heroin or morphine, but this drug, too, can be manipulated by active addicts in an abusive manner.

76 At the dawn of doctors' recognition: Asa P. Maylert, *Notes on the Opium Habit*, 3rd ed. (New York: G. P. Putnam's Sons, 1885); and J. P. Gavit, *Opium* (London: George Routledge and Sons, 1925).

76 The great microbiologist Louis Pasteur: Louis Pasteur, "Inaugural Lecture, University of Lille, December 4, 1854," quoted in John Bartlett, *Bartlett's Familiar Quotations*, ed. Justin Kaplan, 16th ed. (Boston: Little, Brown, 1992), p. 502.

76 Like Moses: Freud's final book, *Moses and Monotheism* (New York: Vintage Books, 1967), was first published in 1939.

76 Writing about the conversation: Freud to Martha, May 29, 1884, Freud, *Letters*, pp. 109–12 (Letter 44).

77 On the nights he sat: Jones, *Life*, vol. 1, p. 91.

77 "I admire and love him": Ibid., p. 90.

77 Fleischl-Marxow eagerly consented: Siegfried Bernfeld, "Freud's Studies on Cocaine, 1884–1887," *Journal of the American Psychoanalytic Association* 1 (1953): 581–613.

78 The four men eventually procured: Jones, *Life*, vol. 1, p. 90.

78 In the time span of less than three months: Late-nineteenth-century dollars were converted into 2010 values using a formula based on the consumer price index from the economic history–focused website Measuring Worth, www.measuringworth.com/index.html (accessed February 25, 2010).

78 This does not even account: Jones, *Life*, vol. 1, p. 91.

78 Freud recalled it: Ibid.

78 A guilt-ridden Sigmund: Ibid., pp. 80–81, 89–96.

79 In the days immediately following: George M. Beard, "Neurasthenia or Nervous Exhaustion," *Boston Medical and Surgical Journal* 80 (1869): 217–21; George M. Beard, *American Nervousness: Its Causes and Consequences; A Supplement to Nervous Exhaustion* (New York: G. P. Putnam's Sons, 1881); H. A. Bunker, "From Beard to Freud: A Brief History of the Concept of Neurasthenia," *Medical Review of Reviews* 36 (1930): 108–14; Charles E. Rosenberg, "The Place of George Miller Beard in American Psychiatry," *Bulletin of the History of Medicine* 36 (1962): 245–59; and Edward Shorter, *A History of Psychiatry: From the Era of the Asylum to the Age of Prozac* (New York: John Wiley and Sons, 1997), pp. 129–130. Beard defined this entity as a bridge of sorts between organic causes and symptoms that affected one's mood, thinking, and feelings. It was marked by fatigue and exhaustion, depression, headaches, dyspepsia, insomnia, paralysis, neuralgia, and a number of other symptoms. The diagnosis fell out of favor beginning in the early twentieth century.

79 In one 1884 publication: The original version of this paper was published in the November 1884 issue of *Klinische Monatsblatter fur Augenheilkunde, Zeherder* and appeared a few months later as E. Merck, "Cocaine and Its Salts," trans. W. M. Smith, *Chicago Medical Journal and Examiner* 50 (February 1885): 157–63. The Latin prescription in Merck's disclaimer is "Muriatic solution of Cocaine, Merck."

79 Budgeting 33 kreuzer: Jones, *Life,* vol. 1, p. 80; late-nineteenth-century dollars were converted into 2010 values using a formula based on the consumer price index from the economic history–focused website Measuring Worth, www.measuringworth.com/index.html (accessed February 25, 2010).

80 His bad mood: Jones, *Life,* vol. 1, p. 80.

80 Like many inquiring doctors: For a fascinating account of self-experimentation in medicine, see Lawrence K. Altman, *Who Goes First: The Story of Self-Experimentation in Medicine* (New York: Random House, 1987).

80 In May 1884: Jones, *Life,* vol. 1, p. 81.

80 "If all goes well": Ibid.

81 "Woe to you": Freud to Martha, June 2, 1884, quoted at length ibid., p. 84.

81 And as his use of cocaine progressed: Jones, *Life,* vol. 1, 84. See also Freud to Martha, June 29, 1884, Freud, *Letters,* pp. 115–16 (Letter 47); pp. 145–46 (Letter 65); and pp. 200–204 (Letter 94). For example, a packet Sigmund sent in June 1885 included a vial containing a gram of cocaine with instructions to divide the drug into "8 small (or 5 large) doses" for her mental indisposition. See Gay, *Freud,* p. 44.

81 Freud's biographer Ernest Jones: Jones, *Life,* vol. 1, p. 82.

82 He now begins: Freud, "On Coca," in Freud, *Cocaine Papers,* p. 58.

82 "A few minutes after": Ibid.

83 In essence, *Über Coca* introduces: Ibid. In a subsequent paper published in 1885, Sigmund writes a specific disclaimer that he is aware of the problems of objectivity when doing such self-experiments; Freud, "Contribution to the Knowledge of the Effect of Cocaine (1885)," in Freud, *Cocaine Papers,* pp. 98–99.

83 By midsummer, Freud saw: Jones, *Life,* vol. 1, p. 93; Sigmund Freud, "Über

Coca," *Centralblatt für die gesammte Therapie* 2 (1885): 289–314. Late-nineteenth-century dollars were converted into 2010 values using a formula based on the consumer price index from the economic history–focused website Measuring Worth, www.measuringworth.com/index.html (accessed February 25, 2010).

85 As early as the second century A.D.: Howard Markel, "Who's on First? Medical Discoveries and Scientific Priority," *New England Journal of Medicine* 351 (2004): 2792–94; and Galen, *On the Natural Faculties,* trans. A. J. Brock, book 3, sec. 10 (Cambridge, Mass.: Loeb's Classical Library, 1916), pp. 279–81.

85 Carl, incidentally: Freud to Martha, January 6, 1885, Freud, *Letters,* pp. 131–32 (Letter 55); quote is from p. 131.

86 "By this time": Hortense Koller Becker, "Carl Koller and Cocaine," *Psychoanalytic Quarterly* 32 (1963): 309–73; Arthur J. Beckhard and William D. Crane, *Cancer, Cocaine and Courage: The Story of Dr. William Halsted* (New York: Julian Messner, 1960), pp. 119–21; Carl Koller, "On the Use of Cocaine for Producing Anesthesia of the Eye," trans. J. N. Bloom, *Lancet,* December 6, 1884; and Carl Koller, "Historical Notes on the Beginnings of Local Anesthesia," *Journal of the American Medical Association* 90, no. 21 (1928): 1742–43.

87 In late 1884: Sigmund Freud, "Contribution to the Knowledge of the Effect of Cocaine," *Wiener medizinische Wochenschrift,* no. 5 (January 31, 1885): 130–33, in Freud, *Cocaine Papers,* pp. 95–104. See also Sigmund Freud, "Addenda to *Über Coca,*" a revised and expanded reprint from the *Centralblatt für die gesammte Therapie,* Vienna, 1885, in Freud, *Cocaine Papers,* pp. 107–09.

87 Freud also claimed: Leopold Königstein conducted some work on cocaine and the eye and later, at Freud's instigation, inserted a letter in *Wiener medizinische Presse,* nos. 42 and 43, asserting Freud's primacy as discoverer of cocaine. Freud, "Beitrag zur Kenntniss," in Freud, *Cocaine Papers,* pp. 95–104. See also L. Königstein, "Über die Anwendung des Cocain am Auge," *Centralbaltt für die gesammte Therapie* (Vienna: Verlag von Mortiz Perles, 1885). Quoted in Jones, *Life,* vol. 1, p. 87.

87 It was an attractive: To make matters more contentious, when Koller published the paper he read to the Vienna Medical Society, he cited Freud's paper as being published in August rather than July. The implication of such erroneous dating, in Freud's view, was to suggest that Koller's work was done before or simultaneously with Freud's rather than after it. In later life, Koller asserted that Freud's work appeared a full year after his own paper. C. Koller, "Nachträgliche Bemerkungen über die ersten Anfäng der Lokalanaesthesie," *Wiener medizinische Wochenschrift,* 1935, p. 7. See also Jones, *Life,* vol. 1, pp. 87–88; and Gay, *Freud,* p. 43.

87 Another barometer of Freud's feelings: Sigmund Freud, *Der Witz und seine Beziehung zum Unbewussten* (Vienna: Deuticke, 1905); published in the United States as Freud, *The Joke and Its Relation to the Unconscious,* trans. Joyce Crick (New York: Penguin Classics, 2002).

87 To Martha, in January 1885: Freud to Martha, January 7, 1885, Freud, *Letters,* pp. 132–33 (Letter 56); and Gay, *Freud,* pp. 44–45. See also Jones, *Life,* vol. 1, pp. 96–97.

87 Later, Freud was said to have inscribed: Becker, "Carl Koller and Cocaine."

87 In 1895, Sigmund reported a dream: Sigmund Freud, *The Interpretation of Dreams*, trans. James Strachey (New York: Penguin Books, 1991), pp. 255–56, 259, 262, 309, 387; and Gay, *Freud*, p. 43.

88 "I may here go back a little": Sigmund Freud, *An Autobiographical Study*, trans. James Strachey (New York: W. W. Norton, rpt. ed., 1989), p. 13.

89 As he read the passage: Fritz Wittels, *Sigmund Freud and His Time* (New York: Liveright, 1931), p. 19. The Freud annotated copy can be found in the Freud Museum and Archives, London; quoted in Gay, *Freud*, p. 45.

89 "I know very well": Jones, *Life*, vol. 1, pp. 83–84; the quote is from a letter from Freud to Wittels, December 12, 1923, cited in Jones. "Allotrion" is a word Sigmund and his teachers used during his schooldays.

Chapter 5. The Accidental Addict

90 At the system's official opening: A. F. Harlow, "Telegraph," in *Dictionary of American History*, vol. 5, ed. J. T. Adams and R. V. Coleman (New York: Charles Scribner's Sons, 1940), p. 238; and Paul Starr, *The Creation of the Media: Political Origins of Modern Communications* (New York: Basic Books, 2004), pp. 153–89.

90 The primary focus: Carl Koller, "Über die verwendung des cocain zur Anasthesierung am Auge," *Wiener medizische Wochenschrift* 34, nos. 43 and 44 (1884); and Carl Koller, "Vorlaufige Mitteilung über Lokale Anestheiserung am Auge," manuscript of a speech delivered for Dr. Koller by Dr. Josef Brettauer at the meeting of the German Ophthalmological Society at Heidelberg, September 15, 1884. Also in the room was Dr. Henry Noyes, of New York City, who immediately wrote a dispatch of this talk for the *New York Medical Record*, "The Ophthalmological Congress in Heidelberg," *New York Medical Record* 26 (October 11, 1884): 417–18. It was likely this paper that introduced Halsted to cocaine. In this dispatch, Noyes stated that "the momentous value of the discovery seems likely to be in eye practice of more significance than has been the discovery of anesthesia by chloroform or ether in general surgery and medicine."

91 The scientific details: Koller's discovery was briefly reported in the major New York newspapers around this time as well. See, for example, "A Costly Anesthetic," *New York Times*, October 23, 1884, p. 8; and "The New Anesthetic: Interesting Experiments with the Discovery in Albany," *New York Times*, October 29, 1884, p. 2. Both of these articles refer to experiments with cocaine already being done in New York after Koller's announcement.

91 The price of cocaine: "The New Anaesthetic: Interesting Experiments with the Discovery in Albany," *New York Times*, October 29, 1884, p. 2; late-nineteenth-century dollars were converted into 2010 values using a formula based on the consumer price index from the economic history–focused website, Measuring Worth, www.measuringworth.com/index.html (accessed February 25, 2010).

91 The 1846 discovery: To be sure, surgical advancement also required an understanding of the concept of surgical shock, intravenous fluids and blood transfusions, and a number of twentieth-century innovations that facilitated more and more invasive surgery, but it was the "discovery" of anesthesia that set this

process in motion. See Sherwin B. Nuland, *The Origins of Anesthesia* (Birmingham, Ala.: Classics of Medicine Library, 1983); Howard Markel, "Not So Great Moments: The 'Discovery' of Ether Anesthesia and Its 'Re-discovery' by Hollywood," *Journal of the American Medical Association* 300 (2008): 2188–90; R. Fulop-Miller, *Triumph over Pain,* trans. E. Paul and C. Paul (New York: Literary Guild of America, 1938); Jurgen Thorwald, *The Century of the Surgeon* (New York: Bantam Books, rpt. ed., 1963); and Martin S. Pernick, *A Calculus of Suffering: Pain, Professionalism and Anesthesia in Nineteenth-Century America* (New York: Columbia University Press, 1985).

91 Although practiced since the days of antiquity: Mirko Grmek, *Diseases in the Ancient World* (Baltimore: Johns Hopkins University Press, 1991), p. 14; H. E. Sigerist, *A History of Medicine,* vol. 1, *Primitive and Archaic Medicine* (New York: Oxford University Press, 1951), p. 334.

92 "It was like a red-hot needle": Florence Emily Hardy, *Early Life of Thomas Hardy, 1840–1891* (New York: Macmillan, 1928), p. 200. Hardy is describing the experience of an old man he met on his travels in the early 1880s.

92 "One can perhaps imagine": William G. MacCallum, *William Stewart Halsted, Surgeon* (Baltimore: Johns Hopkins University Press, 1930), pp. 44–45.

93 He performed the death-defying procedure: Ibid., pp. 43–44. Halsted discovered his mother to be suffering from the classic "Charcot's triad" of gallstones: fever, right upper quadrant pain, and jaundice. This procedure has been credited by some historians of surgery as one of the first gallbladder operations, cholecystostomy, performed in the United States, although it is difficult to ascertain this definitively. Nevertheless, cholecystostomy became a standard surgical procedure Halsted was to perfect and report on in the years to come.

94 He was especially perturbed: "Aseptic Surgery in New York in 1884," in William S. Halsted, *Surgical Papers in Two Volumes,* ed. Walter C. Burket (Baltimore: The Johns Hopkins Press, 1924), vol. 1, p. 46.

94 Convinced by Dr. Joseph Lister's argument: Joseph Lister, *The Collected Papers of Joseph, Baron Lister,* 2 vols. (Oxford: Clarendon Press, 1909).

95 Writing to a colleague in 1921: Letter from William S. Halsted to Rudolph Matas, May 30, 1921, Box 59, Folder 9, W. S. Halsted Papers, Alan Mason Chesney Archives, Johns Hopkins Medical Institutions, Baltimore; and Allan E. Dumont, "Halsted at Bellevue, 1883–1887," *Annals of Surgery* 172, no. 6 (1970): 929–35.

96 Yet when one of them: Simon Flexner and James T. Flexner, *William Henry Welch and the Heroic Age of American Medicine* (New York: Viking Press, 1941), p. 119; and Howard Markel, *When Germs Travel: Six Major Epidemics That Have Invaded America Since 1900 and the Fears They Have Unleashed* (New York: Pantheon, 2004), pp. 207–08.

96 Welch, a frequent houseguest: Alan M. Chesney, *The Johns Hopkins Hospital and the Johns Hopkins University School of Medicine,* vol. 1, *Early Years, 1867–1893* (Baltimore: Johns Hopkins University Press, 1943), p. 111.

96 Halsted's demonstrable success: R. Dunglison and R. J. Dunglison, *A Dictionary of Medical Science,* new ed. (Philadelphia: Henry C. Lea, 1874), p. 874.

96 Welch occupied his days: Welch was an intern at Bellevue beginning in 1876;

Halsted joined the house staff in 1878. See Robert J. Carlisle, ed., *An Account of Bellevue Hospital with a Catalogue of the Medical and Surgical Staff from 1736 to 1894* (New York: Society of the Alumni of Bellevue Hospital, 1893), pp. 333–34.

97 "The patient's mouth filled with blood": Transcript of a letter to William Osler from Halsted, August 25, 1918. Titled "Complete copy for Dr. J. F. Fulton of a handwritten letter of Halsted inserted by Osler in a reprint of Cushing's 'Some conservative jottings apropos of spinal anesthesia,' " *New York Medical Journal* 42 (1895): 483–85, and 488; no. 1800 in *Bibliotheca Osleriana,* 1929, where an abstract is printed; and George J. Heuer Papers, Box 2, File 14, Item 1, Weill Cornell Medical College, Medical Center Archives, New York, N.Y.

97 Thanks to the surgeon's quick packing: Wilder Penfield, "Halsted of Johns Hopkins: The Man and His Problems as Described in the Secret Records of William Osler," *Journal of the American Medical Association* 210 (1969): 2214–18; and Lawrence K. Altman, *Who Goes First: The Story of Self-Experimentation in Medicine* (New York: Random House, 1987), pp. 53–85. See also William S. Halsted, "Practical Comments on the Use and Abuse of Cocaine," *Surgical Papers,* vol. 1, pp. 167–77 (the quote regarding operating in his bedroom is on p. 172); and R. Hall, "Hydrochlorate of Cocaine," *New York Medical Journal* 40 (1884): 643–44.

98 Theater events, dances: MacCallum, *Halsted,* pp. 53–54.

98 "Once we happened to speak": [Sergius Pankejeff], *The Wolf-Man by the Wolf-Man,* ed. Muriel Gardiner (New York: Hill and Wang, 1991), p. 146; and M. Rohrwasser, *Freuds Lektüren: Von Arthur Conan Doyle bis zu Arthur Schnitzler* (Freud's Reading: From Arthur Conan Doyle to Arthur Schnitzler) (Giessen: Psychosozial Verlag, 2005).

99 "Sherlock Holmes took his bottle": Arthur Conan Doyle, *The Sign of the Four* (1890), in *The New Annotated Sherlock Holmes,* ed. L. S. Klinger, vol. 3 (New York: W. W. Norton, 2005), p. 213. At his worst, according to Holmes's second banana, Dr. John Watson, Sherlock self-injected cocaine three times a day for many months. Some have credited Freud's papers on cocaine with inspiring Conan Doyle's interest in using the drug as a literary device in his work. This is likely an overstatement. Conan Doyle probably read *Über Coca,* given his prodigious reading habits and propensity to keep up with the medical literature, but as noted earlier, cocaine was one of the hottest medical topics during this era, both before and after Carl Koller's pathbreaking paper on the drug's anesthetic powers. See also David F. Musto, "Sherlock Holmes and Sigmund Freud," in Sigmund Freud, *Cocaine Papers,* ed. Robert Byck (New York: Stonehill, 1974), pp. 357–70; Alvin E. Rodin and Jack D. Key, *Medical Casebook of Doctor Arthur Conan Doyle* (Malabar, Fla.: Robert E. Krieger Publishing, 1984), pp. 249–99; Andrew Lycett, *The Man Who Created Sherlock Holmes* (New York: Free Press, 2007); Jon Lellenberg, Daniel Stashower, and Charles Foley, eds., *Arthur Conan Doyle: A Life in Letters* (New York: Penguin Press, 2007); and Howard Markel, "The Medical Detectives," *New England Journal of Medicine* 353 (2005): 2426–28.

100 "My dear Halsted": R. J. Hall to Halsted, September 2, 1895. Box 11, Folder 3, W. S. Halsted Papers, Alan Mason Chesney Medical Archives, Johns Hopkins

Medical Institutions, Baltimore. See also R. J. Hall, "Hydrochlorate of Cocaine," *New York Medical Journal* 40 (1884): 643–44.

Chapter 6. Cocaine Damnation

102 The resulting chemical reaction: Dominic Streatfeild, *Cocaine: An Unauthorized Biography* (New York: Picador, 2001), pp. 271–323.

102 Cocaine users soon flocked: National Institute of Drug Abuse, *Research Report: Cocaine Abuse and Addiction,* www.nida.nih.gov/researchreports/Cocaine/ cocaine3.html (accessed May 28, 2009). A more dangerous form of freeing the cocaine from the salt was freebasing cocaine, a popular method of abuse in the early 1980s. When a user smoked the drug in a pipe containing ether, the alkaloid or base portion of the drug was "freed" from the chloride salt, resulting in faster delivery of cocaine molecules to the brain. But the mixture was highly flammable and explosive, leading to a number of injuries and deaths from its use by inebriated people. Most infamous were the severe body burns experienced by the comedian Richard Pryor in 1980; he was smoking freebase cocaine, drinking 150-proof rum, and experiencing a cocaine-induced psychosis.

103 Cocaine can also wreak havoc: M. F. Weaver and S. H. Schnoll, "Stimulants: Amphetamines and Cocaine," in *Addictions: A Comprehensive Guidebook,* ed. B. S. McReady and E. E. Epstein (New York: Oxford University Press, 1999), pp. 105–20; L. L. Cregler and H. Mark, "Medical Complications of Cocaine Abuse," *New England Journal of Medicine* 315 (1986): 1495–1500; F. H. Gawin and E. H. Ellinwood Jr., "Cocaine and Other Stimulants," *New England Journal of Medicine* 318 (1988): 1173–82; and F. H. Gawin, "Cocaine Addiction: Psychology and Neurophysiology," *Science* 251 (1991): 1580–86.

103 After arriving at the brain's prefrontal cortex: M. D. Lemonick and A. Park, "The Science of Addiction," *Time,* July 16, 2007, pp. 42–48; Richard F. Thompson, *The Brain: A Neuroscience Primer,* 3rd ed. (New York: Worth Publishers, 2000), pp. 168–75; Margaret Haney, "Neurobiology of Stimulants," in *The American Psychiatry Publishing Textbook of Substance Abuse Treatment,* 4th ed., ed. Marc Galanter and Herbert D. Kleber (Washington, D.C.: American Psychiatry Press, 2008), pp. 143–55; and D. A. Gorelick, "The Pharmacology of Cocaine, Amphetamines and Other Stimulants," in *Principles of Addiction Medicine,* 4th ed., ed. R. A. Ries, D. A. Fiellen, S. C. Miller, and R. Saitz (Philadelphia: Wolters Kluwer/Lippincott Williams and Wilkins, 2009), pp. 133–57. Others argue that the nucleus accumbens has more to do with the memory, anticipation, and motivation for reward than with appreciation for the reward itself. Hence, this frequent comment from addicts: "I don't even feel that good when I do it, but I cannot stop myself."

103 Under normal circumstances: To be neuroanatomically correct, the dopamine transporter proteins are located in the nucleus accumbens. They sit on the nerve terminals of neurons that originate in the ventral tegmental area and end in the nucleus accumbens; hence, the cocaine acts pharmacologically on or in the nucleus accumbens.

104 A pharmacological version: Alan I. Leshner, "What We Know: Drug Addiction

Is a Brain Disease," in *Principles of Addiction Medicine,* 2nd ed., ed. Allan W. Graham and Terry K. Schultz (Chevy Chase, Md.: American Society of Addiction Medicine, 1998), pp. xxix–xxxvi; N. Volkow and T.-K. Li, "Drug Addiction: The Neurobiology of Behavior Gone Awry," in *Principles of Addiction Medicine,* 4th ed., pp. 3–12; C. V. Dobrin and D.C.S. Roberts, "The Anatomy of Addiction," in *Principles of Addiction Medicine,* pp. 27–38; Robert L. Dupont, *The Selfish Brain: Learning from Addiction* (Minneapolis: Hazelden Publishing Co., 2000); N. D. Volkow, J. S. Fowler, and G. J. Wang, "The Addicted Human Brain: Insights from Imaging Studies," *Journal of Clinical Investigation* 111, no. 10 (2003): 1444–51; G. F. Koob and M. Le Moal, "Plasticity of Reward Neurocircuitry and the 'Dark Side' of Drug Addiction," *Nature Neuroscience* 8, no. 11 (2005): 1442–44; P. W. Kalivas and N. D. Volkow, "The Neural Basis of Addiction: A Pathology of Motivation and Choice," *American Journal of Psychiatry* 162, no. 8 (2005): 1403–13; and B. J. Everitt and T. W. Robbins, "Neural Systems of Reinforcement of Drug Addiction: From Actions to Habits to Compulsion," *Nature Neuroscience* 8, no. 11 (2005): 1481–89.

104 Ecstatic arousal and desire: Haney, "Neurobiology," in *Textbook of Substance Abuse,* 4th ed., pp. 143–55; Gorelick, "Pharmacology of Cocaine," in *Principles of Addiction,* pp. 133–57.

105 Specifically, such crashes: F. S. Hall, X. F. Li, I. Sora, F. Xu, M. Caron, K. P. Lesch, D. L. Murphy, and G. R. Uhl, "Cocaine Mechanisms: Enhanced Cocaine, Fluoxetine and Nisoxetine Place Preferences Following Monoamine Transporter Deletions," *Neuroscience* 115, no. 1 (2002): 153–61. I am grateful to my colleagues Dr. David McDowell, clinical assistant professor of psychiatry at Mount Sinai Medical Center of New York, and Dr. Kirk Brower, professor of psychiatry and medical director of the University of Michigan Addiction Treatment Service, for helping me sort out the complex neurochemistry of cocaine.

105 In time, cocaine abuse: The frontal cortex also contains sensory, reinforcement, and associative circuitry that can be damaged by chronic cocaine abuse. See W. M. Freeman, K. Brebner, K. M. Patel, W. J. Lynch, D. C. Roberts, and K. E. Vrana, "Repeated Cocaine Self-administration Causes Multiple Changes in Rat Frontal Cortex Gene Expression," *Neurochemical Research* 27, no. 10 (2002): 1181–92; C. A. Biggins, S. MacKay, W. Clark, and G. Fein, "Event-Related Potential Evidence for Frontal Cortex Effects of Chronic Cocaine Dependence," *Biological Psychiatry* 42, no. 6 (1997): 472–85; and J. A. Matochik, E. D. London, D. A. Eldreth, J. L. Cadet, and K. Bolla, "Frontal Cortical Tissue Composition in Abstinent Cocaine Abusers: A Magnetic Resonance Imaging Study," *NeuroImage* 19, no. 3 (July 2003): 1095–102.

105 A month later: Streatfeild, *Cocaine,* p. 88; J. H. Woods and C. R. Schuster, "Reinforcement Properties of Morphine, Cocaine, and SPA as a Function of Unit Dose," *International Journal of the Addictions* 3 (1968): 231–37; A. Etternberg, H. O. Pettit, F. E. Bloom, and G. F. Koob, "Heroin and Cocaine Intravenous Self-administration in Rats: Mediation by Separate Neural Systems," *Psychopharmacology* 78 (1982): 204–09; and J. H. Woods, "Behavioral Pharmacology of Drug Self-administration," in *Psychopharmacology: A Generation of Progress,* ed. M. A. Lipton, A. DiMascio, and K. F. Killam (New York: Raven, 1978).

106 McBride was said to have spent: MacCallum, *Halsted,* pp. 45–46.

106 It was likely a close and loving relationship: For social and cultural historical analyses of gender roles, masculinity, femininity, and sexuality during this era, see Gail Bederman, *Manliness and Civilization: A Cultural History of Gender and Race in the United States, 1880–1917* (Chicago: University of Chicago Press, 1996); Carroll Smith-Rosenberg, *Disorderly Conduct: Visions of Gender in Victorian America* (New York: Oxford University Press, 1986); Michael Kimmel, *Manhood in America: A Cultural History* (New York: Free Press, 1996); E. Anthony Rotundo, *American Manhood: Transformations in Masculinity from the Revolution to the Modern Era* (New York: Basic Books, 1993); and John D'Emilio and Estelle B. Freedman, *Intimate Matters: A History of Sexuality in America* (Chicago: University of Chicago Press, 1997).

106 After examining a laborer: Allan E. Dumont, "Halsted at Bellevue, 1883–1887," *Annals of Surgery* 172, no. 6 (1970): 929–35; Wilder Penfield, "W. Halsted of Johns Hopkins," *Journal of the American Medical Association* 210 (1969): 2214–18; and Allen O. Whipple, "Halsted's New York Period," *Surgery* 32 (1952): 542–50. The May 5, 1885, episode is described in detail in the prologue of this book.

106 Instead, the editor lists: William S. Halsted, *Surgical Papers in Two Volumes,* ed. Walter C. Burket (Baltimore: The Johns Hopkins Press, 1924), vol. 1, p. 167. This short notice is followed by a series of letters and documents attesting to Halsted's discovery of nerve blockade, the basis of modern painless dentistry. See also Halsted to Matas, May 24, 1921, Box 59, Folder 9; Halsted to Matas, May 30, 1921, Box 18, Folder 4; Halsted to Matas, July 10, 1921, Box 59, Folder 18; and Halsted from Matas, Box 59, Folder 11, W. S. Halsted Papers, Alan Mason Chesney Archives, Johns Hopkins Medical Institutions, Baltimore.

107 "Neither indifferent as to which": William S. Halsted, "Practical Comments on the Use and Abuse of Cocaine Suggested by Its Invariably Successful Employment in More Than a Thousand Minor Surgical Operations," *New York Medical Journal* 42 (September 12, 1885): 294–95.

107 In the summer of 1885: Halsted to Welch, July 14, 1922, Series II, Notes, Box 31, William S. Halsted Papers, Alan Mason Chesney Archives, Johns Hopkins Medical Institutions, Baltimore.

108 To the end of his life: These events are recounted in a letter Halsted wrote to William Osler on August 23, 1918; it is reprinted in George J. Heuer, "Dr. Halsted," *Johns Hopkins Hospital Bulletin,* Supp. 90 (1952): 21.

108 Every time the urologist: A. P. Stout, "William Stewart Halsted," Notes, Series II, June 9, 1924, Box 49, William Stewart Halsted Papers, Alan Mason Chesney Archives, Johns Hopkins Medical Institutions, Baltimore; Daniel B. Nunn, "Dr. Halsted's Addiction," *Johns Hopkins Advanced Studies in Medicine* 6, no. 3 (2006): 106–10; and Daniel B. Nunn, "William Stewart Halsted: Transitional Years," *Surgery* 121, no. 3 (1997): 343–51.

110 It was a short time: Howard Markel, "The Accidental Addict," *New England Journal of Medicine* 352 (2005): 966–68.

111 Regardless of the veracity: Arthur J. Beckhard and William D. Crane, *Cancer, Cocaine and Courage: The Story of Dr. William Halsted* (New York: Julian Messner, 1960). The authors interviewed a number of New York City doctors and members of the New York Academy of Medicine in the late 1950s who either

knew Halsted personally or knew of him once removed (such as a friend's spouse). Sadly, the authors do not list the book's precise sources or the textual means for verification. Another title in this series of "juvenile biographies" is on Sigmund Freud: Rachel Baker, *Sigmund Freud* (New York: Julian Messner, 1952).

111 Butler was a well-known insane asylum: MacCallum, *Halsted*, pp. 55–57, 58–71. Dr. Vander Poel first suggested Butler Hospital to Halsted a few months earlier, but such an intervention obviously failed.

112 If he could only recover: Ibid., pp. 55–71.

113 How lost and abject: Peter D. Olch, "William S. Halsted's New York Period, 1874–1886," *Bulletin of the History of Medicine* 60 (1966): 495–510; Peter D. Olch, "William S. Halsted and Local Anesthesia: Contributions and Complications," *Anesthesiology* 42, no. 4 (1975): 479–86.

Chapter 7. Sigmund in Paris

114 Soon after its appearance: Ernest Jones, *The Life and Work of Sigmund Freud*, vol. 1 (New York: Basic Books, 1955), pp. 92–94.

114 Around this same time: Sigmund Freud, "Contribution to the Knowledge of the Effect of Cocaine," *Wiener medizinische Wochenschrift*, no. 5 (January 31, 1885): 130–33, in *Cocaine Papers*, ed. Robert Byck (New York: Stonehill, 1974), pp. 97–104.

114 A mealymouthed Sigmund concluded: Sigmund Freud, "Addenda to *Über Coca*," a revised and expanded reprint from the *Centralblatt für die gesammte Therapie*, Vienna, 1885, in Freud, *Cocaine Papers*, pp. 107–09.

115 One of the most intriguing aspects: Freud, "On the General Effect of Cocaine," *Medicinisch-chirurgisches Centralblatt*, no. 32 (August 1885): 374–75, in Freud, *Cocaine Papers*, pp. 111–18.

116 In fact, Sigmund garnered: Jones, *Life*, vol. 1, pp. 92–96. Fleischl-Marxow, apparently, began injecting cocaine subcutaneously (under the skin) at the onset and may well have graduated to intravenous injections.

116 At other times: Sigmund Freud to Martha Bernays, January 6, 1885–September 1, 1886, Ernst L. Freud, ed., *Letters of Sigmund Freud* (New York: Basic Books, 1960), pp. 131–218.

116 Although this arrangement: His mentors Brücke, Meynert, and Nothnagel wrote strong letters of support on Freud's behalf for this grant. See George Makari, *Revolution in Mind: The Creation of Psychoanalysis* (New York: Harper Perennial, 2009), pp. 26–27.

117 Ever the scientific investigator: Freud to Martha, October 12, 1885; quoted in Jones, *Life*, vol. 1, pp. 183–84.

117 Upon returning from her performance: Quote is from Jones, *Life*, vol. 1, pp. 177–78.

117 Beyond Freud's love: Peter Gay, *Freud: A Life for Our Time* (New York: W. W. Norton, 1998), p. 48.

118 "possessed of a thousand demons": Ibid., pp. 47–48; Freud to Martha, October 19, 1885, Freud, *Letters*, pp. 171–74 (Letter 81), and December 3, 1885, pp. 187–88 (Letter 87).

118 In one of these dank hospital wards: Henry Sigerist, *The Great Doctors: A Bio-graphical History of Medicine* (New York: W. W. Norton, 1933), pp. 276–82; P. Pinel, *A Treatise on Insanity,* trans. D. D. Davis (Sheffield, U.K.: W. Todd for Caddell and Davies of London, 1806); Michel Foucault, *Madness and Civiliza-tion: A History of Insanity in the Age of Reason* (New York: Vintage, 1988), pp. 36–38, 72–74; Erwin H. Ackerknecht, *Medicine at the Paris Hospital, 1794–1848* (Balti-more: Johns Hopkins University Press, 1967), pp. 150–51, 168–69; and Dora B. Weiner, *The Citizen-Patient in Revolutionary France* (Baltimore: Johns Hopkins University Press, 2001).

119 Dr. Pinel's removal: Weiner, *The Citizen-Patient;* Ackerknecht, *Medicine.*

120 Neurology, as a clinical specialty: Anne Harrington, *Medicine, Mind and the Double Brain* (Princeton, N.J.: Princeton University Press, 1989); Harrington, *The Cure Within: A History of Mind-Body Medicine* (New York: W. W. Norton, 2008); and Stanley Finger, *Origins of Neuroscience: A History of Explorations into Brain Function* (New York: Oxford University Press, 1994).

121 Instead, they were critical tools: Fielding H. Garrison, *History of Medicine,* 4th ed. (Philadelphia: W. B. Saunders and Co., 1929), pp. 639–41; R. D. Shryock, *The Development of Modern Medicine* (New York: Alfred A. Knopf, 1949), pp. 151–69; and Ackerknecht, *Medicine,* p. 63.

121 A valued collaborator: Freud to Martha, October 21, 1885, Freud, *Letters,* pp. 175–77 (Letter 82); and Garrison, *History of Medicine,* p. 641.

122 But there was never a doubt: Gay, *Freud,* pp. 46–53.

122 To Sigmund's great delight: Freud to Martha, October 21, 1885, Freud, *Letters,* pp. 175–76 (Letter 82).

122 He described Charcot: Ibid.

123 The young physician was bedazzled: Ibid.; and Jones, *Life,* vol. 1, pp. 187–88.

123 "I am really very comfortably installed now": Freud to Martha, November 24, 1885, Freud, *Letters,* pp. 184–85 (Letter 86); and Gay, *Freud,* p. 49.

123 At the same time: In an unpublished letter Ernest Jones wrote to Siegfried Bern-feld on April 28, 1952, Jones confessed, "I am afraid that Freud took more cocaine than he should [during this period] though I am not mentioning that [in the biography]." When Bernfeld pressed him on this issue, Jones wrote another letter a few months later, on June 1, 1952, stating, "No I don't think he ever had ill effects from cocaine." These letters are in the S. Bernfeld Papers at the Library of Congress and are quoted by Peter Swales in his compelling essay "Freud, Cocaine and Sexual Chemistry: The Role of Cocaine in Freud's Con-ception of the Libido," in *Sigmund Freud: Critical Assessments,* ed. Laurence Spurling, vol. 1 (London: Routledge, 1989), pp. 273–301 (see, in particular, pp. 278–79, 290). For a description of the extent Freud, Martha, and Jones endeavored to minimize Freud's cocaine use, and the letters he wrote to Martha documenting it, see Harry Trosman and Ernest S. Wolf, "The Bernfeld Collaboration in the Jones Biography of Freud," *International Journal of Psycho-Analysis* 54 (1973): 227–33.

124 "[Charcot] invited me": Freud to Martha, January 18, 1886, Freud, *Letters,* pp. 192–93 (Letter 91). Dr. Ricchetti was an Austrian physician who practiced in Venice. He and his wife befriended Freud during this period.

124 To complete the picture: Freud to Martha, January 20, 1886, Freud, *Letters,* pp. 193–97 (Letter 92); quote is from p. 195.

124 Sigmund swooned at the sight: Ibid.; quote is from p. 194; and Jones, *Life,* vol. 1, pp. 186–87. The "Gobelins," of course, refer to the famous Parisian-made tapestries that often adorned the walls of the well-to-do during this period.

125 "The bit of cocaine": Freud to Martha, February 2, 1886, Freud, *Letters,* pp. 200–204 (Letter 94); quote is from pp. 201–03.

126 Warmed by the glow: I am indebted to my colleague Professor Daniel Herwitz, director of the University of Michigan Institute for the Humanities, for helping me understand the importance of Sigmund's "Temple" metaphor in his intellectual development.

127 "Thank God, it's over": Freud to Martha, February 2, 1886, Freud, *Letters,* pp. 200–204 (Letter 94).

127 "all kinds of condescending remarks": Freud to Martha, February 10, 1886, Freud, *Letters,* pp. 206–11 (Letter 96); quote is from p. 208.

128 "he rather taken aback": Ibid.

128 The visitor's name: Ibid., p. 209. See also H. Knapp, "On Cocaine and Its Use in Ophthalmic and General Surgery," *Archives of Ophthalmology* 13 (1884): 402–48; and Daniel M. Albert, "Hermann Jakob Knapp," in *American National Biography,* vol. 12, ed. John A. Garraty and Mark C. Carnes (New York: Oxford University Press, 1999), pp. 797–98.

128 "I greeted [Knapp] accordingly": Freud to Martha, February 10, 1886, Freud, *Letters,* pp. 206–11 (Letter 96).

129 For Sigmund, this was one: Ibid., p. 209.

129 Sigmund never saw: Freud not only translated many of Charcot's lectures and quoted the master as an authority in his own works, he also hung an engraving of the painting *Une leçon du Docteur Charcot à la Salpêtrière,* by Pierre André Brouillet, in his consulting room (see page 161). The painting depicts Charcot demonstrating a female hysteric to his students at the Salpêtrière Hospital and was given pride of place by being hung over a bookcase filled with Freud's treasured antique sculpture collection. Moreover, in 1889, Freud named his first son Jean Martin, after the French neurologist, in contradiction to the Jewish tradition of naming a child after a deceased family member. Sigmund Freud picked the names for all of his children and some of his grandchildren but chose to honor people he revered and liked rather than dead relatives. See Gay, *Freud,* pp. 52–53; and Louis Breger Freud, *Darkness in the Midst of Vision* (New York: John Wiley and Sons, 2000), pp. 88–89.

129 The sage teacher: Gay, *Freud,* p. 51.

Chapter 8. Rehabilitating Halsted

130 In the decades that followed: Butler Hospital's first medical director, Dr. Isaac Ray, a pioneer in the American psychiatric profession, was well regarded for his humane and scientific views of caring for the insane; his successor, John Woodbury Sawyer, was equally revered by his colleagues around the nation. F. Way-

land and H. L. Wayland, *A Memoir of the Life and Labors of Francis Wayland, D.D., L.L.D.* (New York: Sheldon and Co., 1867); W. E. Baxter and D. W. Hathcox, *America's Care of the Mentally Ill: A Photographic History* (New York: American Psychiatric Publishing, 1994).

130 Many doctors practiced: Gerald N. Grob, *The Mad Among Us: A History of the Care of America's Mentally Ill* (Cambridge, Mass.: Harvard University Press, 1994); Edward Shorter, *A History of Psychiatry: From the Era of the Asylum to the Age of Prozac* (New York: John Wiley, 1997); and Benjamin Reiss, *Theaters of Madness: Insane Asylums and Nineteenth-Century American Culture* (Chicago: University of Chicago Press, 2008).

130 More broadly, Americans considered: The separation of socially acceptable society from those deemed ill or dangerous is nicely described in Robert H. Wiebe, *The Search for Order, 1877–1920* (New York: Hill and Wang, 1967). See also Allan M. Hamilton, *Recollections of an Alienist: Personal and Professional* (New York: G. H. Doran Co., 1916); Alex Beam, *Gracefully Insane: Life and Death Inside America's Premier Mental Hospital* (New York: Public Affairs, 2001); David J. Rothman, *The Discovery of the Asylum: Social Order and Disorder in the New Republic* (Glenview, Ill.: Scott, Foresman, 1971); Robert Whitaker, *Mad in America: Bad Science, Bad Medicine and the Enduring Mistreatment of the Mentally Ill* (New York: Basic Books, 2002); Nancy Tomes and Lynn Gamwell, *Madness in America: Cultural and Medical Perceptions of Mental Illness Before 1914* (Ithaca, N.Y.: Cornell University Press, 1995); Nancy Tomes, *The Art of Asylum-Keeping: Thomas Story Kirkbride and the Origins of American Psychiatry* (Philadelphia: University of Pennsylvania Press, 1994); Carla Yanni, *The Architecture of Madness: Insane Asylums in the United States* (Minneapolis: University of Minnesota Press, 2007); and Christopher Payne, *Asylum: Inside the Closed World of State Mental Hospitals* (Cambridge, Mass.: MIT Press, 2009).

131 Short-staffed, often filthy: For a fictional account of the sorry state of many insane asylums in the United States as late as the 1940s, see Mary Jane Ward, *The Snake Pit* (New York: Random House, 1946).

131 But it was hardly Bedlam: William Buchan, *Domestic Medicine; or, the Family Physician: Being an Attempt to Render the Medical Art More Generally Useful, by Showing People What Is in Their Own Power Both with Respect to the Prevention and Cure of Diseases, Chiefly Calculated to Recommend a Proper Attention to Regimen and Simple Medicines* (Edinburgh: J. Balfour and W. Creech, 1769); Charles E. Rosenberg, "Medical Text and Social Context: Explaining William Buchan's *Domestic Medicine*," *Bulletin of the History of Medicine* 57 (1983): 22–42.

131 Hence, it is not surprising: Welch and Halsted's mutual and close friends Samuel Vander Poel and George Munroe, both Bellevue physicians, were also aware of Butler and recommended it to Halsted many times in 1885 and 1886. William G. MacCallum, *William Stewart Halsted, Surgeon* (Baltimore: Johns Hopkins University Press, 1930), p. 56.

132 Medical doctrine held that: Vivian Nutton, "Humoralism," in *Companion Encyclopedia of the History of Medicine,* vol. 1, ed. W. F. Bynum and R. Porter (London: Routledge, 1993), pp. 281–91.

133 That said, the *Annual Reports: Annual Report of the Trustees and Superintendents*

of the Butler Hospital for the Insane, January 26, 1887 (Providence, R.I.: Angell and Co., Printers, 1887). See also the annual reports for 1874, 1876, 1877, 1878, 1882, 1883, 1886, and 1888, Collections of the University of Michigan Libraries, Ann Arbor. For further information, see *A Century of Butler Hospital, 1844–1944* (Providence, R.I.: Butler Hospital, 1944).

134 "It has seemed to me best": *Annual Report of the Trustees and Superintendents of the Butler Hospital for the Insane,* pp. 13–16; quote is from p. 16.

134 Nineteenth-century American alienists: George Rosen, *Madness in Society: Chapters in the Historical Sociology of Mental Illness* (Chicago: University of Chicago Press, 1968), pp. 172–228.

134 "Those who study": *Annual Report of the Trustees and Superintendents of the Butler Hospital for the Insane,* p. 9; late-nineteenth-century dollars were converted into 2010 values using a formula based on the consumer price index from the economic history–focused website Measuring Worth, www.measuringworth .com/index.html (accessed February 25, 2010).

135 Typically, these pharmacological morality plays: For a superb discussion of this chapter of medical history, see Joseph E. Spillane, *Cocaine: From Medical Marvel to Modern Menace in the United States, 1884–1920* (Baltimore: Johns Hopkins University Press, 2000).

135 Fleischl-Marxow's addendum: Ernest Jones, *The Life and Work of Sigmund Freud,* vol. 1 (New York: Basic Books, 1955), pp. 90–91. For the original source, see Sigmund Freud, "Coca," trans. S. Pollak, *St. Louis Medical and Surgical Journal* 47, no. 6 (December 1884): 502–05; see also Freud, *Cocaine Papers,* pp. 85–89.

136 "since the use of cocaine": H. Obersteiner, "Über Intoxicationpsychosen," *Wein Med Presse* 24, no. 4 (1886): 24. Translated and cited in Siegfried Bernfeld, "Freud's Studies on Cocaine, 1884–1887," *Journal of the American Psychoanalytic Association* 1 (1953): 581–613; quote is from p. 602.

136 Sounding an alarm: J. A. A. Erlenmayer, "Ueber die Wirkung des Cocain bei der Morphimentziehung," *Centralbaltt d. Nervenheiljunde* 8 (July 1885): 288–99; J. A. A. Erlenmeyer, "Über Cocainsucht," *Deutsche Medizinalzeitung* 7 (1886): 44, translated and cited in Bernfeld, "Studies," 1 (1953): 602. See also Erlenmeyer's full-length book on morphine addiction: *Die Morphiumsucht und ihre Behandlung,* 3rd ed. (Berlin and Leipzig: Louis Heuser, 1887; 1st ed. published 1885).

137 That same year: E. W. Holmes, "*Erythroxylum coca* and Its Alkaloid Cocaine," *Detroit Therapeutic Gazette* 10 (3rd ser., 2, no. 8) (1886): 531.

137 "All reports of addiction": Sigmund Freud, "Contributions About the Applications of Cocaine. Second Series. I. Remarks on Craving for and Fear of Cocaine with Reference to a Lecture by W. A. Hammond," *Wiener medizinische Wochenschrift* 28 (July 9, 1887): 929–32, in Sigmund Freud, *Cocaine Papers,* ed. Robert Byck (New York: Stonehill, 1974), pp. 169–76; quote is from pp. 173–75.

138 In 1888, Charles Bunting: Charles A. Bunting, *Hope for the Victims of Alcohol, Morphine, Cocaine and Other Vices* (New York: Christian Home Building, 1888).

138 Similarly, in 1891: H. G. Brainerd, "Cocaine Addiction," *Transactions of the Medical Society of the State of California* n.s. 20 (1891): 193–201; quote is from p. 200.

138 Springthorpe poignantly recalled: J. W. Springthorpe, "The Confessions of a Cocainist," *Quarterly Journal of Inebriety* 19 (1897): 55–59.

139 "the people in the house": C. C. Stockard, "Some Cases of Drug Habit," *Atlanta Medical and Surgical Journal* 15 (1898–99): 83.

139 "cocaine is probably": T. D. Crothers, "Cocaine-Inebriety," *Quarterly Journal of Inebriety* 20 (1896): 370.

139 With respect to cocaine: Sigmund Freud, "Contributions About the Applications of Cocaine," pp. 929–32, in Freud, *Cocaine Papers,* pp. 169–76; and William A. Hammond, "Volunteer Paper," *Transactions of the Medical Society of Virginia* (1887): 212–26, reprinted in Freud, *Cocaine Papers,* pp. 178–93.

139 But it is also important to note: "Treatment for Past Year Depression Among Adults," *The NSDUH (National Survey on Drug Use and Health) Report,* January 3, 2008, U.S. Department of Health and Human Services/Substance Abuse and Mental Health Adminstration, www.oas.samhsa.gov/2k8/depression/depressionTX.htm (accessed May 28, 2008).

139 Furthermore, evidence is being uncovered: M. D. Li and M. Burmeister, "New Insights into the Genetics of Addiction," *Nature Reviews/Genetics* 10 (2009): 225–31; G. R. Uhl and R. W. Grow, "The Burden of Complex Genetics in Brain Disorders," *Archives of General Psychiatry* 61, no. 3 (2004): 223–29; N. Volkow and T. K. Li, "The Neuroscience of Addiction," *Nature Neuroscience* 8, no. 11 (2005): 1429–30; and G. R. Uhl, "Molecular Genetic Underpinnings of Human Substance Abuse Vulnerability: Likely Contributions to Understanding Addiction as a Mnemonic Process," *Neuropharmacology* 47, Supp. 1 (2004): 140–47.

142 Halsted made excellent progress: Some have suggested that Halsted may have continued to abuse cocaine while at Butler by bribing attendants to procure the drug for him; others have suggested that the morphine was not prescribed but also procured in a more illicit manner. I cannot find any definitive documentation for either of these claims. Given the state of treatment for drug addiction during this time as well as the fact that Halsted had few financial resources to draw upon while a patient at Butler, they appear unlikely. See, for example: A. P. Stout, "William Stewart Halsted," Notes, Series II, June 9, 1924, Box 49, William Stewart Halsted Papers, Alan Mason Chesney Archives, Johns Hopkins Medical Institutions, Baltimore; Daniel B. Nunn, "Dr. Halsted's Addiction," *Johns Hopkins Advanced Studies in Medicine* 6, no. 3 (2006): 106–08; and Daniel B. Nunn, "William Stewart Halsted: Transitional Years," *Surgery* 121, no. 3 (1997): 343–51.

143 Less debatable was the enormous impact: D. B. St. John Roosa, "Thomas Alexander McBride: An Account of His Last Illness," *New York Medical Journal,* October 2, 1886, pp. 265–66; Sherwin B. Nuland, *Doctors: The Biography of Medicine* (New York: Vintage Books, 1988), p. 398; Ralph Colp Jr., "Notes on Dr. William S. Halsted," *Bulletin of the New York Academy of Medicine* 60, ser. 2 (1984): 876–87; and MacCallum, *Halsted,* p. 45.

143 "I've seen enough": Arthur J. Beckhard and William D. Crane, *Cancer, Cocaine and Courage: The Story of Dr. William Halsted* (New York: Julian Messner, 1960), p. 154.

143 There, Welch was charged: Nineteenth-century dollars were converted into

2010 values using a formula based on the consumer price index from the economic history–focused website Measuring Worth, www.measuringworth.com/index.html (accessed February 25, 2010).

145 Underneath its spire: John S. Billings, *Description of the Johns Hopkins Hospital* (Baltimore: Publications of the Johns Hopkins Hospital/Press of J. Friedenwald, 1890). Billings was one of five experts asked by the trustees to help design the hospital in 1875, and his design was considered the best. He remained an adviser to the hospital through its opening in 1889. See also J. S. Billings, N. Folsom, J. Jones, C. Morris, and S. Smith, *Hospital Plans: Five Essays Relating to the Construction, Organization and Management of Hospitals Contributed by Their Authors for the Use of the Johns Hopkins Hospital of Baltimore* (New York: William Wood and Co., 1875); and Gert H. Brieger, "The Original Plans for the Johns Hopkins Hospital and Their Historical Significance," *Bulletin of the History of Medicine* 39 (1965): 518–28.

145 Ever the benevolent puller of strings: Peter D. Olch, "William S. Halsted: The Antithesis of William Osler," in *The Persisting Osler*, ed. J. A. Barondess, J. P. McGovern, and C. G. Roland (Baltimore: University Park Press, 1985), pp. 199–204.

146 "Nobody knows where Popsy eats": Michael Bliss, *William Osler: A Life in Medicine* (New York; Oxford University Press, 1999), p. 211. See also Bert Hansen, "Public Careers and Private Sexuality: Some Gay and Lesbian Lives in the History of Medicine and Public Health," *American Journal of Public Health* 92, no. 1 (2002): 36–44; and Bert Hansen, "American Physicians' 'Discovery' of Homosexuals, 1880–1900: A New Diagnosis in a Changing Society," in *Framing Diseases: Studies in Cultural History*, ed. Charles E. Rosenberg and Janet Golden (New Brunswick, N.J.: Rutgers University Press, 1992). For further information, see D. R. Mendenhall Memoirs, Mendenhall Papers, Sophia Smith Collection, Smith College, Item 3, E, 25, Northhampton, Mass.; Hugh A. Young, *A Surgeon's Autobiography* (New York: Harcourt, Brace, 1940), p. 65; and Simon Flexner and James T. Flexner, *William Henry Welch and the Heroic Age of American Medicine* (New York: Viking Press, 1949), pp. 162, 170.

147 For the next four decades: A. M. Harvey, G. H. Brieger, S. L. Abrams, and V. A. McKusick, *A Model of Its Kind*, vol. 1, *A Centennial History of Medicine at Johns Hopkins* (Baltimore: Johns Hopkins University Press, 1989); and Samuel J. Crowe, *Halsted of Johns Hopkins: The Man and His Men* (Springfield, Ill.: C. C. Thomas, 1957).

147 There, about a mile away: Flexner and Flexner, *Welch*, p. 155. Welch was so devoted to Mrs. Simmons that he moved with her twice, over the years, once to 935 St. Paul Street and later to 807 St. Paul Street.

147 On most evenings: Peter D. Olch, "William S. Halsted and Local Anesthesia: Contributions and Complications," *Anesthesiology* 42, no. 4 (1975): 479–86.

148 If you were wealthy and white: Francis F. Beirne, *The Amiable Baltimoreans* (Baltimore: Johns Hopkins University Press, 1984); and MacCallum, *Halsted*, pp. 62–63.

148 Baltimore did not offer: Joseph H. Pratt, *A Year with Osler, 1896–1897: Notes Taken at His Clinics in the Johns Hopkins Hospital* (Baltimore: Johns Hopkins

University Press, 1949), pp. 191–201; Harvey Cushing, *The Life of Sir William Osler,* vol. 1 (Oxford: Oxford University Press, 1925), p. 378; and Jon Teaford, *The Unheralded Triumph: City Government in America, 1870–1900* (Baltimore: Johns Hopkins University Press, 1984), pp. 140, 156, 219–21, 224, 246–47, 249.

149 He adorned his muscular frame: MacCallum, *Halsted,* p. 106.

149 Heroin addicts have an odd slang term: *Random House Historical Dictionary of American Slang,* ed. J. E. Lighter (New York: Random House, 1997), vol. 2, p. 313.

150 Elsewhere on the second floor: MacCallum, *Halsted,* pp. 58–71.

151 William could always come to him: We have excellent evidence of what William H. Welch sounded like, albeit in old age. In 1932, Welch made a short informational film to commemorate the fiftieth anniversary of the discovery of the tubercule bacillus, or *Mycobacterium tuberculosis,* the causative organism of tuberculosis. I was first introduced to this film in 1989, while in graduate school at the Johns Hopkins Institute for the History of Medicine, by the late professor Jerome Bylebyl. A few years ago, in 2007, Dr. Barry Silverman of Atlanta, Georgia, kindly sent me a DVD recording of the film. Thanks to the digital efforts of the Alan Mason Chesney Archives of the Johns Hopkins Medical Institutions, this film is now available for viewing at www.medicalarchives.jhmi.edu/welch/welcome.htm (accessed May 4, 2010).

152 And it was then: The vial story appears in Beckhard and Crane's young-adult biography of Halsted, *Cancer, Cocaine and Courage,* pp. 155–57.

152 It is unknown how William acquired: For example, decades later, W. T. Councilman recalled experiencing a tooth abscess around this time that required Halsted to inject his mouth with cocaine before Councilman could muster the courage to seek a dentist for a painful extraction. Councilman to MacCallum, February 2, 1928, in William Stewart Halsted Papers, Series II, Notes, Box 49, Alan Mason Chesney Archives, Johns Hopkins Medical Institutions, Baltimore.

152 There he remained: *Annual Report of the Trustees and Superintendents of the Butler Hospital for the Insane;* Peter D. Olch, "William S. Halsted: The Antithesis of William Osler," in *The Persisting Osler,* ed. J. A. Barondess, J. P. McGovern, and C. G. Roland (Baltimore: University Park Press, 1985), pp. 199–204.

Chapter 9. The Interpretation of Dreams

154 In an agate font: "Kleine Chronik," *Neue Freie Presse,* April 25, 1886. A translated version appears in Peter Gay, *Freud: A Life for Our Time* (New York: W. W. Norton, 1998), p. 53.

154 "In the time span": Sigmund Freud, *An Autobiographical Study,* trans. J. Strachey (New York: W. W. Norton, rpt. ed., 1989), p. 17.

154 Among his publications: Sigmund Freud, *On Aphasia: A Critical Study,* trans. E. Stengel (New York: International Universities Press, 1953, originally published in 1891); and Sigmund Freud, *Infantile Cerebral Paralysis,* trans. L. A. Russin (Coral Gables, Fla.: University of Miami Press, 1968; originally published in 1897). For more than ten years (1886–96), Freud worked part-time at the Vienna First Public Institute for Sick Children, or, as it came to be known, the Kassowitz

Institute; he served without pay as he built his private practice. During this period, he put in many thousands of hours, examined many thousands of pediatric patients, and published nine papers and case studies on various neurological topics. See Ernest Jones, *The Life and Work of Sigmund Freud*, vol. 1 (New York: Basic Books, 1955), pp. 211–17. See also Andre Bolzinger, "Freud pédiatre et antipédiatre," *Le Coq-Héron* 146 (1997): 61–69; Carolo Bonomi, "Why Have We Ignored Freud the 'Paediatrician'?" *Cahiers psychiatriques genèvois,* special issue (1994): 55–99; J. Gicklhorn and R. Gicklhorn, *Sigmund Freuds akademische Laufbahn* (Vienna-Innsbruck: Urban & Schwarzenberg, 1960); C. Hochsinger, *Die Geschichte des ersten öffentlichen Kinder-Kranken-Institutes in Wien während seines 150 jährigen Bestandes 1788–1938* (Vienna: Verlag des Kinder-Kranken-Institutes, 1938); P. J. Accardo, "Freud on Diplegia: Commentary and Translation," *American Journal of Diseases of Children* 136, no. 5 (1982): 452–56; L. D. Longo and S. Ashwal, "William Osler, Sigmund Freud and the Evolution of Ideas Concerning Cerebral Palsy," *Journal of the History of the Neurosciences* 2, no. 4 (1993): 255–82; C. W. Wallesch and C. Bartels, "Freud's Impact on Aphasiology, Aphasiology's Impact on Freud," *Journal of the History of the Neurosciences* 5, no. 2 (1996): 117–25; and D. Galbis-Reig, "Sigmund Freud, MD: Forgotten Contributions to Neurology, Neuropathology and Anesthesia," *Internet Journal of Neurology* 3, no. 1 (2004); ISSN 1531–295X; at www.ispub.com/ostia/index .php?xmlFilePath=journals/ijn/vol3n1/freud.xm (accessed February 6, 2009).

155 Specializing in the nascent arena: As time went on, Freud began to distance himself from Charcot's (and, later, Hippolyte Bernheim's) theories on the clinical uses of hypnotism. Beginning in the 1890s, he found that psychotherapy freed him—and his patients—from the need for this method. See Gay, *Freud,* pp. 50–51; and George Makari, *Revolution in Mind: The Creation of Psychoanalysis* (New York: Harper Perennial, 2008), pp. 27–34.

155 The flat leased for 1,600 gulden: Frederic A. Morton, *A Nervous Splendor: Vienna, 1888–1889* (New York: Penguin, 1980), pp. 27–29, 87–88. Morton calls Freud "the first specialist in bourgeoisie angst." See also Carl E. Schorske, *Fin de Siècle Vienna: Politics and Culture* (New York: Vintage Books, 1981), pp. 181–207. The apartment building where Sigmund and Martha Freud first lived was called the Sühnhaus, or the House of Atonement, and the rents collected were contributed to charitable causes. Maria H. Lansdale, *Vienna and the Viennese* (Philadelphia: Henry T. Coates, 1902), p. 41.

156 There were many days: Morton, *Nervous Splendor,* p. 89.

156 As the cultural historian Frederic Morton: Ibid. See also Gay, *Freud,* pp. 53–54.

157 In face-to-face conversations: Morton, *Nervous Splendor,* pp. 138–39.

157 He frequently described his mood: Gay, *Freud,* pp. 75–80.

158 In 1896, a year after: Ibid., pp. 59, 163; Peter Gay, "Sigmund and Minna? The Biographer as Voyeur," *New York Times,* January 29, 1989, p. 44. It is also interesting to note that the letters that do exist between Martha and Freud during these years are mostly centered on the running of the household and the welfare of their children, in distinct contrast to the love letters of their engagement. Martha and Sigmund's sexual pact may have originated as an ultimate measure of birth control. Apparently, Freud detested using condoms.

159 "She was very much bothered": J. M. Billinksy, "Jung and Freud (the End of a Romance)," *Andover Newton Quarterly* 10 (1969): 39–43; quote is from p. 42.

159 "some dreams that bothered him": Ibid., p. 42.

159 "He looked at me": Ibid. Jung went on to tell Billinsky that it was this incident that signaled the end of his storied friendship with Freud. Jung suggested that Freud should have completed analysis and that there was evidence of significant neuroses over the situation, such as several psychosomatic problems and trouble controlling his bladder during the trip to America. "If Freud would have tried to understand consciously the triangle," Jung explained in recollection, "he would have been much, much better off." In subsequent years, many have asserted that it was Jung's rejection of Freud's theory that the libido or inner drive was singularly related to sex, in contrast to the energy or life forces espoused by Jung. But in this article, as well as his autobiography, Jung reported that Freud's inability to be completely truthful about his affair and his need to maintain an authoritative hegemony over his student was really at the root of the relationship's demise. See also Carl G. Jung, *Memories, Dreams, Reflections* (New York: Vintage Books, 1989), p. 149. The dating of Jung's initial visit to Vienna differs in Jones's biography and Jung's autobiography, but according to the correspondence between Jung and Freud, their first in-person visit occurred in March 1907; see W. McGuire, ed., *The Freud/Jung Letters: The Correspondence Between Sigmund Freud and C. G. Jung* (London: Hogarth Press and Routledge and Kegan Paul, 1974), p. 24. I am indebted to Dr. James Harris, professor of psychiatry at the Johns Hopkins University School of Medicine, for helping me to sort out this complex episode in Freud's life.

159 With the practiced duplicity: Franz Maciejewski, "Freud, His Wife, and His 'Wife': Freud and Minna Bernays," *American Imago* 63, no. 4 (2006): 497–506; Franz Maciejewski, "Minna Bernays as 'Mrs. Freud': What Sort of Relationship Did Sigmund Freud Have with His Sister-in-Law?" *American Imago* 65, no. 1 (2008): 5–21; R. Blumenthal, "Hotel Log Hints at Illicit Desire That Dr. Freud Didn't Repress," *New York Times,* December 24, 2006; Albrecht Hirschmüller, "Freud and Minna Bernays: Evidence for a Sexual Relationship Between Sigmund Freud and Minna Bernays?" *American Imago* 64, no. 1 (2007): 125–29; Gay, "Sigmund and Minna?"; and Peter J. Swales, "Freud, Minna Bernays, and the Conquest of Rome," *New American Review* 1 (1982): 1–23.

159 Sigmund was particularly captivated: Gay, *Freud,* p. 52.

160 The diagnosis of hysteria: See, for example, American Psychiatric Association, *Diagnostic and Statistical Manual of Mental Disorders,* 4th ed. (New York: American Psychiatric Publishing, 2000). The fifth edition of the *DSM* is scheduled for May 2013.

160 Before the advent of modern gynecology: Rachel P. Maines, *The Technology of Orgasm: "Hysteria," the Vibrator, and Women's Sexual Satisfaction* (Baltimore: Johns Hopkins University Press, 1998); and Mark S. Micale, *Hysterical Men: The Hidden History of Male Nervous Illness* (Cambridge, Mass.: Harvard University Press, 2008). The Greek root *hystero* means "womb" or "uterus." The suffix *ectomy* comes from the root *ecto* and means "outside" or "removal."

160 As *The Oxford Companion to Medicine* succinctly notes: "Hysteria," in J. Wal-

ton, P. B. Beeson, and R. B. Scott, eds., *The Oxford Companion to Medicine,* vol. 1 (New York: Oxford University Press, 1986), p. 573.

160 These poor souls: Micale, *Hysterical Men,* pp. 117–61; and Andrew Scull, "Prisoners of Gender," *Times Literary Supplement,* January 23, 2009, p. 25.

161 "It was easy to see": Freud, *Autobiographical Study,* p. 12.

162 Still, it is important to recall: "It's always a question of the genitals . . . always . . . always . . . always." See Roy Porter, *The Greatest Benefit to Mankind: A Medical History of Humanity* (New York: W. W. Norton, 1997), p. 515; and Eli Zaretsky, *Secrets of the Soul: A Social and Cultural History of Psychoanalysis* (New York: Alfred A. Knopf, 2004), p. 34.

163 Sigmund reciprocated by sharing: Freud, *Autobiographical Study,* p. 19.

163 In what many members of the audience: The title of Freud's controversial paper to the Vienna Medical Society was "On Male Hysteria." The actual lecture has been lost to posterity but has been pieced together from the society's official minutes and medical newspaper reports of the meeting. See *Anzeiger der k. k. Gesellschaft der Ärzte in Wien* 25 (1886): 149–52; *Allgemeine Wiener medizinische Zeitung* 31 (1886): 506–07; *Wiener medizinische Presse* 27 (1886): 1407–09; *Wiener medizinische Wochenschrift* 36 (1886): 1444–47; *Munchener medizinische Wochenschrift* 33 (1886): 768; and *Wiener medizinische Blatter* 9 (1886): 1292–94. These articles have been gathered together and reprinted in *Luzifer-Amor: Zeitschrift zur Geschichte der Psychoanlyse* 1 (1988): 156–75. Five years later, in 1891, Theodor Meynert made a deathbed request to see Freud. At their final interview, Professor Meynert confessed that he'd fought Sigmund's theories so hard because "I was always one of the clearest cases of male hysteria." See Morton, *Nervous Splendor,* p. 315; Micale, *Hysterical Men,* p. 241; and Sherwin B. Nuland, "Macho Misery," *New Republic,* April 15, 2009, pp. 40–43.

163 Five weeks later: Sigmund Freud, "Beobachtund einer hochgradigen Hemianästhesie bei einem hysterishen Manne," *Wiener medizinische Wochenschrift* 36 (December 1886): 1633–38.

164 "Hysterics suffer for the most part": Josef Breuer and Sigmund Freud, *Studies in Hysteria,* trans. N. Luckhurst (New York: Penguin Books, 2004), p. 11.

164 One of the most fascinating cases: For the case of Anna O., see Breuer and Freud, *Studies in Hysteria,* pp. 25–50. Bertha Pappenheim went on to a prominent career as a social worker, feminist, and Jewish activist. See Lucy Freeman, *The Story of Anna O.: The Woman Who Led Freud to Psychoanalysis* (New York: Jason Aronson, rpt. ed., 1994).

164 But by the summer of 1882: A. Orr-Andrawes, "The Case of Anna O.: A Neuro-Psychiatric Perspective," *Journal of the American Psychoanalytic Association* 35, no. 2 (1987): 387–419; and S. de Paula Ramos, "Revisiting Anna O.: A Case of Chemical Dependence," *History of Psychology* 6, no. 3 (2003): 239–50. Bertha's complex partial seizures, for example, may well have emerged from her drug dependence on morphine or from a preexisting case of epilepsy. In later years, she was able to recover from her morphine abuse. She was readmitted to mental health facilities several times between 1882 and 1887. See also Makari, *Revolution,* pp. 39–41, 44.

165 He hypothesized that talking at length: Jones, *Life,* vol. 1, pp. 222–26; and

William M. Johnston, *The Austrian Mind: An Intellectual and Social History, 1848–1938* (Berkeley: University of California Press, 1972), pp. 221–37.

165 Breuer and Freud went their separate ways: The original text appeared as Sigmund Freud and Josef Breuer, *Studien über Hysterie* (Leipzig and Vienna: Franz Deuticke, 1895).

165 Breuer heatedly disagreed: Eventually Sigmund would revise his theories to abandon the primacy of "seduction theory" and expand the concept to include all sexual frustrations and conflicts, real or imagined, encountered by many a civilized man or woman living in late-nineteenth-century bourgeois Western culture. Paul R. McHugh, *Try to Remember: Psychiatry's Clash over Meaning, Memory and Mind* (New York: Dana Press, 2008).

166 In his later years: Louis Breger, *A Dream of Undying Fame: How Freud Betrayed His Mentor and Invented Psychoanalysis* (New York: Basic Books, 2009); and Saul Rosenzweig, *The Historic Expedition to America (1909): Freud, Jung, and Hall the King-Maker* (St. Louis: Rana House, 1994), p. 108.

167 "My emotional life": Sigmund Freud, *The Interpretation of Dreams*, trans. James Strachey (New York: Penguin Books, 1991), p. 622.

168 This now famous second-story apartment: Louis Breger, *Freud: Darkness in the Midst of Vision* (New York: John Wiley and Sons, 2000), p. 88.

168 "My letter of today": Freud to Fliess, November 24, 1887, Jeffrey M. Masson, ed., *The Complete Letters of Sigmund Freud to Wilhelm Fliess, 1887–1904* (Cambridge, Mass.: Belknap Press of Harvard University Press, 1985), p. 15.

168 As their novel notions: Peter Gay, "Freud: A Brief Life," in Sigmund Freud, *The Ego and the Id*, trans. Joan Riviere, part of *The Standard Edition of the Complete Psychological Works of Sigmund Freud* (New York: W. W. Norton, 1989), p. xiv.

168 Careful nasal examinations: See, for example, W. Fliess, *The Relationship Between the Nose and the Female Sexual Organs* (Berlin: Verlag von Franz Deuticke, 1897); Sander Gilman, *The Jew's Body* (London: Routledge, 1991); Sander Gilman, *The Case of Sigmund Freud: Medicine and Identity at the Fin de Siècle* (Baltimore: Johns Hopkins University Press, 1994); Sander Gilman, *Difference and Pathology: Stereotypes of Sexuality, Race and Madness* (Ithaca, N.Y.: Cornell University Press, 1985); and Janet Malcolm, *In the Freud Archives* (New York: New York Review Books, 1997), pp. 46–49.

169 More intriguing, they explored: Jeffrey M. Masson, "Freud and the Seduction Theory: A Challenge to the Foundations of Psychoanalysis," *Atlantic Monthly*, February 1984, www.theatlantic.com/issues/84feb/masson.htm (accessed May 4, 2010); and Jeffrey M. Masson, *The Assault on Truth: Freud's Suppression of the Seduction Theory* (New York: Harper Perennial, 1992).

170 In another still: Zaretsky, *Secrets*, p. 49; and P. Newton, "Freud's Mid-Life Crisis," *Psychoanalytic Psychology* 9, no. 4 (1992): 447–75. See, for example, Fliess to Freud, July 15, 1896, *Complete Letters*, pp. 2–4, 194–95. Zaretsky notes that while Masson translates the phrase *"befruchtenden Stromes"* as "stimulating current," *befruchten* also means "fertilize" or "pollinate." Freud refers to the homoerotic component of his relationship with Fliess in a letter to Ferenczi; see Ernest Jones, *The Life and Work of Sigmund Freud*, vol. 2, *1901–1919* (New York: Basic

Books, 1955), pp. 83–84. See also Malcolm, *Freud Archives,* p. 47; Gay, *Freud,* pp. 55–58; and Zaretsky, *Secrets,* pp. 49–51.

170 While recuperating: A peritonsillar abscess is a collection of pus that forms in the soft tissue of the throat, next to one of the tonsils. It is the result of an infection and can cause pain, swollen tissues, and, if severe enough, actual blockage of the throat and difficulty swallowing and breathing. Freud to Fliess, May 15, 1893, *Complete Letters,* p. 48.

170 Freud reported feeling especially better: Freud to Fliess, May 30, 1893, *Complete Letters,* pp. 49–50.

171 "The last letter I was able to produce": Freud to Fliess, November 27, 1893, *Complete Letters,* pp. 61–62; quote is from p. 61.

171 Incidentally, it was not the last time: See, for example, Freud to Fliess, April 20, 1895, *Complete Letters,* p. 126. In this letter Freud notes that he was able to pull himself out of "a miserable attack" only with cocaine but might require cauterization or galvanization to open his blocked nasal passages.

171 "Less obvious, perhaps, is the state": Freud to Fliess, April 19, 1894, *Complete Letters,* pp. 67–68; quote is from p. 67.

172 Initially, Sigmund diagnosed: Freud to Fliess, April 25, 1894, and May 6, 1894, *Complete Letters,* pp. 69–71. "Rheumatic myocarditis" is an antiquated term referring to the inflammation of the heart that can follow a bacterial, viral, or fungal infection of the heart. The key symptoms include chest pain, discomfort, and, potentially, congestive heart failure.

172 Interestingly, in 1897: In 1897, Freud wrote Fliess: "The insight has dawned on me that masturbation is the one major habit, the 'primary addiction,' and it is only as a substitute and replacement for it that the other addictions—to alcohol, morphine, tobacco, etc.—come into existence." Freud to Fliess, December 22, 1897, *Complete Letters,* pp. 287–89. Freud makes this point more explicitly in his 1898 essay "Sexuality in the Aetiology of the Neuroses": "Left to himself, the masturbator is accustomed, whenever something happens that depresses him, to return to his convenient form of satisfaction. . . . For sexual need, when once it has been aroused and has been satisfied for any length of time, can no longer be silenced; it can only be displaced along another path. . . . Not everyone who has occasion to take morphia, cocaine, chloral-hydrate . . . acquires in this way an 'addiction' to them. Closer inquiry usually shows that these narcotics are meant to serve—directly or indirectly—as a substitute for a lack of sexual satisfaction." In Sigmund Freud, *Three Essays on the Theory of Sexuality* (New York: Basic Books, 1962), pp. 275–76. See also Breger, *Darkness,* pp. 168–69.

173 Yet most established smokers: Robert H. Julien, *A Primer of Drug Action: A Concise Nontechnical Guide to the Actions, Uses, and Side Effects of Psychoactive Drugs* (New York: Holt/Owl Books, 2001), pp. 154–56.

173 Such quibbles aside: Freud to Fliess, April 19, 1894, and June 22, 1894, *Complete Letters,* pp. 67–69, 83–86.

174 "I would be endlessly obliged": Freud to Fliess, June 22, 1894, *Complete Letters,* pp. 83–86; quote is from pp. 85–86. Sigmund wrote a similar letter on July 14, 1894, complaining of Fliess's order that he stop smoking cigars; *Complete Letters,* pp. 87–88.

174   "I must hurriedly write to you": Freud to Fliess, January 24, 1895, *Complete Letters,* pp. 106–07; quote is from p. 106.

174   "I need a lot of cocaine": Freud to Fliess, June 12, 1895, *Complete Letters,* pp. 131–32; quote is from p. 132.

175   Freud began composing: Sigmund Freud, *Project for a Scientific Psychology,* in *The Complete Psychological Works of Sigmund Freud,* vol. 1, ed. and trans. J. Strachey (London: Hogarth, 1910); see also Masson, *Complete Letters.* Many scholars have noted that this project contains some precursor, or at least explanatory, sections of what ultimately became *The Interpretation of Dreams.*

175   He would then rewrite: Makari, *Revolution,* pp. 74–84.

176   And most important: Gay, "Freud: A Brief Life," pp. xiv–xv.

176   As he had jovially informed Fliess: Freud to Fliess, April 16, 1896, *Complete Letters,* pp. 180–81.

177   In January, he told Fliess: Freud to Fliess, January 16, 1899, *Complete Letters,* pp. 340–41.

177   In mid-June: Freud to Fliess, June 16, 1899, *Complete Letters,* pp. 355–56.

177   A few weeks later: Freud to Fliess, June 27, 1899, *Complete Letters,* pp. 356–57.

177   That he did: Freud to Fliess, July 8, 1899, *Complete Letters,* pp. 359–60.

177   Eventually, Sigmund realized: Freud describes his drinking to Fliess as a "new vice" in early December 1898. December 5, 1898, *Complete Letters,* pp. 335–36; and Gay, *Freud,* p. 100.

177   "In the pages that follow": Freud, *Interpretation of Dreams,* p. 57.

178   "The whole thing is laid out": Freud to Fliess, August 6, 1899, *Complete Letters,* pp. 365–66; and Gay, *Freud,* p. 106.

178   Cradling a newly published copy: The book first appeared in print in November 1899, but its publication on the title page of the first edition was postdated into the new century, 1900. Freud, *Interpretation of Dreams,* p. 34.

178   "After last summer's exhilaration": Freud to Fliess, March 11, 1900, *Complete Letters,* pp. 402–04; quote is from p. 403. Decades later, Sigmund described *The Interpretation of Dreams* as his greatest work. In the preface to the third English edition of the book, published in 1931, Freud noted, "It contains, even according to my present-day judgment, the most valuable of all the discoveries it has been my good fortune to make. Insight such as this falls to one's lot but once in a lifetime" (p. 56).

179   Despite Freud's grand hopes: Gay, *Freud,* p. 3.

179   After all, *The Interpretation of Dreams:* Zaretsky, *Secrets,* p. 31.

179   "Do you think that one day": Freud to Fliess, June 12, 1900, *Complete Letters,* pp. 417–18.

179   It was based on a series: Freud, *Interpretation of Dreams,* p. 187. As we shall see, this period coincides with the point when Freud was having so much difficulty with his nasal passages and sinuses that he underwent a surgical or cauterization procedure of the nasal turbinates performed by Fliess, following which "cocaine, in which Fliess was a great believer, was constantly prescribed." See Jones, *Life,* vol. 1, p. 309; Harry C. Leavitt, "A Biological and Teleological Study of 'Irma's Injection' Dream," *Psychoanalytic Review* 43 (1956): 440–47; and Stanley K. Kaplan, "Narcissistic Injury and the Occurrence of Creativity: Freud's Irma Dream," *Annual of Psychoanalysis* 12 (1984): 367–76.

179 Immortalizing her as "Irma": Some of the physical features of "Irma" are also based on another patient of Freud's named Anna Lichtheim, and Freud always insisted that the figure of Irma was a *sammelperson*, or composite figure. Freud, *Interpretation of Dreams*, pp. 187, 192, 194, 197, 255–56, 259, 262, 297, 309, 387. Cocaine continued to be on Freud's mind, or at least in his dreams. A few nights later he had a dream about his monograph on coca, the botanical nature of the drug, his father's glaucoma operation, and the whole episode of Koller's scooping him on the utility of the drug. Freud makes a point, in his interpretation of this dream, to again assert his role in the discovery. Even though he would never gain primary credit for realizing cocaine's potential as an anesthetic agent, the monograph on dreams he was about to compose would be his greatest accomplishment. Freud, *Interpretation of Dreams*, pp. 256, 258–62, 387–88; and Siegfried Bernfeld, "Freud's Studies on Cocaine, 1884–1887," *Journal of the American Psychoanalytic Association* 1 (1953): 581–613. Many of the documentary details of the event, as recounted by Freud to Fliess, were so incriminating that Freud's daughter Anna and two devoted colleagues redacted them from the first historical volume of the origins of psychoanalysis. See Sigmund Freud, *The Origins of Psychoanalysis: Letters to Wilhelm Fliess, Drafts and Notes, 1887–1902*, ed. Marie Bonaparte, Anna Freud, and Ernst Kris (New York: Basic Books, 1954); see also Malcolm, *Freud Archives;* Masson, *Complete Letters;* and Jeffrey M. Masson, *The Assault on Truth: Freud's Suppression of the Seduction Theory* (New York: Harper Perennial, 1992).

179 "I was making frequent use": Freud, *Interpretation of Dreams*, p. 187. Although Freud "slips" here in dating when he first recommended cocaine—it was 1884, not 1885—the friend he is referring to is, of course, Fleischl-Marxow.

180 Descriptions of scabrous turbinate bones: It was Fliess who taught Freud about this organic compound. Freud, *Interpretation of Dreams*, pp. 193, 401–2. Some scholars have also suggested that the smell of trimethylamine is similar to that created by burning coca leaves.

181 "this group of thoughts": Freud, *Interpretation of Dreams*, p. 198.

181 "When the work of interpretation": Ibid., pp. 198–99.

182 In many cases: For an elegant discussion of the triumphs and pitfalls of surgical decision making, see Atul Gawande, *Complications: A Surgeon's Notes on an Imperfect Science* (New York: Metropolitan Books, 2002); and Atul Gawande, *Better: A Surgeon's Notes on Performance* (New York: Metropolitan Books, 2007).

182 Upon leaving Vienna: Breger, *Darkness*, pp. 131–32.

182 Moreover, Emma's nostrils: Freud to Fliess, March 4, 1895, *Complete Letters*, pp. 113–15.

183 "Before either of us had time": Freud to Fliess, March 8, 1895, *Complete Letters*, pp. 116–18; quote is from p. 117. This is one of the most controversial letters in the Freud collections and for many years was suppressed and unpublished, perhaps because it presented the great Freud in such an unfavorable light. For the story of the discovery and publication of these letters, along with the downfall of the historian-archivist who uncovered them, see Malcolm, *Freud Archives*.

183 After the bloody event: Freud to Fliess, March 8, 1895, *Complete Letters*, p. 117.

184 He reassured Fliess: Ibid., p. 118.

184 Sigmund also informed Fliess: Freud to Fliess, March 28, 1895, *Complete Letters,* pp. 122–23; quote is from p. 123.

184 On April 20, Freud wrote Fliess: Freud to Fliess, April 20, 26, and 27, 1895, *Complete Letters,* pp. 125–26, 126–27, and 127–28.

184 "an unfailing means of rearousing": Freud to Fliess, May 4, 1895, *Complete Letters,* pp. 185–86; quote is from p. 185.

185 A father's death: Preface to the second edition, 1908, Freud, *Interpretation of Dreams,* p. 47.

186 Freud interpreted this: Freud, *Interpretation of Dreams,* pp. 428–29; this dream was reported by Sigmund to Fliess on November 2, 1898. In his book, Freud states the dream occurred the night before the funeral; in the letter to Fliess, he places it on the night after the funeral, which occurred on October 25, 1896; *Complete Letters,* p. 202. For a short time after his father's death, Sigmund worried about if he was repressing a memory of Jacob sexually abusing him or his siblings. He later concluded that this was not the case. See, for example, D. Grubin (writer, director, and producer), *Young Dr. Freud: A Film by David Grubin* (New York: Public Broadcasting Service, 2002).

186 Distraught by his loss: Freud to Fliess, October 15, 1897, *Complete Letters,* p. 270.

186 It is the last extant letter: Freud to Fliess, October 26, 1896, *Complete Letters,* p. 201.

186 One assumes that Freud's clinical experiences: Bernfeld, "Freud's Studies on Cocaine, 1884–1887," p. 611.

Chapter 10. "The Professor"

187 Decades later, a colleague recalled: George J. Heuer, "Dr. Halsted," *Johns Hopkins Hospital Bulletin,* Supp. 90 (1952): 51.

188 "In Halsted's little operating room": The eminent internist Dr. William Sydney Thayer made this observation. See W. S. Thayer, "The Chief," *New England Journal of Medicine* 207, no. 13 (1932): 563–70. Thayer hailed from a rather distinguished Massachusetts family that included several colonial settlers, Harvard professors, and clergymen. Among his most interesting distant relatives were Ralph Waldo Emerson; Ernest Thayer, author of the poem "Casey at the Bat"; and Scofield Thayer, a poet and editor of the famed *Dial* magazine and one of Sigmund Freud's many patients. Thayer was an 1890 graduate of the Harvard Medical School and quickly rose at the Hopkins to be one of Osler's favorite resident physicians and, ultimately, Osler's successor as professor of medicine at Johns Hopkins. See also Edith G. Reid, *The Life and Convictions of William Sydney Thayer, Physician* (London: Oxford University Press, 1936), pp. 1–56; and Alex Beam, *Gracefully Insane: Life and Death Inside America's Premier Mental Hospital* (New York: Public Affairs, 2001), pp. 100–108.

189 Virtually all of his now universally practiced techniques: William S. Halsted, "The Employment of Fine Silk in Preference to Catgut and the Advantages of Transfixing Tissues in Controlling Hemorrhage; Also an Account of the Introduction of Gloves, Gutta-Percha Tissue, and Silver Foil," *Journal of the American Medical Association* 60 (1913): 1119–26.

189 Dr. William Mayo: Michael Bliss, *William Osler: A Life in Medicine* (New York: Oxford University Press, 1999), p. 212; and J. Scott Rankin, "William Stewart Halsted: A Lecture by Dr. Peter D. Olch," *Annals of Surgery* 243 (2006): 418–25.

189 "[His] fingers are engaged": Sherwin B. Nuland, "The Art of Incision: In Praise of the Greatest Surgeon Ever," *New Republic*, August 13, 2008.

190 Those of us who are not surgeons: William G. MacCallum, "William Stewart Halsted," *Biographical Memoirs of the National Academy of Sciences of the United States of America* 57 (1937): 151–70; and Fielding H. Garrison, "Halsted," *American Mercury* 7 (April 1926): 396–401.

190 Given Halsted's history: Heuer, "Dr. Halsted"; Sigmund Freud, *Cocaine Papers*, ed. Robert Byck (New York: Stonehill, 1974); William Golden Mortimer, *History of Coca: The Divine Plant of the Incas* (New York: J. H. Vail, 1901); and George Andrews and David Solomon, eds., *The Coca Leaf and Cocaine Papers* (New York: Harcourt Brace and Jovanovich, 1975).

191 Two years later: Samuel J. Crowe, *Halsted of Johns Hopkins: The Man and His Men* (Springfield, Ill.: C. C. Thomas, 1957), pp. 37–38.

191 At the opening of the twentieth century: Robert Aronowitz, *Unnatural History: Breast Cancer and American Society* (New York: Cambridge University Press, 2007), pp. 87–88. Aronowitz makes particularly good use of the W. S. Halsted Papers, Alan Mason Chesney Archives of the Johns Hopkins Medical Institutions, in documenting Halsted's breast cancer work during the first two decades of the twentieth century, as well as the copious correspondence Halsted maintained with doctors around the world. The procedure Halsted developed, the radical mastectomy, removed so much tissue beyond the breast that it caused serious disability, lymphedema, and cosmetic problems. Still, Dr. Halsted predicted that his successors would find more precise and less debilitating treatments for breast cancer. He was right. Today, thanks to a host of new treatment modalities, the radical mastectomy is no longer performed. Even its less radical procedure, the "modified radical mastectomy," is rarely performed as physicians and patients work to recognize signs of this terrible disease earlier and thanks to the development of new diagnostic methods in the form of frequent breast examinations and mammography, as well as improved treatments in the form of chemotherapy, radiation, and less invasive surgical procedures. That said, breast cancer remains one of the leading causes of death among women in the United States, and this battle is far from over. See also Ellen Leopold, *A Darker Ribbon: A Twentieth-Century Story of Breast Cancer, Women, and Their Doctors* (Boston: Beacon Press, 2000); and Barron H. Lerner, *The Breast Cancer Wars: Hope, Fear, and the Pursuit of a Career in Twentieth-Century America* (New York: Oxford University Press, 2001).

191 During these years, he perfected: For example, goiter and hypothyroidism were among the leading causes for disqualifying young men from entering the U.S. Army in 1918. For a history of this once-common problem and its medical amelioration, see Howard Markel, " 'When It Rains It Pours': Endemic Goiter, Iodized Salt, and David Murray Cowie, M.D.," *American Journal of Public Health* 77 (1987): 219–29.

191 He also created: William G. MacCallum, *William Stewart Halsted, Surgeon* (Baltimore: Johns Hopkins University Press, 1930), pp. 84–93, 139–49.

192 As a result of his renown: Heuer, "Dr. Halsted"; MacCallum, *Halsted,* pp. 84–102; and William S. Halsted, *Surgical Papers in Two Volumes,* ed. Walter C. Burket (Baltimore: The Johns Hopkins Press, 1924). The papers Halsted wrote during the years 1889–95 are particularly helpful for understanding the variety of surgical problems he was encountering in the operating room. A huge collection of Halsted's letters to his colleagues around the world can be found in the Halsted papers at the Alan Mason Chesney Archives of the Johns Hopkins Medical Institutions in Baltimore.

193 For procedures requiring local anesthesia: Heuer, "Dr. Halsted," p. 47; according to an unsigned obituary published in *Science* in 1922 and likely written by Harvey Cushing, Halsted often used a simple salt solution, insisting that even water and sodium chloride could numb the skin; his residents preferred cocaine solutions. "William Stewart Halsted, 1852–1922," *Science* 56, no. 1452 (1922): 461–64. Manuscript copy of this obituary can be found in George J. Heuer Papers, Box 2, File 19, Item 5, Weill Cornell Medical College, Cornell Medical Center Archives, New York. See also: James F. Mitchell, "Memories of Dr. Halsted," *Surgery* 32 (1952): 451–60.

193 Such daily proximity: One of the strangest rumors about Halsted's addiction is a purported reason behind his habit of sending his soiled shirts to Paris for laundering, on an annual basis. According to Heuer, Halsted did so because he considered the laundries in the United States to be inferior to the quality of those in France; Heuer, "Dr. Halsted," p. 69. The rumor mill suggested that the French launderers sent along packets of morphine and cocaine in the return packages. The historian Peter Olch documents the scores of receipts for laundering of shirts in the Halsted papers but does not go as far as to state drugs were sent back to Baltimore for Halsted's consumption; Rankin, "Halsted," pp. 418–25. Indeed, this route seems especially fantastic when one considers that Halsted had such ready access to morphine and cocaine in his own operating room and surgical clinic. The drugs-with-laundry claim has appeared in several accounts over the years; see, for example, Ralph Colp Jr., "Notes on Dr. William S. Halsted," *Bulletin of the New York Academy of Medicine* 60, ser. 2 (1984): 876–87.

194 The fastidious Dr. Halsted: Antiseptic surgery refers to methods where the surgeon kills germs before operating, such as by the use of strong disinfectants. In the decades that followed, surgeons developed aseptic techniques whereby all the instruments, drapes, and gowns were sterilized by means of steam, as opposed to the powerful antiseptics that not only destroyed microbes but also harmed living tissue. In aseptic surgery, as practiced in modern operating rooms around the world, living bacteria are not allowed near open wounds. For the techniques used in Halsted's operating room, see Heuer, "Dr. Halsted," pp. 46–53. The permanganate tended to turn the skin a dark chocolate brown, the oxalic acid oxidized the permanganate and turned the skin back to its natural color, and the bichloride of mercury (1:1000) was known to be extremely rough on the hands and caused terrible dermatitis; for a more general discussion, see Gert H. Brieger, "American Surgery and the Germ Theory of Disease," *Bulletin of the History of Medicine* 40 (1966): 135–45.

194 Armed with drawings of prototypes: MacCallum, *Halsted,* pp. 81–82; and

S. Halsted, "The Employment of Fine Silk." Several historians have presented evidence that Dr. Hunter Robb, an obstetrics-gynecology resident of Howard Kelly's during this period, not Halsted, was the first to advocate the use of rubber surgical gloves for aseptic technique. Historians have parsed the discovery to note that Halsted developed them for his wife-to-be for avoiding dermatitis but Robb and, likely, Halsted's chief surgical resident, Joseph Bloodgood, began using them for purposes of asepsis. Regardless, soon after their introduction, everyone in the operating room eventually adopted the gloves as routine practice, and it caught on across the globe. See Joseph C. Bloodgood, "Halsted Thirty-six Years Ago," *American Journal of Surgery* 14 (1931): 89–148; A. C. Barnes, "A Comment on Historical 'Truth,' " *Perspectives in Biology and Medicine* (Autumn 1977): 131–38; C. Proskauer, "Development and Use of the Rubber Glove in Surgery and Gynecology," *Journal of the History of Medicine and Allied Sciences* 13 (1958): 373–81; and Rankin, "Halsted," pp. 418–25.

194 "I know that you will be astounded": Halsted to Franklin P. Mall, March 25, 1890, Box 28, Folder 20, W. S. Halsted Papers, Alan Mason Chesney Medical Archives, Johns Hopkins Medical Institutions, Baltimore. Booker refers to William D. Booker, a physician and physiologist who helped organize the clinical pediatrics service at Johns Hopkins in 1889 and served as the chair of clinical pediatrics there for six years. He later became a prominent Baltimore pediatrician and a member of the hospital's advisory board. *Semi-Centennial Volume of the American Pediatric Society, 1838–1938* (Menasha, Wisc.: George Banta Publishing, 1938), p. 20.

195 Before the nuptials, Caroline resigned: MacCallum, *Halsted,* p. 82.

195 Theirs was a type of relationship: For elegant discussions of separate spheres, sexuality, and companionate and same-sex relationships during this era, see Caroll Smith-Rosenberg, *Disorderly Conduct: Visions of Gender in Victorian America* (New York: Oxford University Press, 1986); and John D'Emilio and Estelle B. Freedman, *Intimate Matters: A History of Sexuality in America* (Chicago: University of Chicago Press, 1998).

196 According to those familiar: Nip and Tuck were the Halsteds' most famous dogs, most likely because of their charming names. In some accounts, Sisly's name is spelled Sisley. See MacCallum, *Halsted,* pp. 119–20; Heuer, "Dr. Halsted," pp. 65–70; and Judith Robinson, *Tom Cullen of Baltimore* (London: Oxford University Press, 1949), p. 237.

196 William's ceaseless search: MacCallum, *Halsted,* pp. 106–07; Colp, "Notes," pp. 876–87; Sherwin B. Nuland, *Doctors: The Biography of Medicine* (New York: Vintage Books, 1988), pp. 415–16; and Daniel B. Nunn, "Caroline Hampton Halsted, an Eccentric but Well-Matched Helpmate," *Perspectives in Biology and Medicine* 42, no. 1 (1998): 83–93.

196 In 1898, Harvey Cushing: Harvey Cushing to his mother, Betsey Cushing, February 20, 1898, Harvey Cushing Papers, Microfilm Reel 15, p. 03, Sterling Library, Yale University, New Haven; Michael Bliss, *William Osler: A Life in Medicine* (New York: Oxford University Press, 1999), p. 254; Michael Bliss, *Harvey Cushing: A Life in Surgery* (New York: Oxford University Press, 2005), p. 116; and MacCallum, *Halsted,* pp. 103–20.

197 Once his castle's heavy door: Heuer, "Dr. Halsted," pp. 61, 67–70. Although the telephone was initially conceived of as a business tool, by the 1920s, more and more American homes contained the new invention. Leading the way in this new market were wealthy families and the homes of physicians. See C. S. Fischer, "Telephone," *The Oxford Companion to American History*, ed. P. S. Boyer (New York: Oxford University Press, 2001), p. 769; and D. J. Boorstin, *The Americans: The Democratic Experience* (New York: Random House, 1973), p. 391.

197 The small suite of rooms: MacCallum, *Halsted*, pp. 81–82.

197 Rigorous, entirely exhausting: William S. Halsted, "The Training of the Surgeon," *Bulletin of the Johns Hopkins Hospital* 15, no. 162 (1904): 267–75. The typical time frame for training included six years as an assistant followed by two more years as house surgeon. Halsted added in his report that "I know from applications which have been made to me this year that men of the desired quality would gladly serve 10 years on the surgical staff in order to obtain the experience which the house surgeonship and the training leading to it affords." For a recent review on the state of residency training in the United States after the reforms in duty hours, see Institute of Medicine, *Resident Duty Hours: Enhancing Sleep, Supervision, and Safety* (Washington, D.C.: Institute of Medicine/ National Academies of Science, 2008).

198 His visits might last: Heuer, "Dr. Halsted," pp. 53–60.

199 But even among the very rich: Ibid., pp. 56–58.

199 Years later, in 1940: Harvey C. Cushing, *The Medical Career and Other Papers* (Boston: Little, Brown, 1940), p. 225.

199 At the dawn of the Gay Nineties: H. L. Mencken, *Happy Days* (New York: Alfred A. Knopf, 1940), p. 55.

200 Before the century turned: Kenneth M. Ludmerer, *Learning to Heal: The Development of American Medical Education* (New York: Basic Books, 1985); *The Education of American Physicians*, ed. Ronald L. Numbers (Berkeley: University of California Press, 1980); Thomas N. Bonner, *Becoming a Physician: Medical Education in Great Britain, France, Germany, and the United States, 1750–1945* (New York: Oxford University Press, 1995); Ronald L. Numbers, ed., *The History of Medical Education* (Los Angeles: University of California at Los Angeles, 1970).

200 Almost immediately, the Hopkins: Alan M. Chesney, *The Johns Hopkins Hospital and the Johns Hopkins University School of Medicine: A Chronicle*, vol. 1, *Early Years, 1867–1892* (Baltimore: Johns Hopkins University Press, 1943).

200 At the laboratory bench: This organism, if ingested or introduced into an open wound, can cause damage to the gut or gas gangrene in the wound. Ubiquitous and found in decaying vegetation and marine sediment, this bacterium is currently known as *Clostridium perfringens*.

201 Every year until his retirement: Simon Flexner and James T. Flexner, *William Henry Welch and the Heroic Age of American Medicine* (New York: Viking Press, 1949); Donald Fleming, *William H. Welch and the Rise of Modern Medicine* (Baltimore: Johns Hopkins University Press, 1987); Alan M. Chesney, *The Johns Hopkins Hospital and the Johns Hopkins University School of Medicine*, vol. 2, *1893–1905* (Baltimore: Johns Hopkins University, 1958); and A. M. Harvey,

G. H. Brieger, S. L. Abrams, and V. A. McKusick, *A Model of Its Kind*, vol. 1, *A Centennial History of Medicine at Johns Hopkins* (Baltimore: Johns Hopkins University Press, 1989), pp. 19–22.

202 Once there, he approached: Audrey W. Davis, *Dr. Kelly of Hopkins: Surgeon, Scientist, Christian* (Baltimore: Johns Hopkins Press, 1959), pp. 142–74; and "Testimonial Dinner to Howard Atwood Kelly on his 75th Birthday," *Bulletin of the Johns Hopkins Hospital* 53, no. 2 (1933): 65–109.

202 In 1926, Kelly wrote: Howard A. Kelly, *A Scientific Man and the Bible* (Philadelphia: Sunday School Times Co., 1925); and H. L. Mencken, "*Fides Ante Intellectum,*" *American Mercury* 7, no. 26 (1926): 251–52.

202 In discussing Kelly's dual devotion: John F. Fulton, *Harvey Cushing: A Biography* (Springfield, Ill.: C. C. Thomas, 1946), p. 681.

202 "effulgent as an X-ray tube": Quoted in Bliss, *William Osler*, p. 215.

202 The undisputed star of the faculty: Howard A. Kelly, "Osler as I Knew Him in Philadelphia and in the Hopkins," *Johns Hopkins Hospital Bulletin* 30, no. 341 (1919): 215–16; and Harvey Cushing, *The Life of Sir William Osler* (Oxford: Oxford University Press, 1925).

203 He was always impeccably dressed: Howard Markel, "Dr. Osler's Relapsing Fever," *Journal of the American Medical Association* 295 (2006): 2886–87; and Bliss, *William Osler*, pp. 208–58.

203 Having gathered this critical intelligence: Harvey et al., *Model of Its Kind*, vol. 1, pp. 23–25.

203 By insisting that his pupils observe: John Dewey, *Democracy and Education: An Introduction to the Philosophy of Education* (New York: Echo, 2007); Ludmerer, *Learning to Heal*, pp. 43–71; and Henry M. Thomas, "Some Memories of the Development of the Medical School and of Osler's Advent," *Bulletin of the Johns Hopkins Hospital* 30, no. 341 (1919): 214–15.

203 After greeting them: T. M. Boggs, "Osler as Bibliophile," *Bulletin of the Johns Hopkins Hospital* 30, no. 341 (1919): 216.

203 But he always concluded: William Osler, "Books and Men," in *Aequanimitas, with Other Addresses to Medical Students, Nurses and Practitioners of Medicine* (Philadelphia: P. Blakiston's Sons, 1904), pp. 209–15; quote is from p. 211.

204 "part of the permanent hospital record": Heuer, "Dr. Halsted," pp. 26–28; Harvey et al., *Model of Its Kind*, vol. 1, pp. 36–38; quote is from Heuer, p. 26.

204 "it was an impressive demonstration": Heuer, "Dr. Halsted," p. 28.

205 Other medical students: Bliss, *William Osler*, p. 215.

205 Rarely, if ever: "Johns Hopkins Hospital Board of Trustees Minutes," December 10, 1895–March 10, 1896, Alan Mason Chesney Medical Archives, Johns Hopkins Medical Institutions, Baltimore; Welch to Mall, January 11, 1896, Franklin Mall Papers, Alan Mason Chesney Medical Archives, Johns Hopkins Medical Institutions, Baltimore; Chesney, *Johns Hopkins Hospital*, vol. 2, pp. 38, 81–83; and Bliss, *William Osler*, pp. 209, 214–15.

205 During many of the Friday afternoon dry clinics: Bliss, *William Osler*, p. 215.

206 Halsted gruffly stated: Heuer, "Dr. Halsted," pp. 33, 56–68.

206 Indeed, many seasoned Johns Hopkins doctors: R. Matas, J. T. F. Finney, W. H. Welch, and M. Reid, "Memorial Meeting for Dr. William Stewart Halsted, Late

Professor of Surgery in the Johns Hopkins Medical School," _Bulletin of the Johns Hopkins Hospital_ 36, no. 1 (1925): 1–59.

206 In fact, Halsted's absenteeism: "The Matter of Dr. Halsted's Absence," a list of hospital board minutes regarding Halsted's absences from the Johns Hopkins Hospital, Box 69A, W. S. Halsted Papers, Alan Mason Chesney Archives of the Johns Hopkins Medical Institutions, Baltimore. One bone of contention between Halsted and the board had to do with his annual summer vacations, from June 1 to about October 1. The Halsteds escaped the humid heat of Maryland for High Hampton, Caroline's family estate in North Carolina, where she attended to her stable of fine horses. There are also multiple letters in the Halsted papers where, as early as 1891, William requests leaves of absences because of "poor health." His colleagues were also concerned about his appearance during this period. For example, William D. Booker wrote Franklin Mall on May 3, 1891, "He was looking dreadful when he left, but recent letters from him are very encouraging"; Booker to Mall, May 3, 1891, Franklin P. Mall Papers, Series I, Correspondence, Alan Mason Chesney Archives, Johns Hopkins Medical Institutions, Baltimore. For a superb summary of Halsted's many absences, see Daniel B. Nunn, "William Stewart Halsted: Transitional Years," _Surgery_ 121, no. 3 (1997): 343–51. See also Heuer, "Dr. Halsted," pp. 70–78.

206 The flimsy excuse Halsted offered: Bliss, _William Osler_, p. 213.

206 "with the scalpel in his hand": Heuer, "Dr. Halsted," p. 25; a similar account of this behavior was expressed by Roy D. McClure, the surgeon-in-chief at the Henry Ford Hospital in Detroit and one of Halsted's former chief residents, in a letter to Heuer on October 22, 1948; George J. Heuer Papers, Box 2, File 13, Item 8, Cornell Medical Archives, Weill Cornell Medical School, New York.

207 "This gave me an extraordinary amount": H. L. Mencken, _The Diary of H. L. Mencken_, ed. C. A. Fecher (New York: Alfred A. Knopf, 1989), p. 10 (diary entry for January 14, 1931). In a biography of the Hopkins obstetrician Thomas Cullen, published nearly two decades later, Mencken noted that Halsted "would start an operation, go on for a bit, then seem to get tired and say to his assistant, 'You see what I want to do, you finish it,' and walk away. But Max Broedel [a medical illustrator and a great friend of H. L. Mencken's], who worked with them all, always said Halsted was the pick of the Big Four. He knew things"; Robinson, _Tom Cullen_, p. 238. Joseph Colt Bloodgood came to Johns Hopkins as an assistant resident surgeon in 1892 and stayed there, rising to the rank of clinical professor of surgery, until his death in 1935. He was also chief of surgery at Baltimore's St. Agnes Hospital. For a surgical memoir of Bloodgood's tenure under Halsted, see Joseph C. Bloodgood, "Halsted Thirty-six Years Ago," _American Journal of Surgery_ 14 (1931): 89–148.

210 The volume was elaborately bound: William Osler, "The Inner History of the Johns Hopkins Hospital," ed. D. G. Bates and E. H. Bensley, _Johns Hopkins Medical Journal_ 125 (1969): 184–94. For descriptions of the fabled Osler Library, which contains the bulk of William Osler's extensive rare book collection, see C. Lyons and D. S. Crawford, "Whatever Happened to William Osler's Library?," _Journal of the Canadian Health Library Association_ 27, no. 1 (2006): 9–13; C. Gray, "The Osler Library: A Collection That Represents the Mind of Its Col-

lector," *Canadian Medical Association Journal* 119 (1978): 1442–45; and *Bibliotheca Osleriana: A Catalogue of Books Illustrating the History of Medicine and Science* (Oxford: Clarendon Press, 1929); see also Colp, "Notes," pp. 876–87.

210 Some have speculated: For fascinating accounts of this medical librarian's life, see Thomas E. Keys, "Osler's Librarian, Dr. W. W. Francis," in *The Persisting Osler*, ed. J. A. Barondess, J. P. McGovern, and C. G. Roland (Baltimore: University Park Press, 1985), pp. 213–22; and Marian F. Kelen, "Memories of My Librarian Father, W. W. Francis, M.D.," in *The Persisting Osler*, pp. 223–27. Francis died in 1959.

210 The historical record trumped privacy: Osler, "Inner History," pp. 184–94.

210 The speech was widely reported: William Osler, "The Fixed Period," in *Aequanimitas, with Other Addresses*, pp. 375–93; and Bliss, *William Osler*, pp. 321–28.

211 Not surprisingly, he waxes a tad envious: Osler's substantial income is discussed in W. Bruce Fye, "William Osler's Departure from North America: The Price of Success," *New England Journal of Medicine* 320 (1989): 1425–31.

211 He did add, however: Osler, "Inner History," pp. 184–94; nineteenth-century dollars were converted into 2010 values using a formula based on the consumer price index from the economic history–focused website Measuring Worth, www .measuringworth.com/index.html (accessed February 25, 2010).

211 "He had never": Osler, "Inner History," p. 190. On the original manuscript, after the word "daily" there is an asterisk, but no elucidating comments or writing follow. See also John L. Cameron, "William Stewart Halsted: Our Surgical Heritage," *Annals of Surgery* 225, no. 5 (1997): 445–58; and Peter D. Olch, "William S. Halsted: The Antithesis of William Osler," in *Persisting Osler*, pp. 199–204. One can only speculate here, but I believe Welch knew about these issues all too well.

212 "Subsequently he got the amount down": Osler, "Inner History," p. 193, footnote 32. The notation of 1912 is especially curious; given the date of the amendment, one wonders if it was an error for 1902 or actually refers to the later date.

213 At such moments: This sentiment was best expressed by the noted physician, author, and director Jonathan Miller with respect to cigarettes and nicotine addiction. See D. Cavett, "Why Can't We Talk Like This?," *New York Times*, May 29, 2009, http://cavett.blogs.nytimes.com/2009/05/29/why-cant-we-talk-like-this/?apage=8 (accessed May 4, 2010).

Chapter 11. Dr. Freud's Coca Coda

214 A year later, Freud admitted: Freud to Fliess, August 7, 1901, Jeffrey M. Masson, ed., *The Complete Letters of Sigmund Freud to Wilhelm Fliess, 1887–1904* (Cambridge, Mass.: Belknap Press of Harvard University Press, 1985), pp. 446–48; quote is from p. 447. In this letter, Freud expresses resentment of Fliess's wife, who is jealous of the two men's relationship; Josef Breuer, for planting such a seed of jealousy in her mind; and Fliess's habit of taking sides against Freud in terms of criticizing his work.

214 Taken immediately to the Krankenhaus: Fliess to Freud, July 20, 1904, *Complete*

Letters, p. 463; Peter Gay, *Freud: A Life for Our Time* (New York: W. W. Norton, 1998), pp. 101–02, 154–56; Otto Weininger, *Geschlecht und Charakter: Eine prinzipielle Untersuchung* (Vienna: Wilhelm Braumüller, 1903); and Wilhelm Fliess, *Die Beziehungen zwischen Nase und weiblichen Geschlechtsorganen (In ihrer biologischen Bedeutung dargestellt)* (Saarbrücken: Verlag Dr. Müller, rpt. ed., 2007).

215 *Sex and Character* is a sprawling, racist treatise: Chandak Sengoopta, *Otto Weininger: Sex, Science, and Self in Imperial Vienna* (Chicago: University of Chicago Press, 2000), p. 1.

215 Consequently, in the summer of 1904: Fliess to Freud, July 20, 1904, *Complete Letters*, p. 463.

215 Astoundingly, Freud went as far as to imply: Freud to Fliess, July 23, 1904, *Complete Letters*, p. 464. Freud denies Fliess's claim that Swoboda was one of his students; rather, he rationalizes a bit by introducing him as a patient. In a subsequent letter, he does call him a student, and, of course, Fliess picked up on this slip rather angrily.

216 "I believe," he wrote angrily: Fliess to Freud, July 26, 1904, *Complete Letters*, pp. 465–66. The source who told Fliess was Dr. Oscar Rie, the Freud children's pediatrician and a colleague of Sigmund's at the Vienna First Public Institute for Sick Children. Dr. Rie's wife was the sister of Ida Bondy, who married Fliess in 1892.

216 "I do not believe": Freud to Fliess, July 27, 1904, *Complete Letters*, pp. 466–68.

216 Some historians have generously suggested: *Complete Letters*, p. 460. Freud admits that he borrowed one of Fliess's concepts on bisexuality for his book *The Psychopathology of Everyday Life,* but there he curiously refers to Fliess only as a "friend with whom I used at that time to have a lively exchange of scientific ideas. . . . Since then I have grown a little more tolerant when, in reading medical literature, I come across one of the few ideas which my name can be associated, and find that my name has not been mentioned." Sigmund Freud, *The Psychopathology of Everyday Life,* part of *The Standard Edition of the Complete Psychological Works of Sigmund Freud* (New York: W. W. Norton, 1990), pp. 143–44. This book is also the volume that introduced an explanation of verbal slips and lapses now known as the "Freudian slip."

216 In her dotage, Anna Freud: *Complete Letters*, p. 4.

217 "The friendship with Fliess": Quoted from Bonaparte's unpublished notebook in *Complete Letters*, p. 3; Marie's paternal grandfather was Pierre Napoleon Bonaparte, who was the son of Lucien Bonaparte, one of Napoleon's younger and less cooperative brothers, who was eventually disinherited. For this reason, Marie was not considered a member of the branch of the family that made claim to the French throne. Her maternal grandfather, François Blanc, was one of the chief real estate developers of what became Monte Carlo, and this was the source of Marie's immense fortune. See Célia Bertin, *Marie Bonaparte: A Life* (New Haven: Yale University Press, 1982). To Freud's request to destroy the letters, Princess Marie responded, "How much would be lost if . . . the Platonic dialogues had been destroyed just to protect the reputation of Socrates, the pederast!" Quoted in Gay, *Freud,* p. 614.

217 Only a decade later: For example, in 1909, Freud was invited to give five major lectures on psychoanalysis at Clark University, in Worcester, Massachusetts, by the great American psychologist G. Stanley Hall. Freud also traveled to Boston, where he met with Harvard professors William James, James Jackson Putnam, and many other luminaries; to New York City, where he explored Chinatown and the Jewish ghetto; and through Albany to Buffalo to see Niagara Falls. Unfortunately, Freud did not venture south to Baltimore and the Johns Hopkins Hospital, where Halsted was still practicing. These lectures appear in Saul Rosenzweig, *The Historic Expedition to America (1909): Freud, Jung, and Hall the King-Maker* (St. Louis: Rana House, 1994); see also J. Harris, "The Clark University Vicennial Conference on Psychology and Pedagogy," *Archives of General Psychiatry* 67, no. 3 (2010): 218–19. In 1909 and 1910, Freud published second editions of *Studies in Hysteria, The Interpretation of Dreams,* and *Three Essays on Sexuality;* George Makari, *Revolution in Mind: The Creation of Psychoanalysis* (New York: Harper Perennial, 2008), pp. 234–35.

218 "You have not only noticed": The italics are Freud's and appear in his letter. Freud to Ferenczi, October 6, 1910. Quoted in Ernest Jones, *The Life and Work of Sigmund Freud,* vol. 2, *1901–1919* (New York: Basic Books, 1955), pp. 83–84. "Cathexis" is a Freudian term referring to the investment of emotional significance in an object, activity, or notion.

218 "You probably imagine": Unpublished letter, Freud to Ferenczi, October 17, 1910, quoted in *Complete Letters,* p. 4.

219 "I have now overcome": Unpublished letter, Freud to Ferenczi, December 16, 1910, quoted in *Complete Letters,* p. 4.

219 "any particular predilection": Sigmund Freud, *An Autobiographical Study,* trans. James Strachey (New York: W. W. Norton, rpt. ed., 1989), p. 6.

220 "We are doctors": J. Turner, "The Otto Gross–Frieda Weekley Correspondence," *The D. H. Lawrence Review* 22, no. 2 (1990): 137–227; quote is from p. 143. See also Makari, *Revolution in Mind,* p. 226. This comment, made in 1908, was in response to Dr. Otto Gross's grandiose compliment that Freud was a scientific revolutionary who broke the mythologies of past attempts to understand human psychology.

220 "That you surmised": Freud to Ferenczi, October 6, 1910; quoted in Jones, *Life,* vol. 2, pp. 83–84. This is the same letter where Freud makes his veiled confession about a possible homosexual relationship with Fliess.

222 Writing to Jung: Freud to Carl Jung, June 21, 1908, in W. McGuire, ed., *The Freud/Jung Letters: The Correspondence Between Sigmund Freud and C. G. Jung* (London: Hogarth Press and Routledge and Kegan Paul, 1974), pp. 157–60; quote is from p. 158. Freud eventually dismissed Gross from the psychoanalytic movement because of his addictions, a series of sexual scandals, his unorthodox medical practices, and a desire to convert psychoanalysis into a philosophy of revolution. Starving and living on the streets of Berlin, Gross died of pneumonia in 1920.

222 Only a few months earlier: Freud to Ferenczi, June 1, 1916, and February 13, 1916, in Jones, *Life,* vol. 2, p. 189.

223 More often than not: Jones, *Life,* vol. 2, pp. 381–86.

224 Dr. Schur administered: Both Jones's and Gay's biographies poignantly document Sigmund Freud's valiant last years as he slowly succumbed to the ravages of oral cancer. Ernest Jones insists that during Freud's fatal battle with cancer he avoided all painkillers save aspirin. Jones delicately states that at the very end, Freud was given "adequate sedation" for his severe cancer pain, but he avoids concluding that the situation was more akin to an assisted suicide; Ernest Jones, *The Life and Work of Sigmund Freud,* vol. 3, *1919–1939* (New York: Basic Books, 1957), pp. 218–48. Peter Gay, on the other hand, documents rather conclusively that while Sigmund probably was not using opiate painkillers during his long bout with cancer, he did receive morphine to end his life in September 1939; Gay, *Freud,* pp. 649–51, 739–40. Gay bases his conclusions on a review of Max Schur's unpublished manuscript "The Medical Case History of Sigmund Freud," which is dated February 27, 1954; Max Schur Papers, Library of Congress, Washington, D.C. See also Max Schur, *Freud: Living and Dying* (New York: International Universities Press, 1972); and S. Aziz, "Sigmund Freud: Psychoanalysis, Cigars, and Oral Cancer," *Journal of Oral and Maxillofacial Surgery* 58, no. 3 (2000): 320–23.

225 In a book entitled *Freud and Cocaine:* E. M. Thornton, *Freud and Cocaine: The Freudian Fallacy* (London: Blond and Briggs, 1983), pp. 1–10.

225 In recent years: For other accounts on the relationship between Freud's cocaine abuse from 1884 to 1896 and his thoughts and theories, see Frederick C. Crews, ed., *Unauthorized Freud: Doubters Confront a Legend* (New York: Viking, 1998); Frederick C. Crews, *The Memory Wars: Freud's Legacy in Dispute* (New York: New York Review Books, 1995); Frederick C. Crews, *Follies of the Wise: Dissenting Essays* (New York: Counterpoint, 2007); J. Lilly, "From Here to Alterity and Beyond," in *Mavericks of the Mind: Conversations for the New Millennium,* ed. D. J. Brown and R. M. Novick (Freedom, Calif.: Crossing Press, 1993), pp. 203–25; Robert C. Fuller, "Biographical Origins of Psychological Ideas: Freud's Cocaine Studies," *Journal of Humanistic Psychology* 32 (1992): 67–86; R. Karmel, "Freud's Cocaine Papers (1884–1887): A Commentary," *Canadian Journal of Psychoanalysis* 11 (2003): 161–69; Jürgen vom Scheidt, "Sigmund Freud und das Kokain," *Psyche* 27, no. 5 (1973): 385–430; R. Dadoun, "Un 'Sublime Amour' de Sherlock Holmes et de Sigmund Freud," *Littérature* 49 (1983): 69–76; and Stanley E. Hyman, "Freud and Boas: Secular Rabbis? Vienna Gaon, Tsaddik of Morningside Heights" (a book review of Ernest Jones's *Life and Work of Sigmund Freud,* vol. 1, and M. J. Herskovits's biography *Franz Boas*), *Commentary* 17, no. 3 (1954): 264–67. Preceding all these works by several decades is the superb essay by Siegfried Bernfeld, "Freud's Studies on Cocaine, 1884–1887," *Journal of the American Psychoanalytic Association* 1 (1953): 581–613. Bernfeld also notes the "guilty" dreams Freud had about Fleischl-Marxow during this period.

225 Most intriguing is a theory: Peter Swales, "Freud, Cocaine and Sexual Chemistry: The Role of Cocaine in Freud's Conception of the Libido," in *Sigmund Freud: Critical Assessments,* ed. Laurence Spurling, vol. 1 (London: Routledge, 1989), pp. 273–301; quote is from p. 274. Freud defined the libido—or sexual drive—as an instinctual energy that constitutes the "id," or unconscious portion of one's psyche. He posits that one's libido often is in conflict with the behaviors

acceptable to a given society (which is represented in the psyche as the "super-ego") and that such conflicts can lead to significant tension and disturbances, which require a variety of ego defenses to counterbalance the tensions. If too excessive, the ego defenses can lead to a neurosis. Indeed, one of the goals of psychoanalysis was to allow the libidinal drives to enter one's conscious thought and, thus, allow the patient to confront them directly and limit the need to rely on ego defenses. Swales also asserts that Freud's experience with cocaine is the source of his early views about somatic sexual neuroses. As Swales notes, at several points in Freud's writings on neuroses, particularly his 1905 essay on sexuality and the etiology of neuroses (*A Case of Hysteria, Three Essays on Sexuality, and Other Works,* in *Standard Edition of the Complete Psychological Works of Sigmund Freud,* vol. 7, p. 279), Freud likens a neurosis to the use of a chemical substance, such as "the use of certain alkaloids" (i.e., cocaine), which is damaging when taken to excess or during withdrawal. At other points, Freud describes a "toxicological theory" of neuroses. It is also important, however, to consider the late-nineteenth-century concept of autointoxication—an excess of toxic chemicals resulting from either constipation or lack of sexual activity. Such endogenous toxins represent a different entity than an exogenous "toxin" such as cocaine. Nevertheless, this observation is fascinating in suggesting how Freud may have used his cocaine experiences to elaborate and explain some of his concepts.

226 For all the reasons enumerated: Peter Gay, "Freud: A Brief Life," in Sigmund Freud, *The Ego and the Id,* trans. Joan Riviere, part of the *Standard Edition of the Complete Psychological Works of Sigmund Freud* (New York: W. W. Norton, 1989), p. xviii.

226 The clinical odds: D. D. Simpson, G. W. Joe, and K. M. Broome, "A National 5-Year Follow-up of Treatment Outcomes for Cocaine Dependence," *Archives of General Psychiatry* 59 (2002): 538–44. There may be a genetic explanation for cocaine addiction. Recently scientists have demonstrated that cocaine use can actually alter the gene expression, causing changes in neuronal morphology and behavior; see I. Maze, H. E. Covington, D. M. Dietz, Q. LaPlant, W. Renthal, S. J. Russo, M. Mechanic, E. Mouzon, R. L. Neve, S. J. Haggarty, Y. Ren, S. C. Sampath, Y. L. Hurd, P. Greengard, A. Tarakhovsky, A. Schaefer, and E. J. Nestler, "Essential Role of the Histone Methyltransferase G9a in Cocaine-Induced Plasticity," *Science* 327 (2010): 213–16.

Chapter 12. Dr. Halsted in Limbo

228 In 1905 Mary Elizabeth Garrett: In late 1892, Mary Elizabeth Garrett, whose father once ran the Baltimore and Ohio Railroad Company, made a major gift of over $300,000 (or almost $7.5 million in 2010 dollars) that allowed the Johns Hopkins Medical School to open its doors in 1893, provided women medical students were admitted. In tribute to her work, the Hopkins trustees commissioned Sargent to paint her portrait and provided half of the fee, with Garrett paying the rest; in return, she donated the funds to pay for the group portrait. Both paintings hang in the Welch Medical Library in Baltimore. *The Four Doc-*

tors was formally unveiled in 1907. Although the son of a Philadelphia eye surgeon, Sargent had lived in Europe since boyhood. One of the premier portraitists of his day, the artist made his home in London and found his muse in the persons of the rich and famous. He charged $5,000 or more a portrait ($125,000 in 2010 dollars), and the majority of his customers hailed from the gentry of Great Britain and the Continent. A smaller number of well-heeled Americans anxious to be so sumptuously captured for the ages happily crossed "the pond" at their own expense to sit patiently in Sargent's studio. See A. M. Harvey, G. H. Brieger, S. L. Abrams, J. M. Fishbein and V. A. McKusick, *A Model of Its Kind*, vol. 2, *A Pictorial History of Medicine at Johns Hopkins* (Baltimore: Johns Hopkins University Press, 1989), pp. 68–69; Nancy McCall, ed., *The Portrait Collection of Johns Hopkins Medicine: A Catalog of Paintings and Photographs at the Johns Hopkins University School of Medicine and the Johns Hopkins Hospital* (Baltimore: The Johns Hopkins University School of Medicine, 1993); Stanley Olsen, *John Singer Sargent: His Portrait* (New York: St. Martin's Press/ Griffin, 2001); and Elaine Kilmurray and Richard Ormond, *John Singer Sargent* (Princeton, N.J.: Princeton University Press, 1998). To convert 1905 dollars into 2010 values, I used a formula based on the consumer price index from the economic history–focused website Measuring Worth, www.measuringworth.com/ index.html (accessed February 25, 2010). I am indebted to Nancy McCall, chief archivist of the Alan Mason Chesney Archives at the Johns Hopkins Medical Institutions, for sharing her knowledge and research on this great painting.

228 There they reunited: Harvey Cushing, *The Life of Sir William Osler*, vol. 2 (Oxford: Oxford University Press, 1925); and Michael Bliss, *William Osler: A Life in Medicine* (New York: Oxford University Press, 1999).

228 Sargent was said to have pulled: Royal Cortissoz, *The Johns Hopkins University Circular*, February 1907; quoted in "The Four Doctors," *Johns Hopkins Alumni Magazine* 2 (1913–14): 23–26.

229 Legend has it: D. Geraint James, "John Singer Sargent and 'The Four Doctors,' " *Journal of Medical Biography* 15, Supp. 1 (2007): 5; and Stefan C. Schatzki, "The Four Doctors," *American Journal of Radiology* 169 (1997): 504. The entire painting underwent restoration in 2001.

231 After the war: R. B. Wallace, "Historical Perspectives of the American Association for Thoracic Surgery: George J. Heuer, M.D. (1882–1950)," *Journal of Thoracic and Cardiovascular Surgery* 130, no. 4 (2005): 1194–95. Heuer had a close filial relationship with Halsted and even dined with the surgeon in his home. He recalls, in his biography, charming stories of Halsted's consideration for him as a guest, to the extent of running out to the market to make sure Heuer had a fresh grapefruit for breakfast and how jovial and pleasant Halsted could be among the company of one or two close friends at the dining table and in his study.

232 "In the pages of this narrative": William H. Welch, "Introduction," in William G. MacCallum, *William Stewart Halsted, Surgeon* (Baltimore: Johns Hopkins University Press, 1930), pp. v–xiii; quote is from p. ix.

233 "Dr. Halsted did not escape": MacCallum, *Halsted*, pp. 55–56.

234 For more than two decades: The George J. Heuer papers are preserved at the Weill Cornell Medical College/New York–Presbyterian Hospital Archives in

New York City. An editor at Macmillan, W. H. Seale, expressed interest in the book in 1940; see W. H. Seale to Heuer, April 10, 1945, Box 2, File 12, Item 7. Two years after Heuer's death in 1950, his biography of Halsted was published as "Dr. Halsted," in the *Johns Hopkins Hospital Bulletin,* Supp. 90 (1952): 1–104.

234 "You are indeed a sturdy friend": Halsted to Matas, May 30, 1921, Box 59, Folder 8, W. S. Halsted Papers, Alan Mason Chesney Archives, Johns Hopkins Medical Institutions, Baltimore.

234 "How can I ever express": Halsted to Matas, April 3, 1922, Box 18, Folder 4, W. S. Halsted Papers, Alan Mason Chesney Archives, Johns Hopkins Medical Institutions, Baltimore. These letters were also published in William S. Halsted, "Practical Comments on the Use and Abuse of Cocaine," *Surgical Papers,* vol. 1, pp. 167–77; and MacCallum, *Halsted,* pp. 224–25.

235 "All said there was no direct evidence": Heuer to MacCallum, December 9, 1940, and MacCallum to Heuer, December 18, 1940. George J. Heuer Papers, Box 2, File 13, Item 3, Weill Cornell Medical College Archives, New York.

235 Similarly, two of Mrs. Halsted's nieces: Heuer, "Dr. Halsted," p. 25; see also Dr. Heyward Gibbs of Columbia, South Carolina, to Heuer, March 11, 1941. Gibbs had heard from a mutual colleague, Harry Slack, about Heuer's biography and the "whispering campaign to the effect that the Professor had resumed the taking of cocaine, or some other sedative, after he had succeeded in ridding himself of the habit in early years." Gibbs goes on to categorically deny such an occurrence based on his intimate association with Mrs. Halsted's nieces Lucy Bostick and Gertrude Barringer. The former stated that "she feels perfectly positive that there was noever [*sic*] the slightest indication of Dr. Halsted using drugs of any nature during the time that she knew him." Interestingly, Gibbs admits to having only "casual contacts" with Halsted and his wife. George J. Heuer Papers, Box 2, File 13, Item 5, Weill Cornell Medical College Archives, New York. Heuer replied on March 21, 1941, thanking Gibbs for his concern and to assure him that he was simply trying to run down every item, adding, "I can find no evidence thus far that Dr. Halsted continued to use drugs"; Box 2, File 13, Item 6, Heuer Papers, Weill Cornell Medical College Archives, New York.

236 So powerful and controversial: Heuer, "Dr. Halsted," pp. 22–23.

236 Moreover, Cushing labored: Cushing was a great admirer of Osler's and for a time rented the house next to Osler's on Franklin Street in Baltimore. He spent considerable time basking in the glow of this charismatic medical professor, even though he was a surgeon assigned to Halsted's service. There is no evidence that William Osler told anyone about his sealed "Inner History of the Johns Hopkins Hospital." See Cushing, *Sir William Osler;* Michael Bliss, *Harvey Cushing: A Life in Surgery* (New York: Oxford University Press, 2005), pp. 84–203; John F. Fulton, *Harvey Cushing: A Biography* (Springfield, Ill.: C. C. Thomas, 1946); J. A. Barondess, "Cushing and Osler: The Evolution of a Friendship," in *The Persisting Osler II,* ed. J. A. Barondess and C. G. Roland (Malabar, Fla.: Krieger Publishing, 1994), pp. 95–120; and A. M. Harvey, "Harvey Williams Cushing: The Baltimore Period, 1896–1912," in *Research and Discovery in Medicine: Contributions from Johns Hopkins,* ed. A. McGehee Harvey (Baltimore: Johns Hopkins University Press, 1981), pp. 71–91.

238 "Here I am, a youth": Quoted in Bliss, *William Osler,* p. 254; Cushing to Kate Crowell, March 15, 1898, Harvey Cushing Papers, Microfilm Reel 17, p. 343, Sterling Library, Yale University, New Haven.

238 "In a discussion of MacCallum's book": "Notes on Dr. Halsted from Harvey Cushing, March 1, 1931, Given to me (G.J.H.) by Elliott Cutler, November 10, 1939," George J. Heuer Papers, Weill Cornell Medical College Archives, Box 2, File 14, Item 5. Apparently, Cushing had had a similar conversation nine years earlier with his Yale colleague and future biographer, the neurophysiologist John F. Fulton, on December 5, 1930. In a brief note in the Cushing papers at Yale, Fulton mentions that Cushing had been in the Halsted home only twice in fifteen years and that "he never suspected the cocaine habit, and only with difficulty was he led to accredit it many years later." Cited in Sherwin B. Nuland, *Doctors: The Biography of Medicine* (New York: Vintage Books, 1988), p. 398. Fulton had long suffered from a serious drinking problem and wrote his 1945 biography of Cushing in "a kind of alcoholic haze." See Bliss, *Harvey Cushing,* p. 520. Cushing died on October 7, 1939.

Reid Hunt (1870–1948) was a prominent pharmacologist and a colleague of Halsted's at Johns Hopkins before becoming the chairman of pharmacology at Harvard. Heuer wrote Hunt a letter asking for confirmation of this point on December 4, 1940, but Hunt did not reply. In the published version, Hunt's name is omitted and he is, instead, referred to as an "eminent scientist." Heuer does quote in the published version the letter he wrote Hunt but notes, "No reply to my letter was received and he has since died." Heuer also adds, without evidence or explanation, that he does not believe Hunt was close enough to Halsted to rule in or out such an assertion. Heuer, "Dr. Halsted," p. 25; see also Heuer to Reid Hunt, December 9, 1940, George J. Heuer Papers, Box 2, File 13, Item 1, Weill Cornell Medical College Archives, New York.

The mention of De Quincey in the first paragraph of this document, of course, refers to the great English poet, journalist, and author of *Confessions of an Opium Eater,* Thomas De Quincey (1785–1859).

239 "an abundance of putty-like material": Samuel J. Crowe, *Halsted of Johns Hopkins: The Man and His Men* (Springfield, Ill.: C. C. Thomas, 1957), pp. 232–33.

239 On August 21: Heuer, "Dr. Halsted," pp. 70–78.

240 Dr. Karl Schlaepfer, the surgeon: Karl Schlaepfer, M.D., to Matas, September 8, 1922; W. S. Halsted Papers, Box 59, Folder 13, Alan Mason Chesney Archives, Johns Hopkins Medical Institutions, Baltimore.

240 "was certain that [Halsted]": Heuer, "Dr. Halsted," p. 25. Dr. Mont Reid died in 1943, leaving this particular thread untied.

240 Halsted, Crowe claims: Halsted's final illness and hospital chart are summarized in Crowe, *Halsted of Johns Hopkins,* pp. 232–33.

241 Consequently, his patients: Ibid., p. 233.

241 Conversely, there exists: Several scholars have suggested that Halsted may have been taking quite a bit more morphine at this time than he admitted. See, for example, Nuland, *Doctors,* p. 421.

241 "Although it has been widely reported": Emile Holman, "Sir William Osler and William Stewart Halsted—Two Contrasting Personalities," *Pharos* 34, no. 4

(1971): 134–39, 144. Sprong, who became a professor of urology at UCLA, wrote the letter containing Welch's statement to Holman on May 29, 1968. Sprong added, "I do not remember that Dr. Welch mentioned how long these relapses might last, or even how they occurred, but he felt pretty strongly that the facts should be on the record." The original letter resides in the Emile Holman Papers, Box 13, Archives and Modern Manuscripts Division, History of Medicine Division, National Library of Medicine, Bethesda, Maryland; see also Daniel B. Nunn, "Dr. Halsted's Addiction," *Johns Hopkins Advanced Studies in Medicine* 6, no. 3 (2006): 106–08; and Daniel B. Nunn, "William Stewart Halsted: Transitional Years," *Surgery* 121, no. 3 (1997): 343–51.

241 "The real truth": "Notes on Dr. Halsted from Harvey Cushing."

243 Such episodes also may have included: Before his premature death, the pathologist and medical historian Peter Olch worked on the life and addictions of Halsted. According to the journalist Scott Shane, during the 1960s Dr. Olch interviewed some of the living caretakers of Halsted's North Carolina summer home. Shane writes that one of them suggested to Dr. Olch a suspicion that the surgeon was often incapacitated from drug use during his summer vacations. Unfortunately, Olch died prematurely, before he could process and publish such testimony. Scott Shane, "A Casualty of Cocaine," *Baltimore Sun Magazine,* January 30, 1994, pp. 6–15; and J. Scott Rankin, "William Stewart Halsted: A Lecture by Dr. Peter D. Olch," *Annals of Surgery* 243 (2006): 418–25. This account is also mentioned in a fine essay by Daniel B. Nunn, "Caroline Hampton Halsted: An Eccentric but Well-Matched Helpmate," *Perspectives in Biology and Medicine* 42, no. 1 (1998): 83–93. In it, Nunn describes a correspondence with Dr. Olch, who interviewed Douglas Bradley, the former caretaker at High Hampton. Bradley recounted an episode where Mrs. Halsted became very upset when a package from Parke, Davis did not arrive at their home and, consequently, sent him to a local practitioner to procure some morphine. Parke, Davis, of course, sold both cocaine and morphine. Bradley also suggested to Olch in a phone interview that Mrs. Halsted may have been addicted to morphine. The proof of such a statement, however, has yet to be definitively found.

244 Sadly, the ashamed, guarded, and lonely Halsted: Shane, "Casualty of Cocaine," pp. 6–15; and "The Matter of Dr. Halsted's Absence," a list of board minutes regarding Halsted's absences from the Johns Hopkins Hospital, Box 69A, W. S. Halsted Papers, Alan Mason Chesney Archives of the Johns Hopkins Medical Institutions, Baltimore.

Epilogue

245 His body progressively demands: N. D. Volkow, J. S. Fowler, G. J. Wang, and J. M. Swanson, "Dopamine in Drug Abuse and Addiction: Results from Imaging Studies and Treatment Options," *Molecular Psychiatry* 9, no. 6 (2004): 557–69; N. D. Volkow, J. S. Fowler, G. J. Wang, J. M. Swanson, and F. Telang, "Dopamine in Drug Abuse and Addiction: Results from Imaging Studies and Treatment Options," *Archives of Neurology* 64, no. 11 (2007): 1575–79; and J. S.

Fowler, N. D. Volkow, C. A. Kassed, and L. Chang, "Imaging the Addicted Human Brain," *Science & Practice Perspectives* 3, no. 2 (2007): 4–16.

245 The addict's luck: Alan I. Leshner, "What We Know: Drug Addiction Is a Brain Disease," in *Principles of Addiction Medicine,* 2nd ed., ed. Allan W. Graham and Terry K. Schultz (Chevy Chase, Md.: American Society of Addiction Medicine, 1998), pp. xxix–xxxvi; and Robert L. Dupont, *The Selfish Brain: Learning from Addiction* (Minneapolis: Hazelden Publishing, 2000).

246 Even at this late date: For a superb account of a modern-day doctor trapped by addiction but with fatal results, see Abraham Verghese, *The Tennis Partner: A Doctor's Story of Friendship and Loss* (New York: HarperCollins, 1998).

Index